Body Mechanics and Self-Care Manual

MARIAN WOLFE DIXON, MA, LMT

Oregon School of Massage

Prentice
Hall

UPPER SADDLE RIVER, NJ 07458

Library of Congress Cataloging-in-Publication Data
Dixon, Marian Wolfe.
    Body mechanics and self-care manual / Marian
        Wolfe Dixon
        p. cm.
    Includes index
    ISBN 0-8385-0747-6
        1. Masseurs—Health and hygiene. 2. Physical
therapists—Health and hygiene. 3. Overuse injuries—
Prevention. 4. Human mechanics. I. Title.

RM722 .D59 2000
615.8´22 do21

                                        00-035681

Publisher: Julie Alexander
Acquisitions Editors: Barbara Krawiec and Mark Cohen
Director of Production and Manufacturing: Bruce Johnson
Managing Production Editor: Patrick Walsh
Production Editor: Linda Begley, Rainbow Graphics
Production Liaison: Danielle Newhouse
Manufacturing Manager: Ilene Sanford
Creative Director: Marianne Frasco
Director of Marketing: Leslie Cavaliere
Editorial Assistant: Melissa Kerian
Cover Designer: Maria Guglielmo
Composition: Rainbow Graphics
Printing and Binding: Courier/Westford

Prentice Hall International (UK) Limited, *London*
Prentice-Hall of Australia Pty. Limited, *Sydney*
Prentice-Hall Canada, Inc., *Toronto*
Prentice-Hall Hispanoamericana, S.A., *Mexico*
Prentice-Hall of India Private Limited, *New Delhi*
Prentice-Hall of Japan, Inc., *Tokyo*
Prentice-Hall Singapore Pte. Ltd
Editora Prentice-Hall do Brasil, Ltda., *Rio de Janeiro*

Contents

CHAPTER THREE: PRINCIPLES OF PHYSICS—MOVING AND STATIC OBJECTS, WEIGHT AND PRESSURE   33

CHAPTER FOUR: EASTERN INFLUENCES ON BODY MECHANICS   59

CHAPTER FIVE: MOVEMENT REEDUCATION INFLUENCES ON BODY MECHANICS 82

CHAPTER SIX: UNPATTERNING 109

CHAPTER SEVEN: REPETITIVE MOTION AND OTHER COMMON INJURIES 132

CHAPTER EIGHT: TAKING CARE OF YOURSELF—
PART I (PHYSIOLOGICAL) 161

CHAPTER NINE: TAKING CARE OF YOURSELF—
PART II (PSYCHOLOGICAL) 189

CHAPTER TEN: ADAPTATIONS FOR SPECIAL POPULATIONS/CONDITIONS   213

CHAPTER ELEVEN: STRESS AND THE BODYWORKER   248

Preface

Work-related injury is a major reason why bodyworkers drop out of the massage industry. Understanding how to implement body mechanics and self-care techniques (physiological and psychological) helps emerging and established professionals to work smarter, not harder, and to avoid occupational injury, stress, and burnout.

Body Mechanics and Self-Care Manual stresses the importance of becoming an active player in your own health and wellness. The text helps each individual to *prepare* and *renew* for the demanding work of massage therapy.

Identifying sensations of discomfort allows you to make appropriate physical changes to feet better while you work. This skill, in turn, helps facilitate the process of positive emotional change. *Body Mechanics and Self-Care Manual* enhances the ability to sense in the moment when a body position or technique is not comfortable or effective, and provides alternatives for unhealthy patterns.

Learning to relax through simple techniques such as stretching, breathing with attention, and guided imagery help to ease the process of letting go of harmful patterns. Specific relaxation techniques are presented throughout the text, to allow readers to learn these skills at a comfortable pace.

Body Mechanics and Self-Care Manual provides a basic understanding of the *contributing factors* and *self-care options for common injuries and overuse syndromes* that affect bodyworkers, such as thoracic outlet syndrome, carpal tunnel syndrome, low back pain, headaches, stiff neck, temporomandibular joint disorder, sciatic pain, and knee and other joint discomforts. It also provides strategies for preventing the recurrence of these conditions.

Body Mechanics and Self-Care Manual provides a clear, easy to use program that can be followed for a complete course of ergonomic study. The content is comprehensive enough to allow educators to develop a body mechanics class based on the book.

The material can be taught in modules—taking each chapter as a unit. Considering each chapter as a module provides schools with a framework to cover important aspects of body mechanics, while leaving the flexibility to mix and match topics as needed. Specific chapters can be easily integrated into established bodywork classes as students learn basic (or advanced) massage techniques. The material is especially recommended for the beginning student as attention to body mechanics and self-care right from the start makes massage learning easier and more effective.

For practitioners who have never had the opportunity to systematically approach body mechanics as a subject of inquiry, or who may need a refresher course, *Body Mechanics and Self-Care Manual* can serve as a reference manual or as an enlightening way to meet continuing education requirements in the form of a class or support group.

The text is also appropriate as an ergonomic primer for anyone experiencing the stresses of repetitive motion in corporate or health care environments.

The face of massage professionals is changing. Younger students are approaching massage as a viable profession as well as seasoned individuals who are choosing a major mid-life (or later) career change. *Body Mechanics and Self-Care Manual* helps hold the interest of all levels of students, from high school graduate to individuals with advanced degrees. Instructors and students alike will benefit from the complete learning package which includes:

- **Instructor's Guide** containing presentation content, objectives, suggested strategies for teaching, and sample test questions and answers.

- **End of chapter** summaries that highlight the major concepts presented in each section.

- **Kinesthetic exercises** and **questions for discussion** to provide classroom activities and encourage students to think critically and apply unit concepts to real life situations.

- **Body mechanics red flags** and **guidelines** that provide ways to identify unhealthy massage patterns and strategies for improving efficiency and enjoyment during work.

Acknowledgments

I wisk to thank my family for their presence, support, and love, which has sustained me throughout the creation of this book. Thank you Art, Roy, and Sophie Dixon.

I also wish to acknowledge Lisa Ann Kuhnau, L.M.T., the artist, who has spent an enormous amount of time and energy with the illustrations that grace these pages. Thank you for your kindness, patience, and support.

Reviewers

David Kasprzyk, Director
New York Institute of Massage
Williamsville, New York

Nancy Gamboian, MFA, PhD
Desert Institute of Healing Arts
Tuscon, Arizona

Pete Whitridge, NCBTMB Faculty Member and Continuing Education Provider
Florida School of Massage
Gainesville, Florida

Dwight Zieman
Cayce/Reilly School of Massotherapy
Virginia Beach, Virginia

Rosalie Joan Yeager, Certified Instructor, Therapeutic Massage
Fair Oaks, California

Nancy W. Dail, LMT, NCTMB, Director
Downeast School of Massage
Waldoboro, Maine

Peggy Lamb, RMT, Faculty Member
Wellness Skills, Inc.
Dallas, Texas

Chapter One

Introduction to Body Mechanics and Self-Care

CHAPTER OBJECTIVES

Conceptual Objectives The massage student/practitioner who successfully completes this chapter (reading and exercises) will be able to:

- List five or more benefits of using good body mechanics.

- Define *body mechanics.*

- Define *ergonomics.*

- Define *self-care.*

Practical Objective The massage student/practitioner who successfully completes this chapter (reading and exercises) will be able to:

- Give a personal example of the difference between imitative action and kinesthetic experience.

PURPOSE OF THE BOOK

I have wanted to write this book and share this knowledge for a long time. *Body Mechanics and Self-Care Manual* is an expression of the true authentic force inside me. It is about discovering how to practice your craft as a bodyworker in the most free and clear expression of yourself and your own true movement.

Bodyworkers need to utilize proper body mechanics and self-care techniques (both physiological and psychological) to promote ease in working with clients and to avoid occupational injury, stress, and burnout. This text was written to address these concerns.

Body Mechanics and Self-Care Manual stresses the importance of being an advocate and active participant for your own health and wellness. It is the responsibility of each licensed massage therapist (LMT) to learn how to *prepare and renew* ourselves physically and emotionally for the demanding role of massage practitioner. As "helpers," we are often so busy trying to "give" that we do not tune into our own body signals of physical and emotional needs. The importance of preparation and renewal becomes redoubled when performing clinical or deep tissue massage. Achieving deeper pressure requires (1) deep emotional focus and energy, (2) *specific* attention to body positioning and mechanics in order to exercise sufficient pressure and focus on a targeted muscle or muscle group, and (3) a balance between applying specific techniques to effect a physiological change and giving clients the space to heal on their own.

Identifying sensations of discomfort allows you to make appropriate physical changes as you work. The skill operates in the same way when facilitating the process of emotional change. This text aims to enhance your ability to *sense in the moment* when a body position or technique is not comfortable or effective, and will provide alternatives to unhealthy patterns. Your increased awareness and ease will indisputably transfer to clients. You will find that you are serving clients better while empowering yourself to reshape your massage trade to become more effective, potent, and prosperous.

Learning to relax through simple techniques such as stretching, breathing with attention, and guided visualizations eases the process of "letting go" of harmful patterns. Sometimes such processes are familiar to the massage therapist, but we may need a little reminder of the power of and the application of the techniques. Specific relaxation techniques are presented and outlined throughout the text, so that students or professional therapists can follow along at their own pace.

Sometimes, despite our best understanding and intentions, we get hurt. This text provides a basic understanding of the *etiology and treatment options for overuse syndromes* that can affect bodyworkers, such as thoracic outlet syndrome, carpal tunnel syndrome, low back pain, temporomandibular joint (TMD or TMJ) disorder, headaches, sciatic pain, and knee and other joint dysfunctions. It also provides strategies for preventing the recurrence of these conditions.

The text will develop the basic body mechanics skills by providing a theoretical framework and the kinesthetic experience of the theory. It is ideally suited to a classroom environment, where the exercises can form the basis for class experiences and discussion. The aim of this book is to help bodyworkers to kinesthetically understand, that is, to feel in their own bodies, the techniques and practices that are most ergonomically suited to their own individual needs.

A New Approach to Body Mechanics

First as a student of bodywork, then as a teacher and an administrator of academic courses of massage study, I have observed body mechanics inadvertently being taught as dogma. I have seen well-meaning instructors telling students "this is the only right way to hold your hands." Or they might be told "this is the right table height" or "this is how you move exactly to execute the best massage stroke," or even "this is the way you brace yourself against the table." Meanwhile, what I have observed for myself is that mimicking another person's actions without deviation does not feel right inside. Many "expert techniques" are more accurately just the habitual way the instructor learned to do bodywork. For example, tall students will not necessarily want to leverage a stretch in the same way as a short instructor. Students with large hands may not be able to fit their appendages comfortably underneath the client's neck, as the small-boned teacher demonstrates in class. Techniques taught by rote can be harmful to the earnest practitioner who is trying to mold his or her body into a preplanned shape that cannot work for everyone. In my 20-year career as an educator, I saw more and more how training others to reproduce a pattern is not sufficient. This is true not only for massage and specifically body mechanics, but also for efficient action in fields as diverse as physics, dance, and safety education. Doing things the way others tell you to do them without understanding why creates fearful practitioners who do not trust in the value of their own self-expression. Learning solely by imitation, without the inclusion of innovation, creates therapists who are hurting themselves trying to emulate body movements that do not fit their own individual body style.

Imitation versus Initiation

Most classes that teach a physical skill require students to imitate exercises, movements, and postures rather than initiate creative solutions to kinesthetic problems. When the instructor bends his or her knees, you bend yours. The instructor raises his or her left arm, and you follow suit. The instructor demonstrates or explains in detail a complex sequence of movements. Students are expected to learn by imitating each step, and you do your best to duplicate the pattern as it is shown.

Indeed, there is much inherent value in the imitative act. In fact, it is often said, "imitation is the best form of flattery." As children, we learn how to function in society by modeling the actions of others. We learn to talk, walk, spell, read words, add numbers, and balance checkbooks by copying the admired (and sometimes not so admired) traits of those around to teach us. Sometimes special mentors appear in our lives to take us by the hand. Sometimes we turn to professionals for help. These hired helpers can also show us new ways that imitation can be a source for growth. Psychotherapists and other members of the helping professions use modeling to show clients how to deal with situations that they cannot master on their own.

And let us not forget that imitating can be fun! The childhood game of "monkey see–monkey do," although an excruciatingly irritating tease to the one who is mocked, is just as excruciatingly pleasurable to the "monkeys" who copy every act they see and hear the other do.

With so many advantages to learning by imitation, why would anyone want to teach the movements of massage any other way? What can one gain from learning by initiation and interpretation that cannot be absorbed from modeling behavior?

In my own process of trying to answer this question, I have turned to the teachings of two philosophers, or "lovers of learning." Plato and Ram Dass (Richard Alpert) hail from different eras but share similar messages about the value of learning by initiative, interpretation, and innovation.

Ram Dass (1978), a contemporary truth-seeker, relates a story that might shed some illumination on the value of individual interpretation, innovation, and initiation. In this story, God and Satan were walking together along a path when the Lord bent down and picked something up. Satan asked God, "What is it that you have there?" The Lord Almighty gazed at the thing glowing brightly in his hand, and answered, "This is truth." Satan grasped out for the thing and said, "Here, let me have it. I'll organize it for you."

Plato, the classical Greek scholar and mystic, introduced the character of Socrates and his unique method of teaching, known today as the Socratic method. The Socratic method involves continual questioning and probing of the students. Teacher/tutors do not provide information laid out on a platter, but instead act like a midwife to draw the truth out of their students. The quest for inner knowledge and individual understanding is an integral part of the Socratic method of learning. *Eureka* means "Aha! I have found it!" (*The American Heritage Dictionary,* 1985).

Both the Socratic method and the story about Satan indicate that it is indeed possible and quite desirable to learn to know and think as individuals. We can then design our lives and actions from an inner knowing rather than from the external rules, idols, or status symbols imposed on us by the outside world. Learning to trust our bodies and becoming familiar and comfortable with this somatic knowledge can show us that we need not always look to others for help or reassurance with body mechanics, or with anything. When mentally and physically tackling a problem of how to move in the most efficient or relaxed way (with the least amount of external, unneeded tension), at a certain point, it is necessary to let go of the outside help and focus in on our own inner resources. When we mechanically adopt rules prescribed by some outside "expert," we exchange a fuller experience of life for something less. The alternative can be quite "one-derful"— adapting principles with motion and body awareness to our own best use.

Resistance to Learning by Initiation

There is a great deal of resistance toward learning processes that require self-searching and discovery. I have found in over 20 years of teaching in America that there are strong objections to educational methods that do not promise or provide absolute certainty. Self-observation provides qualitative and subjective information, rather than qualitative and objective truth. Public education in this nation has traditionally relied heavily on mere regurgitation of memorized facts. Unfortunately, most of the information is quickly forgotten after the exam.

As a teacher/trainer for many years, I have observed a great opposition to creative learning. Most surprising was the source of the resistance. The loudest protests against problem-solving education did not stem from my fellow instructors, nor did they emerge from parents, administrators, or even from school counselors. Instead, the firmest opposition to learning by innovation came directly from the students themselves. Many students in my university health education classes had rarely, if ever, been encouraged to try to create anything new. These young people rebelled against having to initiate anything that they had not been shown exactly how to do, step by step, inch by inch. They were uncomfortable learning when their answers could not be checked against a correct response. However, I also found that once students got past the initial discomfort of creative problem solving, it was amazing how quickly they opened to the discovery process and how eager they were to meet new challenges head (and hands) on.

How Is Massage Learned?

In today's current market of massage training, learning strokes, protocols, and routines by mirroring may or may not consciously be the case. I believe some of the best massage instruction leaves a space for the creativity and true authentic form of the student practitioners to emerge. I see some of the greatest joy manifesting in my students when they discover their own unique way of interpreting a stroke. The world of massage would certainly be a boring place if everyone massaged in exactly the same way. I never want to see my students routinely aping "Marian's massage." It is much more fulfilling to me as an instructor to see my rendition develop into the modification of "Betsy's spiraling massage" or "Isaiah's compression massage." It would be as if Mozart's and Beethoven's compositions sounded exactly like a Bach concerto, or if all flowers looked and smelled like roses.

Even when learning by initiation is encouraged in massage education, learning by imitation still has its place. Modeling healthy and comfortable massage movements serves as a good starting point for demonstrating good body mechanics. When educators consciously incorporate principles that create freer and stronger body movements into their own practice, this awareness will be reflected in the skill of the next generation of bodyworkers. Freer and more unrestricted motion has far-reaching effects that extend to the clients who will partake of the students' bodywork service. When massage educators supplement the modeling of healthy movement with a description of principles that lie behind the motion, understanding is enhanced. Exploring why we move the way that we do will provide the next generation of bodyworkers with a rationale for adapting touch skills when the situation calls for a change (e.g., working in a smaller studio, on a different massage table, with or without music).

Giving no direction to the novice bodyworker about body mechanics does not work. "Just doing your own thing" is not enough. Too many massage practitioners are injuring themselves and opting out of a profession that they love because it hurts them to continue to massage. Their style of massage consists of a hodgepodge of techniques that they liked plus old habitual ways of moving. These old habits are patterns that massage therapists develop for themselves due to lack of understanding and observation of some basic principles that can be easily taught and understood. Luckily, even world-weary massage practitioners can develop more effective patterns of motion when they understand and feel how their body works. (Greater body awareness, by the way, is just what I hope to encourage in clients during a massage session. Can you see how much more effective massage touch might be when communicated through a body that kinesthetically understands how to be more comfortable, easy, and joyful in its work? It is no accident that when the massage therapist is moving in a way that is free and easy, massage strokes feel better and bring greater relaxation and spasm relief to the client.)

I began this attempt to understand body mechanics by writing down some basic principles to keep bodywork practitioners from injuring themselves. True kinesthetic comprehension of these principles can help you to develop a free authentic style of movement that will not hurt you. Combining a basic grasp of the how and why we move the way we move with a kinesthetic experience of these principles can allow you to improve and to continue to improve your own body mechanics. Improved body mechanics skills that develop out of a kinesthetic understanding will allow you to avoid injury in your practice. Should an occupational injury due to overuse or misuse occur despite your best efforts, this book can guide you to the processes that will speed your healing and keep the injury from occurring again. The text also provides a basic understanding of how and why bodyworkers can become susceptible to thoracic outlet syndrome, carpal tunnel syndrome, low back pain, temporomandibular joint disorders (TMJ or TMD), headaches, sciatic pain, knee problems, and other repetitive motion injuries. It also provides strategies for alleviating and preventing the recurrence of these syndromes.

The skills that arise as you work through the exercises in this book will allow you to be more aware of positions and movements that will and will not work for you and the kind of massage you wish to practice. You need not abandon certain types of massage because they are too difficult on your body. You can instead mold your awareness and intention and body weight to the type of work that you want to do. The self-awareness of what feels right when performing deeper, focused work will be very different than the self-awareness of what feels right when practicing subtle energy techniques. The concepts and principles that are the backbone of this text grew out of some earlier work with kinesthetic understanding. In my previous work, *Bodylessons,* kinesthetic understanding provided the key to realizing that the body and its movement are the key to becoming whoever and whatever you want to be. In that text, I began to explain the process of merging conceptual understanding with kinesthetic experience to produce a deeper and fuller kinesthetic understanding (Dixon, 1992).

THE CONCEPTUAL FRAMEWORK

Concepts presented in this book are not theories I invented anew. They are derived from tried-and-true methods established over eons of moving experiences. To a great extent, the human body functions by rules that are universal to the species. All physical life histories are shaped by a past. They all live in the present and move toward a future. The principles utilized in this text are drawn from established practices for organizing the human body, mind, heart, and spirit. These well-known disciplines include hatha yoga, tai chi, Trager® work, Bartinieff Fundamentals, shiatsu, and Traditional Chinese Medicine. It is important to note that all of these disciplines have emerged with the recognition that to obtain any real knowledge about the body, one must examine one's own physical self. Above all, one must take the self-observations and compare and contrast them against any stated principles or rules.

I have a deep conviction that although all human bodies are shaped by the past, present, and future, the events and influences of each moment in time are unique to each individual. Each body builds its own life history with special combinations of activities and experiences. I am not alone in this belief. This is basic somatic field theory. Whenever possible, I have supplemented universal "rules" about how bodies function as derived from the movement disciplines of hatha yoga, tai chi, and other practices with personal experiences. These are anecdotes about trial-and-error encounters with the kinds of actions that seem to work most easily and effectively in massage practice. I have tried to adapt these most effective movements to a variety of body types. Massage therapists (and clients) come in all shapes and sizes. It is a crucial recognition in this work that each human frame is unique and exquisite in its integrity.

In addition to a background in movement therapies and disciplines, and experience with massage and massage education, I bring a knowledge and comprehension of the laws of human physics to the task. Physics is the study of the nature of objects in the physical world. According to Aristotle, the first reflective thinker to discourse about the cosmos, "Nature is what happens for the most part." I have attempted to observe "what happens for the most part" and formulate practical principles to guide the bodyworker in comfortable and effective body mechanics. I would like the reader to remember that if the exercises and observations elucidated in the book do not work for you, do not use them. Each body is a singular and beautiful creation that works according to its own plan. The foremost principles of this book are meant to teach you how to listen to your own inner body wisdom, which takes precedence over any doctrine that I, or anyone else, may have formulated.

KINESTHETIC EXPERIENCE

Kinesthetic experience is the body awareness that you bring to life experiences, and specifically to your experience of massage. A conceptual approach, by itself, is not enough. As massage therapists, we can certainly sense that to truly understand a mind–body shift, it must be experienced. This applies to physiological shifts to produce a greater sense of ease and comfort as we work. When one asks the question, "What does it mean to be alive?", it is likely that first the intellect will search for concepts, theories, or other words to explain. Our mental center, however, can only *think* about life. Intellect alone is unable to absorb life in all its immediacy, in the here and now. To make a real shift in our body mechanics, we must supplement that understanding with body knowledge. Kinesthetic experience can be considered a shift toward greater body awareness, which can be activated at any instant.

Puppies, kittens, and young children seem to be aware of their lives in this immediate, direct, uncomplicated way. Youngsters and animals seem to respond with whole selves, not just their heads. Sometimes, confronted with the power of the natural world, even adults can get a sense of the immediate contact with life. Deep in the woods, on the top of a mountain, watching the waves of an ocean, or the babbling of a mountain stream, we can feel life pulsing through all things, ourselves included. Here, we can feel pulsations taking on different shapes and forms, yet remaining changeless. Some call this experience "feeling the life force" or "being at one with nature"; others call it "feeling the presence of God." Whatever name we put on the experience, it is the experience, not some abstract notion, that teaches us the deepest truths about being alive.

Combining Conceptual Comprehension with Kinesthetic Experience

Although all creatures can experience life's special moments, only adult human beings can have a deep experience and know that they are having it. This new text about body mechanics, or body awareness, asks readers to pause and reflect on the meaning of their movements in massage in a new way. I hope to share how the most important thing about any kinesthetic experience, including the giving and receiving of massage, is that it shows how we are alive in the here and now. We practice our craft in a world where everything around us is alive also. Our profession bestows on us the extreme honor of touching the pulsation of life in other creatures and the opportunity to see how touch enlivens another being. This book asks massage students and professionals to consider, to sense, and to feel what it is like to live in physical bodies. When you truly consider, sense, and feel, you cannot help but wonder at the wisdom that the human body holds. And when you practice this new form of body-wise, self-aware, self-correcting body mechanics, which is more correctly termed *body awareness,* you cannot help but feel new life infuse into your hands as you work.

Layout of the Text

This first chapter serves as an introduction to the text. Here I explain the purpose and intent for writing the book (as outlined above), describe how to use the text to get the most out of the information provided, and begin to tackle the concepts of body mechanics, ergonomics, and self-care.

Chapter 2 introduces what I term *meta-principles.* These are principles that overlie the insights derived from any particular discipline. They teach any practitioner how to get "MORE" out of their massage. It is an introduction to the MORE system (created by the author) of body mechanics (**M**ovement, **O**bservation, **R**est, and **E**ase and Exploration). These are four easy methods for making massage more enjoyable and fun for the bodywork practitioner (and client).

Chapters 3 through 5 approach the study of body mechanics through knowledge bases and principles derived from three very different perspectives on physicality. Chapter 3 centers on the application of principles borrowed from the science of physics. We look at notions about how and why objects move and/or stay as they are, and examine what is the reality of vague but commonly used concepts like weight and pressure. We take our exploration of these concepts and ask how can we apply this understanding of the physical world to a study of massage (for example, how can we use physical mass to stand, shift weight, and balance during a session? Or how do we use our weight to leverage a bigger one?). Chapter 4 follows the very different paths of traditional Chinese medicine, shiatsu, and tai chi to study, theorize, and kinesthetically experience more about concepts like energy, flow, and resistance. Chapter 5 concentrates on the lessons to be derived from movement-based therapies or reeducation systems like Feldenkrais® work, Alexander work, Trager Mentastics®, and Aston Patterning®. Questions like "How could I make my work easier? What would be more playful? More fun? Lighter?" begin to emerge from this line of study.

Chapter 6 continues the investigation of movement by shifting into the examination of patterns of habitual movement. We will explore how such patterns develop, how to reshape those patterns, and how to get into the patterns presented by clients in their bodies—to "get into our client's skin," so to speak.

Chapter 7 deals with the results of repetitive patterns that are not adaptive. It describes and explains a host of repetitive motion injuries that plague the bodyworker. Along with etiology, Chapter 7 discusses prevention and treatment options for the ailing massage therapist.

Chapters 8 and 9 deal with preparing the physical body for massage. Premassage work involves some amount of physical training. Massage practitioners need to build up muscular tissue so that it is strong enough to exert whatever force is needed in the bodywork session. We also need to stretch muscles before and after massage to protect against undue tension, tearing, and pain.

In Chapter 10, the principles of effective body mechanics are adapted to special populations or conditions that can limit or change our freedom of movement. For example, if you are performing on-site massage in a corporate environment, you will want your clients to be seated in a chair. Using your body weight effectively into a body seated upright in space will be very different from the physical actions required to apply pressure down into a body supported by a massage table.

Premassage preparation also includes psychological grounding. This would encompass establishing boundaries so that clear parameters about payment, cancellation policies, and services rendered exist. Psychological preparation would also include honing up on communications skills for those times when your boundaries are going to be tested (which they will), and keeping yourself fresh and interested in your work, so it does not become just a menial outpouring of physical labor.

As referred to previously, even with the best intentions to use our body efficiently and prevent overuse and misuse of our bodies, it is possible to develop what are known as repetitive motion injuries. Chapter 10 focuses on stresses that attack each joint in the body—spine, shoulder, elbow and wrist, hip, knee, and feet and ankles. Certain syndromes well known to massage therapists and often feared out of context are highlighted and discussed. These include thoracic outlet syndrome, carpal tunnel syndrome, low back pain, midback pain, rotator cuff injuries, sacroiliac immobility and other hip problems, knee joint injuries, and feet problems.

A book on self-care for bodyworkers would be remiss if it did not include a chapter on stress. As therapists, we use physiological techniques (touch, pressure, movement, and sometimes hydrotherapy) to reduce stress and tension. It would be fitting to understand the mechanism of the relaxation response. Understanding how to prevent the buildup of harmful stress effects and subsequent disease in our own bodies will enable us to serve as gatekeepers and health educators to clients. It will also enable us to "walk the talk" of our profession in promoting health and well-being and a higher quality of life for all.

DEFINITIONS

Let us end this introductory chapter with some definitions of body mechanics, ergonomics, and self-care. These definitions will be referred to in every chapter hereafter and will begin to establish a framework for the subject matter of this book.

Body Mechanics

According to *The American Heritage Dictionary* (1985), mechanics is the analysis of the action of forces on matter or material systems. That would make body mechanics the action of forces on the human body. Unfortunately, the term can conjure up notions of the body as a machine that operates (or does not operate) according to strict and unwavering rules. As a child, I often passed by auto body shops on the highways and byways of the eastern shore of Maryland. Seeing these repair facilities, I remember thinking of these businesses as gymnasiums and spas for people to fix their aches and pains. Just as this notion was naive, so is the idea that human bodies are machines with one uniform prescription for operating at peak efficiency—tighten a screw here, hammer down a nail there, and everything will be all right. Maximum output is the goal, no matter what the circumstance. For bodyworkers, nothing could be farther from the truth.

I now believe that a more accurate term and tool for describing the endeavor to achieve efficiency in massage practices would be *body awareness*. Body awareness incorporates a fuller understanding of the action of forces on the human body. This term consolidates a comprehension of the way directional forces work with the kinesthetic lessons and processes described throughout the text. The term body awareness does not reduce the wonderfully unique and vital human body to a machine with interchangeable transmissions, crankshafts, and gears. As you will see in the discussion of ergonomics that follows, an unvarying protocol for a body mechanics dilemma cannot work in isolation of situational and human factors.

Ergonomics

Ergonomics is the use of tools in a way that helps the human body, as opposed to adapting the human body to fit the standard tools. An example of a non–ergonomically designed tool would be the "QWERTY" arrangement of keys on the standard typewriter. Studies have shown that the standard arrangement of the top letters of the keyboard (which reads as QWERTY) is extremely difficult on human wrists and fingers. In fact, the QWERTY system was actually designed to slow down the superiority of human coordination. At the turn of the century, secretaries would routinely break typewriters because they were able to key in letters faster than the machines could handle. Machines would break and businesses would lose valuable typing time and incur the expense of keyboard repair. Unfortunately, the current design for the mechanical typewriter is very stressful on the human wrist joint. As I input this text, I am noticing that in order to hold my hands to type on the keyboard, they must be excessively hyperextended and my fingers become excessively hyperflexed. In addition, my wrists become abnormally abducted (turned to the radial or thumb side) and I can feel the strain from typing just a few paragraphs. A more ergonomically designed keypad would actually separate the letters into a right and left side and be angled down (rather than up) so that a typist's wrists can remain as straight as possible.

For massage therapists, our biggest investment and most important ergonomic tool (besides our own bodies) is the massage table. It provides support for the client and for us as we use our mass to free the client from musculoskeletal pain. How do you utilize a massage table in the most ergonomically supportive way? Perhaps the most obvious answer is to set the table at the correct height. If a table is too high, you end up using your shoulders and upper body strength to do all the work. Since our biggest and most powerful muscles are in the legs and hips, we want to involve them in any use of our force. When the table is too high, the lower extremities are effectively put to sleep, as we lift our shoulders toward our neck. On the other hand, if the table is too low, the lumbar curve increases to compensate and the therapist can excessively strain his or her lower back. Both ways, the results are not good, and the end product is PAIN.

From the previous discussion, setting the table at the correct height seems like a given. The problem with defining even that much of a protocol is that the "correct height" may be more elusive than it first seems. When you are working on the back, for example, you may want to have more leverage into the core of the body than you would want when working on the shins. Thus, you want the table at a lower level to massage the back than what would be optimal for the shins. Another example of the intricacies involved at setting a table at the "perfect" height is that for palpating and releasing a spasm with deep static pressure, you may need to be further above the client than is beneficial to perform gliding effleurage strokes on the legs. What if your client has a thicker body frame? What if the client needs to be in the sidelying position (as would a pregnant client) for the work? It may be the case that for part of the massage session, you want more height over the client, and for another part, you may want to be more even with his or her body level. Aside from buying a $1,000+ hydraulic massage lift, how can you practically take care of your body?

For this problem, sly massage practitioners will look into their grab bag of tools for a variety of solutions. You may want to invest in a small step stool and/or a pair of clogs (at a cost of $10 to $15) that you can easily slip into and out of, in order to adjust your height. You may also want to purchase an office chair with a hydraulic height adjustment (available for about $40 to $60 at office supply stores). And you may want to perform passive stretches when your client has gotten dressed (e.g., hamstring stretches) so that they can be positioned on the floor. Can you see how the ergonomic solution involves knowledge of a variety of mechanical principles, of a variety of tools, and most of all, of yourself?

Let us see how you might apply this reasoning to choosing a width for your massage table. Some "experts" recommend using a 30-inch-wide table; we will take that as a baseline. Taller practitioners may be able to shift their weight over the width of this table without excessive leaning and strain to their backs. Shorter therapists may be tempted to choose a narrower table; however, the client's arms may fall off the sides without some accommodation (like a slip in sidearm piece). For wider clients, the 30-inch rule may not provide enough support for the shoulders and arms. It may be necessary to ask the client to move over gently toward you during the massage, in order to get the leverage you need. Many therapists balk at asking clients to move during the massage; however, I believe strongly that when you coach clients to move in an easy and light way, you are actually helping them to consciously integrate the massage patterns of relaxation into their muscles. When patrons simply lie passively on the table during a massage, they may feel great during and even after the session, but they have no idea how to move in a way that is nonstressful to their bodies. When clients are encouraged to practice moving in a way that is easy on the table, perhaps they can carry that sensorimotor education into everyday life.

Finding an ergonomical answer to the width dilemma may require processing all the data and choosing the best fit for you. Combining the purchase of side extenders for the arms with the adjustment of our own body height (this will affect your reach) *and* asking the client to move when necessary may all be needed. What other tools can you pluck from your bag of tricks?

Self-Care

According to *The American Heritage Dictionary* (1985), *care* means to be concerned or interested. In relation to body mechanics, self-care is turning our concern and interest to maintaining one's own good health, in order to perform bodywork easily and well. For holistic practitioners, it would seem apparent that taking care of the body is inseparable from taking care of the heart, mind, and soul. Thus, psychological self-care, such as finding social support and/or setting good and safe boundaries for yourself and your clients, is as important as a standard regimen of exercise, good nutrition, and adequate rest. These topics will be discussed more fully in Chapters 8 and 9.

It may be clear that good preventive health care involves self-care *during* the massage (e.g., shaking out hands that feel cramped or changing positions when your body says it hurts). Meanwhile, it is important to note that reliable self-care does not begin and end when the client gets on and off the table. It is imperative to make preparations *before* the session (e.g., developing coordination, stretching and strengthening routines to prepare your body to be able to meet the demands of the session). It is also crucial to maintain health care habits after a massage (e.g., icing to relieve inflammation that may have developed due to repetitive motions, and stretching to counteract the effects of habitually curling your upper back.) Self-care becomes a process that begins to shape the massage therapist's way of life. If we can't take care of ourselves, how can we offer good care to others? This book is about learning to care for ourselves as bodywork professionals—in body, mind, heart, and spirit.

SUMMARY

This chapter provides an introduction to the basic structure of the book to follow. It outlines the form and contents of each chapter and presents the importance of supplementing reading with kinesthetic experience. It presents the notion of combining understanding of rules that tend to improve ease of motion with the kinesthetic feedback that is provided by sensing your body as it moves (or does not move) in space. Key terms such as body mechanics, body awareness, ergonomics, and self-care were defined as they are used in the text. Body mechanics is the study of how forces act on the human body. Body awareness incorporates the study of body mechanics with the internal study of how the body feels as it acts. Ergonomics means allowing your body to find tools that help you, rather than adapting your body to fit a so-called tool. Self-care is turning our concern and interest to maintaining one's own good health, in order to perform bodywork easily and well. Self-care is important *during* the massage, as well as preparing your body for its work *before* a session and taking the time to re-create, refresh, and renew *after.*

REFERENCES

The American Heritage Dictionary (1985). Boston: Houghton Mifflin.

Bloom, Allan, *The Republic of Plato* (1968). New York: Basic Books.

Dixon, Marian Wolfe, *Bodylessons* (1992). Portland, OR: Rainbow Press.

Dass, Ram, *Journey of Awakening: A Meditator's Guidebook* (1978). New York: Bantam Books.

Chapter Two

Meta-Principles—
Introduction to the MORE System

CHAPTER OBJECTIVES

Conceptual Objectives The massage student/practitioner who success-fully completes this chapter (reading and exercises) will be able to:

- List five component principles of the MORE system of body mechan-ics.

- Describe each principle and relate the benefit of using it in massage.

Practical Objective The massage student/practitioner who successfully completes this chapter (reading and exercises) will be able to:

- Explain how each principle affects one's personal massage—for better or worse.

This chapter introduces basic concepts to help you begin to understand body me-chanics *from the inside.* These are ways of understanding that are based on how *your* body responds, so that you can feel for yourself what is true. Each concept will be introduced along with movement exercises, which I think of as "body-lessons" because they are lessons that the body can share with the heart, mind, and spirit. Readers need to practice and explore with the movement exercises to truly get a sensibility and a passion for the concepts. Kinesthetic principles do not hold true because an authority pronounces their validity as the authentic gospel, but only because you can sense and validate them as genuine from your core be-ing. The movement exercises or bodylessons provide a way to track daily life from the vantage point of your own body and its unique qualities and capabilities. Learning to trust this knowledge and becoming familiar and comfortable with our bodies can show how we need not always look to others for help and reassurance. When resolving a problem of how to move in the most relaxed or efficient way, at a certain point it is necessary to let go of all outside help and focus on our own strength and resourcefulness. When we automatically adjust ourselves to rules prescribed by some outside expert, we exchange a fuller experience of life for something less. On the other hand, using motion and body awareness to creatively understand our lives and our massage can be a one-derful experience.

So if you run into certain situations in which the MORE system does not seem to work for you, all I ask is that you give the basic concepts of movement, observation, rest, and ease and exploration a fair try. I have heard that it takes approximately 60 repetitions to instate or break a habit. Please realize that the way we move our bodies is learned over many years—with many defenses, reflexes, patterns, and habits to overcome. Therefore, it would be wrong to expect to replace years of habits in just a few attempts. With that caveat in place, we will proceed to the basics of getting more out of your massage.

THE MORE SYSTEM OF BODY MECHANICS

Let us begin with a general discussion of the MORE system of body mechanics—what it is, where it originated, what it was designed to do, and how it has been implemented in the past. MORE is an acronym that I invented to help students remember some basic kinesthetic principles to help bodies move more effectively and efficiently. The four letters spelling out the acronym stand for **M**ovement, **O**bservation, **R**est, and **E**ase and **E**xploration. Notice that the "E" does double duty and actually stands for two body mechanics principles.

Moving more efficiently means that you can do what you have to do (like massaging the six clients in a row that you booked for today) without hurting yourself *or* your clients. It also means that you can find the ways to use what tools you have to "get the most bang for the buck" so that at the end of your day, you will still have some energy left to carry you into your evening activities with family and friends.

In this chapter, I will explain what I mean by each of these concepts and provide critical movement exercises—the bodylessons—for experiencing each concept. The exercises are meant to be practiced and felt in the body. Remember that without kinesthetic experience to corroborate or refute the veracity of a guideline, ideas are merely abstractions without content. I believe that the real basis for understanding body mechanics will be to comprehend each of these concepts in the core of your being. Without this internal understanding, the rest of the information provided in this text will be limited, if not impossible. Without a kinesthetic understanding of movement, observation, rest, and ease and exploration, physical principles provided by any theory of biomechanics have no relationship to physical experience. Concepts without experience provide only fodder for mechanical textbook memorization without thought, consideration, or any real awareness.

I first had the idea of consolidating these four principles when teaching an advanced elective class for massage students, which I called *Bodylessons*. Bodylessons are defined as lessons that the physical body has for the thoughts, emotions, and soul. It seemed to me that massage students, before absorbing other tools for self-understanding, had to engage movement, observation, rest, and ease and exploration. When students utilized and mobilized these features, they reported being able to put more into their massage practices. And when you put more into your work, it naturally follows that you will reap more rewards and benefits back. The benefits were not nebulous at all. These were tangible results, like *more* clientele, *more* money, *more* enjoyment of the massage work, *more* excitement about the process, and falling in love with the profession all over again. I have also observed less injury and quicker recovery from trauma, stress, and burnout to the body as a result of the MORE system. Student response to the MORE system was so great that I found myself teaching experiential seminars for a variety of massage schools and for the national American Massage Therapy Association educational conference on body mechanics, with these four (five) concepts always at the heart and soul of the workshop.

Movement

The first principle of the MORE system is to keep your body *moving*. Clients can feel the difference between the touch of a therapist who is static and stuck in his or her own body, and the touch of one who is comfortable and flowing in his or her own rhythm and power. Even if you do not have a preconceived plan for how to move, the idea is that some movement is better than no activity at all. It may be an infinitesimal inner movement that only you can physically discern, but some sense of movement is crucial to life. From the day we are born to the day we die, the body stays in motion, one way or another, to keep us alive. We would expire without the rising and falling of the diaphragm, as it brings breath and vital force into the body. We cannot continue to exist without the heart beating in its chest cavity, as it propels oxygen and wastes along the circulatory canals, or the chugging away of peristalsis, as it pushes nutrients along the pathways of digestion and assimilation. Voluntary skeletal movement is the means for conveying sensory information about where body parts are in respect to each other and in respect to the space in which we live. Action is the means for making a change in surroundings, situation, or even attitude. When we are hurt, ill, or stop moving for other reasons, the neural circuits that transmit sensory and motor information do not operate as effectively. All life is in motion to some degree. Muscles work best when exercised and allowed to move freely. Inaction is an unnatural state for living animals. Even plants actively reach toward the sun as they grow and move passively with the forces of wind and rain and other acts of nature. And even minerals express the movement of atoms and molecules in a magical chemistry of life.

Synonyms and antonyms for the noun *movement* and the verb *to move* prove illuminating (*Webster's Collegiate Thesaurus,* 1976). Analogues for the noun *movement* include action, transit, change, activity, eventfulness, motion, progress, rhythm, tempo, inclination, tendency, and drift. Words with the equivalent meaning to the verb *to move* include to arouse, excite, agitate, drive, propel, rouse, shake, influence, impress, affect, touch, introduce, propose, recommend, or suggest. Antonyms are much fewer in number. Antipodes of the noun *movement* are inertia, idleness, inactivity, and pause. For the verb *to move,* opposite meanings include to halt, fix, arrest, or cease. Which group of words would you like to associate with your approach to bodywork? Which group of words would be most appealing to a client seeking to benefit from massage therapy?

I wish to make the distinction between "moves" and "movement" in touch. All too often, students focus on massage techniques or "moves" as taught, without any attention paid to the intermediate processes (how the movement proceeds). Some students try to duplicate each procedure exactly as it has been shown, in order to master the tricks of the trade. When these students graduate, they wonder why they are not achieving the amazing effects claimed by their teachers, and feel cheated as a result. Moves, by themselves, are static and dead formulas—recipes without the pizzazz and spice. Movement adds the special touch, the distinctive relish that creates a sensory experience that one can savor and remember for a long time.

In terms of physical well-being, any position, if held for too long a time, will cause injury and strain. When you keep moving during massage, you do not get stuck in uncomfortable, stress-producing, and potentially harmful stances and holds. At least when you make it a habit to continue to move during massage, you will be out of harmful holding patterns soon. When you do happen to find yourself in a nonoptimal posture as described by theoretical biomechanical theory (translation: one that feels bad), any harmful effects on your body will be limited.

I like movement for both the client and the therapist because it is easy, it is fun, and it is empowering. It is easier to move than to continually hold your body in stasis. The movements do not have to be large or forceful but whatever feels right for your body. Many of us have become so detached from our bodies that we no longer can sense what feels right; we no longer have a feeling of what our own authentic movement might be. If so, this first group of movement exercises, or bodylesson, is designed for you. They are derived from the field of dance therapy and are simply known as authentic movement.

Exercise 2.1. Authentic Movement

This exercise involves intending "to move from your inner self," whatever that may mean to you. First of all, it means tuning in to the *you* that you are right now. Today, you may feel expansive and open, or you may feel a little vulnerable and shy. You may want to move with big and flowing motions, or your steps may be small and more protective. Either way is right for you, if it feels right inside. Any style can be wrong if it does not feel authentic. Now that you have checked in on an intellectual level with your kinesthetic self, put on some music that you would enjoy hearing today. (*Hint:* Music with not too strong of a beat will allow you more freedom to find your own body rhythms without the overpowering influence of an outside tempo. The exercise can also be performed very successfully with no music at all.) Lie on the floor, just perceiving the vibrations and sounds of the music (or the silence outside and the inner vibrations inside you). Then allow yourself to perceive sensations of your physical movement. (Start with something small, like "how does it feel to move my little finger?" Or "how does it feel to move my pinkie toe?") Make sure the action feels good and right to you. Allow yourself to imagine the sensations as you rest from the movement. Continue in this way allowing your movements to expand outwardly from you. You can play with opening your attention outward, to the space you are in and the other objects that maintain their space in the room, by opening your eyes. See how the movement becomes different with eyes open and eyes closed. If it feels unsafe at any time, go back to the eyes closed and movements that do feel safe. As you feel your boundaries expand, perhaps you can incorporate moving to a kneeling and crawling base, then exploring sitting, standing, and stepping out as you feel ready to do so.

Questions for Discussion. How did this feel to you? How would you describe the movements that were most easy and comfortable to you today? Are you more aware of a pulse and a respiration that flows through your body, supporting its fluidity and rhythms? How does your body feel after this opportunity to move in any way that it wanted to?

Movement is also fun and empowering. Cortical (brain) involvement allows you to move more efficiently and to bypass autonomic patterns (habits) that may not be optimal for the body. It is both empowering and fun to take conscious control of your muscles. This next exercise, borrowed from creative drama classes, should demonstrate the power and joy that movement can impart to physically fit kids of ages 3 to 93 and beyond.

Exercise 2.2. Explosion Tag

Remember the game of tag you used to play as a kid? This is a new twist on that old favorite. The rules were pretty minimal, if you remember. You need a group of people to play, and within space limitations, the more the merrier. One person is It. It chases after anyone he or she can catch and when another person is caught, he or she becomes It and starts chasing anew. With explosion tag, there are some slight modifications. First, if you are running on a hard surface, you will need lots of cushions, futons, or soft spaces for the floor. Also, secure and mark any barriers, so that people will not run into something hard and inadvertently hurt themselves. Here are the new rules: Whenever a new It is tagged, he or she must "explode." Explode in whatever way feels right—spin like a tornado and make noise; project out like a volcano; chug along and prolong a long, drawn-out fall (onto the pillows of course). Try the game with these new rules for a while, then add a new twist—once It explodes, everyone in the group must mimic the explosion. Then, if you wish, try some more variations; for example, you could run and explode in slow motion, run and explode backwards, repeat the exploding five times in a row, explode one after another in rapid-fire "explode mode," or whatever silly thing you want.

Questions for Discussion. Monitor your heart rate and breathing pulse now. Do you feel vitally alive, with heart bounding and breathing full? Or do you simply feel winded and exhausted? How are you feeling emotionally? Did you laugh and scream during the game? Was it fun? Was it empowering to move? Would you like your massage clients to be able to share this sense of fun and empowerment during a session?

Exercise 2.3. Authentic Movement with a Table and Partner

Begin with the warm-up described in Exercise 2.1, and have a partner and massage table handy. The partner will be performing the same activities as you, but in his or her own unique style. After your authentic movements have taken you to a standing level, allow yourself to gravitate over in the direction of the massage table. Your partner will be gravitating to this meeting place in his or her own time. Allow your movements to interact with your table. Explore the space under, around, and on top of this tool that you depend on so thoroughly in your bodywork practice. Continue to explore your physical relationships with your body and the table. When you feel ready, open up your consciousness to your partner as well. Begin interacting with both the table and your partner and follow the dance. Notice whether one of you (people only) feels like assuming a more active role (like the massage therapist) and one has a tendency today to assume a more passive role (like the client), and see where the dance takes you next. Continue until the music has ended, or the dance feels complete. Switch roles and repeat the exercise.

Questions for Discussion. How did it feel to incorporate movement into your massage as the therapist? As the massage client? Did it feel easy, fun, and/or empowering? What else did you learn from the experience that might translate to how you perform bodywork in the future?

Observation

The second kinesthetic principle of the MORE system is *observing* what you are doing and how it feels when you move. Body mechanics will vastly improve when you watch yourself massaging in the here and now. Observing does not mean daydreaming about what you will do this evening or replaying that silly fight you had with your neighbor yesterday. It does not mean imagining yourself in a tropical beach resort (unless that's where you work already) or in a forest mountain scene—no matter how pleasant these places may sound. Watching in the here and now means putting some commitment into the place and space you occupy in this moment of your life. Once you notice, you can adjust to the feedback. For example, if you witness that a massage stroke or stance causes you pain, then you have the option of changing what you are doing. Pain is a clear signal that something is wrong with the body. Similarly, detecting facial expressions, gestures, or twitches in your clients can signal their pain and a need to adapt what you are doing.

Be aware that observing is not at all the same as judging. Blame should not enter into the equation at any point, either directed toward yourself or toward your client. You are not being "bad" if your body cannot stand a position that another therapist recommended to you. Neither is the client being uncooperative, if for some reason, he or she cannot relax. In fact, if you listen to either of these situations without judging, you get a clue as to how and where to focus your attention next—to relieve the discomfort and pain. See if you can learn to observe without judging, and maintain a double-edge of awareness with one edge pointed on the sensations coming into your self, and the other edge focused on observing the world and especially the client's response to your movements and touch.

One of the most important lessons of bodywork is to maintain an attitude of observation (awareness) while practicing our craft. The art of massage therapy lies in the way that we apply techniques that we have learned. If the technique is not accompanied by awareness, massage becomes a mechanical procedure. Compression, stretching, and effleurage operate better when you are cognizant of what you sense and feel and of how the client is responding to the work. In this way, massage can become a meditation.

During special moments, when the senses are keenly attuned, when motor responses are at their peak, we function at our very best. Athletes report experiencing this kind of heightened awareness as a part of "peak performance" (Millman, 1979; Dychtwald, 1986). For gymnasts, it may be a recognition that their routine just flows. Even before seeing the scores, they know that they have just completed the most exquisite backflip of the season. I have experienced this feeling of being truly aware occasionally when dancing, massaging, and teaching. As a teacher, I notice that when my students and I are working together at a keenly attuned level, I am able to reach beyond the words and to respond accordingly to their questions or comments on an expanded level.

However, peak performance is not a prerequisite for observation. Often, individuals report an expanded perception that accompanies communing with nature. Some remember a field of flowers; others see a mountain peak or waves crashing against a sandy beach. The majesty of nature can spark a "mindfulness" in many of us.

True observation and clear awareness can occur when there is no grand aspect involved whatsoever. Mindfulness can occur while drinking a cup of steaming tea, washing the daily dishes, or even when sitting alone, quiet and still.

It feels good to allow the freedom of simply being aware without judging into our corporeal lives. Self-observation is very different from making self-defeating analytic and judgmental statements like "I am not strong enough to be a massage therapist" or "It is my fault that I am experiencing pain in the lateral epicondyles of my upper arm."

The next four exercises are designed to help you develop your sense of observing without judging. As you try them, be curious and ask many questions. "How do I move? How do I turn and bend? Where do I stop moving? How is the way that I massage different from the way that my teacher(s) and fellow students massage? And how do we both perform our functions in a wonderfully divine, unique and special way?" When we listen for the answers to these questions and work with the observations that follow, our bodywork improves, along with our lives.

Exercises 2.4–2.6. Silent Witnesses

2.4. For an entire day, remember to keep both feet on the floor whenever you are sitting or standing. At first glance, the task may seem easy. But for most people, making the effort to do anything nonhabitual can be somewhat of a shock. The shock helps wake you up to a higher level of awareness, which you can then use in your bodywork practice or for self-development.

2.5. Consciously alter some other physical habit of your choosing. For example, study what it is like to choose to drink nothing but water for one day.

2.6. For one day (or one hour, or for five minutes—you can set the time limits), try to be cognizant of one part of your body, say your left toe, whenever you can remember to do so. Feel whatever sensations you feel in that area—pulsations, "stuckness," tingling, heat, cold, fluidity, or whatever.

Questions for Discussion. What sort of things were you thinking about, as you attempted to perform these three seemingly simple exercises? What brought your attention/observation to the task at hand? What took your attention away? What brings your attention back to the massage when you are working in your studio? What sorts of thought, feelings, or sensations take your attention away?

Exercise 2.7. Progressive Muscular Relaxation (Observation by Relaxing Tension)

Progressive muscular relaxation (PMR) (Jacobsen, 1929) is a tool for becoming more aware of physical tension in your body so that you can consciously release it. Letting go of physical tension amazingly transfers to relaxation of mental tension. You cannot relax your muscles and worry at the same time. The other benefit of this easy-to-learn technique is that once you have learned how to identify tension, you can let it go before it has a chance to develop into pain. (*Caution:* PMR may be contraindicated for people with a history of hypertension because it requires subjects to artificially increase their blood pressure for a short time before letting go.)

The technique itself is easy. Participants report that they do not even have to believe in the efficacy of PMR for it to work. Simply tense the muscles in one area of your body, say your right foot, feel the stress and strain, and then release. Contract your muscles as you inhale and let go as you exhale, to help differentiate the feelings of tension and relaxation. Move up through the calves, knees, and thighs progressively (thus the name) feeling the tension and then letting it go. Continue until you have worked through every part of the body. (See Figure 2.1.)

Questions for Discussion. Were you able to observe tensions in different parts of your body? How did that affect your ability to let go? Do you think that this would be a helpful tool for clients who cannot relax? How do you think that you could use PMR to develop better body mechanics in yourself?

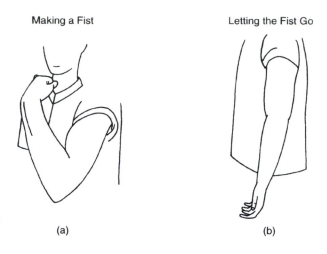

Making a Fist   Letting the Fist Go

(a)   (b)

Figure 2.1 (a–b)   Progressive muscular relaxation involves tensing muscles in one area of the body (e.g., making a fist) and then letting go.

Rest

The word *rest* has a double meaning when it comes to body mechanics and the MORE system. On the one hand, it means allowing your body to rest and restore itself when it becomes fatigued, as evidenced by tiredness, lack of concentration and coordination, or exhibiting symptoms of pain or paresthesia (numbness and/or tingling). Rest may mean lying down and taking a nap, but it also includes restorative movements that help your body to refresh and renew itself. Think of what feels like a restorative activity for you. You may enjoy swimming, talking with friends, walking, waltzing, soaking up the sun, or taking a hot, foamy bubble bath. Also consider what motions your body makes when it wants to restore itself. Many people find that shifting from side to side relieves tension in the low back. Some individuals like to twist their spines to wring out tensions like a sponge. Others prefer to open up their chests and lungs in a big expansive breath. Think of your favorite stretch and do it now, do it often, do it when you need a break from the routine you developed for your massage.

The usual interpretation of rest also encompasses the idea of stopping the kinds of repetitive motions that contribute to injury and pain. For example, if your wrists hurt, you may want to consider splinting the area for your next massage and using your forearms to deliver pressure or rescheduling the session to a time when your wrists feel better. It is important to not overwork areas that bear the brunt of your massage work, such as wrists and thumbs. Resting your body means taking care to avoid nonfunctional (injury-producing) use. In accordance with this notion of rest, massage therapists need to take special care that they are not hyperflexing or hyperextending wrists and thumbs. They also need to watch for angling the wrist toward either the thumb (abduction of the wrist) or toward the little finger (adduction of the wrist). Keep the line of the wrist as straight as possible when executing a stroke or stretch. (See Figure 2.2.)

Another nonphysiological movement that I try to avoid is an extended, abducted, and unsupported thumb. I make it a rule to never use an unsupported thumb. Thumbs are meant to oppose the hands, that is, to squeeze toward the rest of the hand, not to be forced out to the side to bear all the weight of releasing

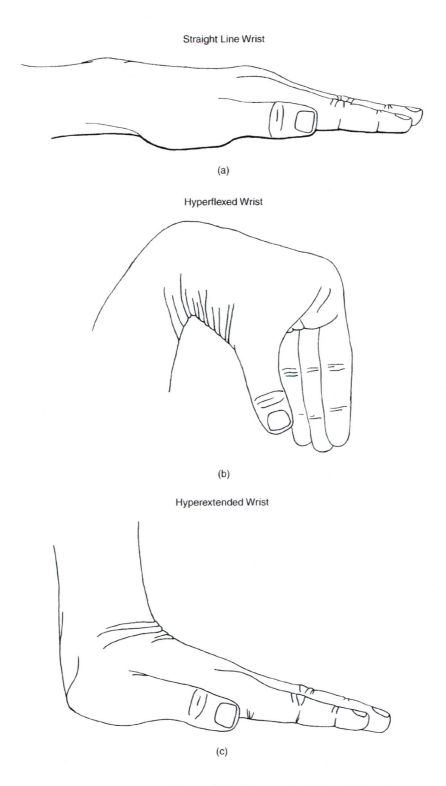

Straight Line Wrist

(a)

Hyperflexed Wrist

(b)

Hyperextended Wrist

(c)

Figure 2.2 (a–c) Keep the wrists in a straight alignment. Avoid hyperflexing, hyperextending, adducting, or abducting the wrists in massage. *(continues)*

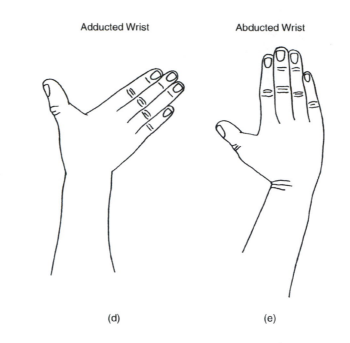

Adducted Wrist   Abducted Wrist

Figure 2.2 (d–e) *(continued)*   (d)   (e)

muscles by themselves. I do not like to see or feel thumbs away from the other fingers. You can use the thumb on the other hand to support the first thumb by interlocking the two. Alternately, you can brace your thumb against the other fingers of the same hand by making a fist. A third option is to brace one finger over another as a focused hand tool instead of using the unsupported thumb. (Most therapists brace the middle finger over the index finger or vice versa.) (See Figure 2.3.)

The other interpretation of rest for the MORE system is to use the rest of your body as bodyworker tools. Besides overused fingers, palms, wrists, and thumbs, you have a myriad of anatomical choices "within reach" for your massage manipulations and strokes. Forearms, elbows (using a guiding anchor of two fingers of the opposite hand on either side of the elbow), backs and sides of hands, closed or loose fists, and knuckles all provide different surfaces for sculpting a massage. Using the rest of your body creates variety and allows your hands to recuperate. You will be surprised at how creative your bodywork can become. I even heard of one student who became proficient in using her chin for frictional massage. (*Disclaimer:* This text does not suggest chin massage as a practice.)

Exercise 2.8. Constructive Rest*

The constructive rest position was developed to allow the body to rest in a way that theoretically requires no muscular effort (Sweigard, 1974). Remember that if a position is not comfortable for you, do not force yourself to endure it. Try the constructive rest position, with modifications if necessary, and observe the effects for you. (See Figure 2.4.)

*Adapted from "Constructive Rest" in Lulu Sweigard, *Human Movement Potential* (1974). Dodd Mead & Co./Rowman and Littlefield: Lanham, MD.

Opposed Thumb

Abducted Thumb

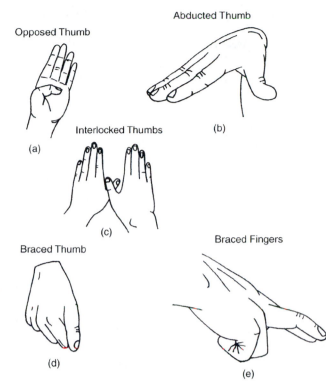

Interlocked Thumbs

(a)

(b)

(c)

Braced Thumb

Braced Fingers

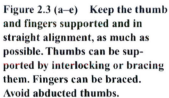

Figure 2.3 (a–e) Keep the thumb and fingers supported and in straight alignment, as much as possible. Thumbs can be supported by interlocking or bracing them. Fingers can be braced. Avoid abducted thumbs.

(d)

(e)

Lie on your back in a comfortable, undisturbed place. Let the soles of your feet stand on the floor. Bend your knees and draw them together to release your quadriceps and psoas muscles. The feet are slightly farther apart than the knees. Drape your arms comfortably across your chest, or rest them on the floor. Allow the weight of your body to be supported by the floor. With arms across the chest, the rhomboids begin to relax. As you release your body weight, the intervertebral discs are less compressed and the spine will begin to lengthen. You may need to lift your head or pelvis and reposition your spine on the floor in order to accommodate this change. Constructive rest is said to be an effective position for total body realignment. It releases tension and allows the skeleton and organs to rest, supported by the earth. Constructive rest can be practiced at any time of the day. Many knowledgeable massage therapists

Constructive Rest Position

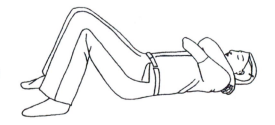

Figure 2.4 The constructive rest position is said to allow the body to rest in a way that requires no muscular effort.

use it in between clients, as a pick-me-up before the next scheduled session.

Modifications to make the pose easier for beginners include the following: Put more padding on the floor. Place a small pillow under the lower part of the pelvis. Place a pillow under the lower back, as well. Let your lower legs rest on a chair seat with the knees directly above the thigh joints. Bring the knees to rest on the chest for a few minutes to relieve pressure on the posterior pelvis. Turn to a sidelying position temporarily and rub any sore areas. If you decide to stay on your side, put more pillows under the head to align it with the torso.

Questions for Discussion. How was this constructive rest position for you? What adaptations did you have to make? How did your skeleton change over time? What muscles were affected? What other soft (ligaments, tendons, or muscles) or hard (bones or vertebral discs) tissues were affected? How was your mental and/or emotional state affected? How could you adapt this position to use as a renewal from the repetitive motions of massage?

Exercise 2.9. Listing Alternate Sources of Renewal and Restorative Movements

(a) Make a list of what you do or what you would do (if you had the time, resources, and money) to take a mini-vacation. Elaborate as much as you want. One of my friends likes to take a bubble bath with candles and incense burning and beautiful pictures that surround her. She shops for and keeps lots of toys, like a rubber ducky and soap crayons, to play with in the tub. The pièce de résistance is the set of little Christmas lights hanging around the room (everything is grounded of course), so when she turns off the overhead lights, it looks like tiny stars blinking all around.

(b) Make a list of the stretches and movements you make (or would make, if you had the time, resources, and money) to restore your body to optimal comfort. If you cannot think of anything your body would like to do, repeat the very first exercise in this chapter on authentic movement to let your body do what it wants without interference from the analytical/critical side of your brain.

Questions for Discussion. What was on your list that surprised you? Pick three items from each list and see if you can find a way to practically incorporate these into your life in the coming month. Make a plan for when (frequency), where (location), and for how long (duration) you will do these restorative activities. From past experience, I have seen that if you do not develop a strategy for change, the activities will not happen.

Exercise 2.10. Using the Rest of Your Body to Perform Massage

You will need a partner and a massage table for this exercise. Put on some music that is a little livelier than the typical new age fare; pick something you would like to listen and dance to. Your mission is to massage for an hour (if this seems too daunting, try a half hour at first) *without* using the palmar surfaces of your hands or the pads of your fingers or thumbs. These are the anatomical surfaces that massage therapists tend to overly depend on in a typical session. When you have completed your allotted time, exchange roles, so that you can experience the session from the receiver's perspective.

Questions for Discussion.   Did you get bored when you tried this new method of performing massage? Did you get bored as a client when you experienced this new technique? Or was the massage fresher, more vital and more fun? What new tools for massage did you discover in your body? Did you incorporate forearms? Knuckles? Backs or sides of hands? Knees? Even your back? What old friends in the form of massage strokes did you rediscover? Were there strokes that you rarely use that became more prominent? Did you find yourself using more *compression* (pumping the muscle against bone), *jostling* (rocking in conjunction with the client's body rhythm), *percussion* and *tapotement* (brisk simultaneous or alternating impact to the surface of the skin), and *stretching* or *traction*? Did you find that it was more difficult, if not impossible, to use effleurage (the long, flowing strokes that most people associate with massage)? How will this experience alter the way you typically think of massage? How does your body feel, especially any areas that have typically been sources of pain and discomfort for you?

Ease and Exploration

Remember that the last letter of the MORE acronym has two parts. E actually stands for two kinesthetic principles to guide your self-study of body mechanics: ease and exploration.

Ease.   Any human body can do a better job, no matter what the task, if it flows from a state of ease, as opposed to one of tension. Use your observation skills as you massage (and as you move through all the tasks of your day) to see just how you can move in a way that is easier. How can you relax other people's muscles in a way that is lighter on your own? How can you move in a way that is simpler? Some muscle contractions are necessary to hold your skeleton in a position or to transport your body structure to act. How can you let go of tensions that are not helping you maintain a posture or movement that you are intending in your massage? If you are a massage practitioner who specializes in deep tissue or other focused work, these questions apply doubly to you. Can you allow the full weight of your frame to make a client's deep release easy on your body, rather than shouldering the brunt of the burden in your upper extremities, joints, or spine (Dychtwald, 1986)? Some specific solutions to this particular question (as applied to specific stretches, compressions, or other techniques and manipulations) will be offered in later chapters, but for now I would like you to get a personal sense of how your body could adapt to make your work easier. Remember that if you hold tensions in your body, this is translated to your clients, which makes it more difficult for them to let go. In order to get some kinesthetic sense of how to incorporate ease into your bodywork, try the following exercise.

Exercise 2.11. Finding Ease of Motion*

Moshe Feldenkrais, a movement reeducator, physicist, and black belt judo master, put together tiny "Awareness through Movement" activities (1977) to allow one to find the easiest way of making a larger motion. The sequence causes you to break the habitual message your brain sends to your muscles. Here is an adaptation from a typical Feldenkrais session (1977). The steps may look complicated, but give it a try. (You may want to read the steps into a tape recorder and play them back to follow your own directions.)

Walk around the room, noticing the relative ease of your movements as you do so. You will compare this baseline feeling after you have completed the exercise. Lie down on your right side, with your knees drawn up in a fetal position and your right arm stretched out in front of you. Your left arm is resting on your buttocks. Move your left shoulder forward, then back to neutral. Do this a few times. (Remember to perform all the actions in the easiest way possible and if you get tired or if any of the actions feel stressful at any time, rest!) Move the left shoulder backward, then back to neutral. Do this a few times. Now combine the motions to move the left shoulder forward and backward a few times. Rest on your side.

Repeat these actions, but this time let your face rotate down as your left shoulder goes forward, and let your face rotate up as your left shoulder goes back. Feel the involvement of the back and of the spine. Put both these motions together; repeat until you feel tired and rest on your back. (See Figure 2.5.)

Now, roll back onto your right side, bringing up the knees a little closer to the head. This time, extend both arms out in front. Allow your left arm to become "longer" than the right by moving shoulders and spine and head and whatever other body parts help the movement, then move it back to neutral. Allow the left arm to draw back and become "shorter" than the right. Combine the actions, repeat a few times, and then rest on your back. (See Figure 2.6.)

Feel the difference between the two sides. Repeat the entire sequence lying on the left side. (If you are listening to this on a tape recorder, you may want to reread the directions above, interposing left and right.) Rest as appropriate. Slowly roll to one side, push up to a seated position, and then slowly stand. Take a little walk around the room, and notice the sway of your arms, head, and spine as you move.

Questions for Discussion. Do you notice a difference in ease as you walk for the second time? If so, to what do you attribute this enhanced ease of motion?

*Adapted from Maureen McHugh, personal communication/Feldenkrais Awareness through Movement® Class, 1990.

Feldenkrais Exercise A—Step 1

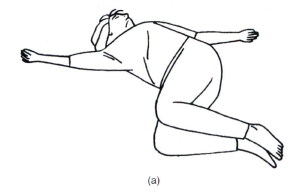

(a)

Feldenkrais Exercise A—Step 2

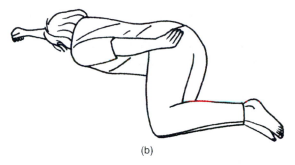

Figure 2.5 (a–b)   Feldenkrais Exercise A—Lie on the right side and move the left shoulder back (2.5a), then forward (2.5b). Repeat on the other side.

(b)

Feldenkrais Exercise B—Step 1

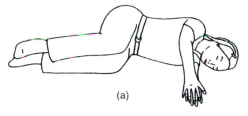

(a)

Feldenkrais Exercise B—Step 2

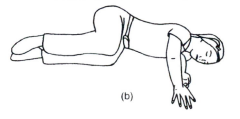

Figure 2.6 (a–b)   Feldenkrais Exercise B—Lie on the right side (2.6a), and move the left arm forward (2.6b). Repeat on the other side.

(b)

Exploration.   As far as exploration goes, the more you can incorporate into massage, the better. I sometimes observe students or practicing therapists who believe that once you get enough techniques under your belt, you should establish a set, unvarying format or protocol for each client problem that you enounter. What is wrong with this strategy? It certainly allows the therapist to develop a plan of action. I believe in developing a plan of action after interviewing my client in the intake procedure. However, once the client lies down on the massage table or sits in the onsite chair, it becomes crucial to adapt and revise the plan, depending on what I discover as I palpate the tissues. If I do not proceed to the second phase of exploration, this freezes each client into a problem to be treated or fixed. Withdrawing attention from what you see and feel during the massage stops your own (and in turn, the client's) inner process of discovery. Massage practitioners who view their work as exciting, exploratory, and full of wonder and joy create a rhythm and flow in massage that is perceived immediately and directly by their clients. Contrast this with a technician who is inherently bored with massage or consumed and concerned by other matters. You can easily see how this, too, can have a direct effect on the client. It also has a direct and clear effect on massage practitioners and their body mechanics. A massage therapist who is not fully engaged in the work is more likely to inadvertently lock the knees or hold the back in an excessive lumbar or cervical curve.

Practitioners may not want to waste time during a session to explore and adjust. This makes them more likely to disregard ergonomics. For example, a hurried therapist may use unsupported thumbs as a quick way to release a spasm, rather that taking the few seconds of time to adjust, shift positions, and avoid injury. Thorough examination coupled with listening is actually a more efficient way to utilize time.

Massage therapists may be reluctant to inquire or explore because they do not want to make a mistake. It feels safe to stick to tried-and-true methods that have released spasms or adhesions in the past. Bodyworkers may also not want to inadvertently perform a movement that may be a little out of the ordinary, for fear of how others will react to something new. In my own practice, I have found that when I regularly ask for feedback, people are extremely helpful and responsive about new approaches. When clients are included in the healing process, they respond far more favorably to the experience as a whole. Perhaps this next experience (plus well-established lines of communication between therapist and client) can alleviate some fears around trying something new.

Exercise 2.12. Exploring the Hand

You will need a partner for this exercise. (*Optional:* Put on some background music. Play a piece without too strong a beat or too many words that could distract you from the exploration at hand.) For the next 10 to 15 minutes, suspend your "knowledge" about your partner's hand, and instead imagine that it is a creature from another planet. You have never seen anything like it and you are trying to gather as much information about this friendly creature (it will not bite or hurt you in any way) as you can. You are encouraged to use all of your sensations to explore the crea-

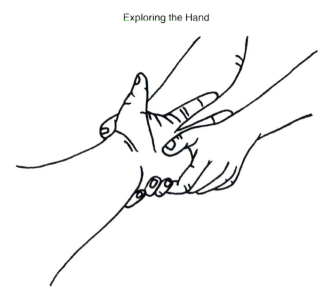

Figure 2.7 Exploring the hand can help you to stay fascinated with bodywork.

ture (except perhaps the sensation of taste) in your investigation, but concentrate especially on the sensation of touch—your primary medium as a massage therapist. If you find yourself either getting bored during the exercise or lapsing into trying to massage or fix this creature, remind yourself that your job is to explore and to stay fascinated with your work. When you have completed the 10- to 15-minute exploration (set an alarm, because time may pass before you are ready and you may not want to stop), exchange roles with your partner. You become the creature, and your partner becomes the explorer for the next 10 to 15 minutes. (See Figure 2.7.)

Questions for Discussion. Discuss the answers to these questions with your partner. When you played the role of explorer, what did you learn about yourself? What did you learn about your partner? In what ways was the creature wonderful? What did you not like about the creature? What sorts of qualities did you find yourself exploring? When you played the role of the creature, what did you learn about yourself? What did you learn about your partner? What role did you enjoy more today? How does your hand feel after being explored in this way?

SUMMARY

This chapter provides an introduction to the key concepts of the MORE (movement, observation, rest, ease and exploration) system. Movement is necessary to keep your body (and the massage) fluid and to allow you pass out of harmful positions before they become set patterns. Observation means paying attention to what you do without judging. Rest

(continued)

means taking the time to recover and renew and restore your energy and stamina. Rest also means using alternate parts of your body to deliver pressure in a massage. Ease reminds us to find the easy and comfortable ways to move our muscles. Exploration involves seeing each new body-work situation as a fresh challenge, finding something in each session that is exciting and new. By providing exercises for each concept—movement, observation, rest, and ease and exploration—the chapter re-inforces the importance of supplementing reading with kinesthetic experience. Think about what you have learned kinesthetically through these basics before proceeding to the next section.

REFERENCES

Dixon, Marian Wolfe, "Awareness—A Bodylesson for Bodyworkers," *Massage and Bodywork Journal* (Spring 1996), pp. 20–22.

Dychtwald, Ken, *Bodymind* (1986). Los Angeles: Jeremy P. Tarcher, Inc.

Feldenkrais, Moshe, *Awareness Through Movement* (1977). New York: Harper & Row.

Jacobsen, E., *Progressive Relaxation* (1929). Chicago: University of Chicago Press.

McHugh, Maureen (1990). Feldenkrais® class personal communication. Arlington, VA.

Millman, Dan, *Body Mind Mastery* (1999). Novato: New World Library CA, www.nwlib.com

Sweigard, Lulu, *Human Movement Potential* (1974). Lanham, MD; Rowman and Littlefield.

Webster's Collegiate Thesaurus (1976). Springfield, MA: G & C Merriam Company.

Chapter Three

Principles of Physics—Moving and Static Objects, Weight and Pressure

CHAPTER OBJECTIVES

The massage student/practitioner who successfully completes this chapter (reading and exercises) will be able to:

- Explain Newton's three laws of motion.

- Describe how Newton's laws relate to efficient body mechanics.

- Explain how Newton's principles affect one's personal massage—for better or worse.

- Explain the law of structural alignment.

- Explain the law of balance.

- Describe how the law of structural alignment and the law of balance relate to efficient body mechanics.

- Explain how the law of structural alignment and the law of balance affect one's personal massage—for better or worse.

- List four guidelines to keep in mind when striving for dynamic alignment.

- List six signs that one's body is not working with efficient body mechanics.

This chapter begins by elucidating principles that govern the behavior of physical objects in the world. You will become acquainted with static forces that help achieve and/or maintain an upper body position or a lower body stance and the dynamic forces that contribute to movement, compressive forces, and leverage (for lifting, used in passive or active and resistive stretching). Kinesthetic awareness (paying attention to how your body feels in the moment) is paramount to putting the principles of good body mechanics into practice. Without the benefit of the kinesthetic exercises described in the previous chapter, these principles cannot be practically applied to fit your particular body frame and style of practice.

WHERE DO RULES FOR BODY MECHANICS COME FROM?

In this section, the laws of human physics are used to establish an understanding of efficient body mechanics. Mechanics is a branch of physics that studies the behavior of objects in the physical world. Physical science is a process of observing the natural world and summing up the observations. For body mechanics, the process of inquiry is the same—observing and summarizing the findings. According to Aristotle, in his discourse about the cosmos, "nature is what happens for the most part." The human body functions by natural physical laws that happen for the most part as well.

This chapter allows you to scrutinize notions about how and why objects move and/or stay as they are. You will also explore the reality of commonly used but unclearly defined concepts like weight and pressure. Taking the examination further, you will apply an understanding of how physical objects behave to the study of massage. For example, how can we efficiently use our weight to stand, balance, and shift positions? Or how do we use our mass as a ballast to leverage a heavier client?

Earlier chapters stressed the importance of testing rules against your own experience. There may be exercises or activities that do not work for you. If nature is indeed "what happens for the most part," then logic dictates that some people will operate outside these parameters. Humans can be remarkably similar in certain aspects, but each body is a singular and beautiful creation that works according to its own plan. Natural body mechanics principles developed in this chapter are intended to be measured against your own kinesthetic experience.

The principles described here will be supplemented with rules derived from alternative perspectives in the next two chapters. Chapter 4 explores Eastern-based systems like traditional Chinese medicine, shiatsu, and tai chi and builds on their concepts of energy, flow, and resistance. Chapter 5 concentrates on the sensorimotor lessons to be derived from movement-based therapies or reeducation systems like Bartenieff Fundamentals, Feldenkrais®, Alexander work, Trager Mentastics®, and Aston Patterning®. In this chapter, you are prompted to ask questions like "How can you make your work easier and lighter? What would be more playful, and fun?" No matter which chapter perspective(s) you adopt for your main organizing principle(s), remember to ask, "How can these guidelines work for my clients and me?"

Comprehending the rules described in these three chapters (or coming up with individual alternatives based on a conceptual understanding of the principles and exercises presented therein) can lead to performing bodywork in a way that will not hurt you. Should an occupational injury take place despite your best efforts, turn to Chapter 10 to guide you to processes that will speed healing and keep the injury from happening again. Chapter 10 covers the etiology and treatment options for major overuse syndromes that can affect bodyworkers, such as thoracic outlet syndrome, carpal tunnel syndrome, low back pain, temporomandibular joint (TMJ) disorder, headaches, sciatic pain, and knee and other joint discomforts. It also provides strategies for preventing the recurrence of repetitive motion conditions.

Standards for bodywork efficiency take us directly back to the concepts of *body awareness, ergonomics,* and *self-care.* In Chapter 1, body awareness was defined as being aware of the body. Body awareness consolidates the study of how forces act on the human body with the internal study of how the body feels as it acts. Ergonomics means allowing your body to find tools that help you, rather than adapting your body to fit a so-called tool. Self-care is turning our concern and interest to maintaining one's own good health. Self-care is important *during* the massage, as well as preparing your body for its work *before* a session and taking the time to "re-create and refresh and renew" *after.*

At first, it may seem unusual to look to the world of traditional physics to establish standards for efficient bodywork. Body mechanics implies understanding of how bodies work. To achieve an understanding of how bodies move in time and space requires study and examination. A good place to begin a scientific inquiry on motion is to borrow from Sir Isaac Newton's (1687) axioms on laws of motion.

The Law of Inertia

Newton's first law states that *"Every body continues in its state of rest, or of uniform motion in a right line unless it is compelled to change that state by forces impressed upon it."* This law is commonly known as the *law of inertia.* The current task is to determine how inertia applies to bodyworkers. In fact, this axiom can apply to several massage situations. Let us examine the law of inertia with regard to the client's body. If the client has an adhesion (a stuck place between or within a muscle), chances are that the "stuck place" will remain the same unless some kind of input (in the form of massage, movement, or hydrotherapy) is added.

The law of inertia can also help to understand the way practitioners' bodies move (or do not move) as they work. For example, a state of inaction, once adopted (such as stabilizing yourself in a horse stance) is apt to continue, unless something stimulates change. Notice that when a particular place in your body is stuck and does not move as you massage, the stoppage tends to block all of your movements. It also requires more impetus and work to shift out of the stable position. Working, for example, with thighs locked against the massage table effectively cuts off the power of the lower extremities and forces you to rely on sheer upper body strength. In response, shoulder, neck, and upper back muscles become overworked and strained. Muscle fibers that attempt to hold onto a position that is no longer efficient are a major cause of fatigue and overuse or misuse syndromes for bodyworkers. That translates into a primary source of injury for the massage practitioner. Lest you think that you are "unselfishly" helping the client by bracing and holding onto an uncomfortable position, check it out with the client—your best expert. Discomfort, a feeling of being stuck, and obstruction of movement are undeniably transferred. My friend, Ingrid, who rides horses, recounts a story that illustrates how this happens. She told me of a riding exercise in which the rider keeps the eyes closed and body relaxed and concentrates on feeling strains that arise in the horse. Another person leads the horse around the ring. According to Ingrid, the rider can actually feel the horse pick up tensions. If the leader is holding the neck forward, the horse will too. It is also true that when the rider holds his or her back rigidly, the horse adopts that same stance. It is not a far stretch to imagine that the same kind of transfer takes place between givers and receivers of massage. When you take the time to move out of a scrunched position, clients can experience touch as more comfortable to receive.

The law of inertia states that a moving object most easily continues in a straight line. Consider the positioning of your body as you deliver a massage stroke. When you are lined up in the direction of your stroke, the move becomes more efficient. When your spatial intent is clear, your whole body can participate in the movement, and the various parts of your body can share in the impetus for change. Know and align your whole self in the direction you want the tissues to move. This is especially important in various dynamic lines of the body, including the head to coccyx line of the spine and the line between the anterior superior iliac spines (ASISs). You can palpate your own ASISs by following your iliac crest to the front and feeling for the bumps. Sometimes in body mechanics, these protrusions are likened to the headlights of the body. It is best to keep them shining in the direction of your work. The direction of your feet is also important. If everything is facing and focusing effort in one direction, but the feet are pointing away, your body cannot help twisting and distorting the force. This tends to divert the power away from your work and to hurt you. (See Figure 3.1.)

The Second Law of Motion

Newton's (1686) second law declares that *force equals mass times acceleration (F = ma or F/m = a); at any instant, the acceleration (change, strictly speaking, the change in direction and speed) of a body is directly proportional to the force applied to it and inversely proportional to its mass.* This means that the bigger a body you are working with, the more effort it requires to change. It also means that how much force you apply directly relates to how much change you get. "F = ma" does not mean that you must bear down like a hammer on clients, especially the larger ones, with all of the pressure you can muster in order to effect any kind of appreciable change. It does mean that clients with denser tissue (providing that they do not have an extremely low pain threshold) will tend to require deeper work. (Remember that pain is always an indication to back off and reassess. Make sure to establish good verbal communications to encourage and understand your clients' signals when pain gets in the way of your work.) F = ma also suggests that a therapist who has learned to apply more force without strain will be better prepared to effect change (providing that the force does not cause trauma or resistance) in a client. Acceleration refers to change in direction as well as speed. Therefore, positioning your body to move in the direction of intended force will increase the accelerative (healthy change) effect. If the client's body resists your effort, the law of action and reaction, as described in the next section, will moderate the second law.

Torqued Body

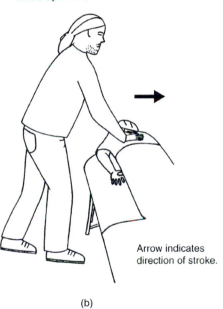

Arrow indicates
direction of stroke.

(a)

Lined Up in Direction of Stroke

Arrow indicates
direction of stroke.

**Figure 3.1 (a–b)   Keep the body
all lined up from feet to head in
the direction of the stroke.**

(b)

The Law of Action and Reaction

Newton's (1686) third law states that *"If one body exerts a force on a second, the second exerts an equal and opposite force on the first."* This axiom is commonly referred to as the law of action and reaction. Does this immutable third law hold true only for machinery and robots or does it apply to living creatures as well? Perhaps the next experience will provide an answer to this question.

Exercise 3.1. Tissue Reaction in the Human Body

This exercise is designed to demonstrate the reaction of the soft tissues in the body to various types of pressure. First, take a baseline measurement by pressing as deeply as you can into the skin and underlying muscles and fascia of your opposite forearm. Now repeat the exercise, but this time allow yourself to "listen" to the tissues of the forearm. This means taking time and sinking in only as far as the structures allow. Do not push past the point of resistance. Wait for the tissue to soften before going further. Take all the time you need to follow the muscles' give before moving out.

Questions for Discussion.   Which way could you get in deeper? Why do you think this phenomenon occurred?

When you push hard against an object, even an object like your own living skin, the first reaction of the tissues is to push you back out. In contrast, when you take the time to let the tissues adjust to your pressure, you find that you can go much deeper into the core structure of the body. In that way, you are setting up a situation in which the tissues can respond, rather than merely react.

Exercise 3.2. Mirroring

In a typical mirroring exercise, partners begin by facing each other. One partner takes the "initiator" role, and the other becomes the "mirror." The initiator moves (with any part of the body and in any direction that he or she chooses), and the follower mirrors the actions. Keep your movements slow enough so that they can be followed. The object of mirroring is for the actions to be successfully duplicated. Continue in your original role for a specified amount of time (e.g., 5 minutes), and then reverse roles. Switching roles allows both participants to assume the responsibility for leading (in the initiator role). It also allows both participants to sense their bodies moving in a way that can seem very foreign to them (in the mirror/follower role). (See Figure 3.2.)

In a more advanced form of mirroring, teams play the two roles. Teams face each other, and one entire crew first takes the initiator role. In this version of the kinesthetic exercise, each person must not only mirror a counterpart, but must also maintain the same relationship to his or her crew members as the counterpart on the other team.

Questions for Discussion.   How did you feel as the initiator? What did you learn from that role? How did it feel to tangibly see the results of your actions, as portrayed by another? How did you feel as the follower? What did you learn from that role? About yourself? About your

Mirroring

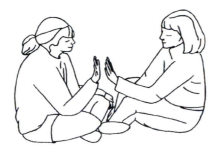

Figure 3.2   In mirroring, one partner initiates a movement and the other follows.

partner(s)? Which role did you like better today? Why? Do you think that would be the same for you on another day? Why or why not?

One major difference between inanimate and living human bodies is that humans have the potential of realizing that they can respond, act, and feel as they choose. Lack of freedom does not come from other people or outside conditions, but from inside yourself. One way to give up your freedom is to not allow yourself to make a choice. You are not free when you give up the choice of how to respond in a given situation. You are not free when you simply react.

Reacting implies merely acting again, without calling forth any new response to meet the challenge. Responding is a higher-level process, which involves knowledge of yourself and the situation at hand, and making a choice. Reacting occurs on a baser, more instinctive level and involves no choice. When a stranger criticizes you, you may react by feeling hurt and angry. The first step to freedom is realizing that you have other options. For instance, it may be that you could think that this stranger is criticizing you only because he or she is having a bad day. Do you want to succumb to a reaction that makes you feel bad about yourself, or do you want to choose a response that makes you feel good? This ability to respond is at the heart of true responsibility.

In the next variation of the mirroring experience, the lines between initiator and follower may become blurred.

Exercise 3.3. Circling Hands

Once again, take a partner for this exercise. Put on some soothing music and face each other. Let your hands come together with your partner's hands, palms to palms, fingers intertwined, or in a handshake hold—whatever is comfortable. Gradually allow your connected hands to make circles in the air. Stay connected to your partner, whatever that means to you. As the music continues to play, allow the circles to evolve into a pattern of movement with each other. Without speaking, take turns becoming the leader and follower. Allow a hand "dance" to emerge out of the shared movement.

Questions for Discussion. As you follow these instructions, you will notice that you may tend to assume the initiator role, or you may tend to assume the role of the follower. Which role did you assume most often? Which did you prefer? Think about the paired roles in terms of leading and following, giving and receiving, speaking and listening, doing and being. Does this partnership relate to the simultaneous act of giving and receiving within a massage? How?

If you experienced a natural unfolding and relaxation of muscles, tendons, and ligaments in either role, answer the following questions. How would a client experience this kind of relaxation? Can you facilitate a change in tissue simply by using your hands to listen? Is this different from acting on and expecting a "fixed" reaction from the soft tissues? How so? Do you utilize massage techniques that encourage and allow clients to heal themselves or do you focus on "fixing" or "treating" complaints?

In addition to Newton's three laws of motion, other natural laws (of mechanical motion) explain additional forces that govern a human body as it moves. Some axioms help explicate static and dynamic *alignment* (shifting weight), or finding and using *balance* and equilibrium and the *center* of the body (grounding). Other principles relate to *breathing* and *support*.

The Law of Structural Alignment

"In any plane, physical or non-physical, structure implies relationship" (Rolf, 1989, p. 30). The law of structural alignment says that structure reflects the relationships and connections within the body. No muscle works alone. For example, to flex the elbow, the biceps (the "make a muscle" muscle on the front of the upper arm) must contract, and the triceps (on the back of the upper arm) must relax. Otherwise, we would find ourselves in a continual struggle to move our elbows. The structure of the skeleton also provides links between our various body parts. Because of the spinal column, the head and coccyx maintain interdependence. Because of the way the shoulder joint connects to the elbow, and the elbow joint in turn connects to the wrist, the scapula affects the hand.

Another way to speak about the alliance of structures within the body is to use the term *dynamic alignment.* This term implies an association that is not fixed and immobile, but one with an ability to form and maintain efficient relationships between body parts. The following guidelines can help maintain dynamic alignment during a massage.

1. *Have the feet facing in the direction of the stroke.* Feet can be slightly turned out, but a right or obtuse angle is too much. When toes are spread at right angles (or greater), the body is split in its intention. The pelvis is positioned to move in two different and mutually exclusive directions. You are very stable, but so much so that you are immobilized. You cannot move. A common error is to let the back foot turn out when there is no weight on it.

Even so, it is important to have the back foot in place, so that the pelvis can move forward with no rotational split. Therefore, the back foot should face the direction of the stroke even when it bears none of your weight.

2. *Keep the spinal curves intact.* The spine holds a natural curvature at the levels of the thorax (kyphosis), neck, and low back (cervical and lumbar lordosis). Looking on anteriorly, the spinal curve demonstrates convexity at the cervical spine, then becomes a concave curve at the rib cage which then turns convex again at the lumbar spine. (The sacrum/coccyx forms a fourth curve that looks concave from the front. However, at this level, the bones are fused together.) When the rib cage gets displaced either forward (hypokyphosis) or backward (hyperkyphosis), disruptions in the normal curve of the thoracic spine tend to disengage the scapula. In a displaced position, the strength of the upper body is lost and the work being done is muscled with the arms. This can prove exhausting, as well as damaging to the structures of the shoulder joint, shoulder girdle, and neck.

   Too much lumbar curve (hyperlordosis of the low back) can overwork the erector spinae muscles and result in low back pain. Too little curve (hypolordosis) results in overstretching and weakness in the low back area.

   It can be tempting for bodywork practitioners to drop the head to look down at the client or to lift the head up too far. Too much cervical curve (hyperlordosis of the neck) results from a neck that juts up and forward. Too little cervical curve (hypolordosis) can have some dramatically bad results for the massage therapist. When the head is compressing down on the thoracic area, many important muscles are compressed and contracted. Two of these, specifically the pectoralis minor and the scalenes can in turn put pressure on the brachial plexus, a braid of nerves that innervate the arm and hand. As you can guess, the outcome would not be beneficial. The syndromes that can result from this kind of impingement are discussed in more depth in Chapter 7.

3. *Line up the body directly behind the hands.* Although every hand is designed a little differently, all therapists should follow this step as much as reasonably possible, in order to bear the weight of the pressure through the bones. (See Chapter 2, section on Rest.) There is a great tendency in massage to hyperextend at the wrist, finger, and thumb joints. To a lesser extent, you may be also tempted to hyperflex or to abduct or adduct your wrist.

   Keep wrists long and extended. Any kind of torque is bad for the wrist joints. Carpal bones are easily susceptible to dislocation. At times, you will need to adapt alignment in the three spinal curves by bending at the waist or knees in order to keep your hands aligned. For example, when performing a shingling stroke (i.e., hand-over-hand effleurage) over the hamstrings, you will need to bend at the knees to keep the wrist in a position that is almost parallel with the surface of the table. To accomplish this, it will help to back away from the table and use your back foot as a lever.

4. *Keep the thumb close to the fingers.* Thumbs also have different shapes. If you use the pads of the thumbs to press down, they have a tendency to hyperextend. Anytime a joint is hyperextended, it puts stress on the tendons

and ligaments and can tear fibers. If this microinjury happens repeatedly, it becomes a source of inflammation, pain, and swelling. Instead keep your thumb close to your fingers so that you are working straight on, and the thumb bears its weight in a vector that moves in line with the rest of the joint. (See Chapter 2, section on Rest).

5. *Avoid hyperextending the elbows and knees.* Both of these hinge joints need to be slightly flexed. This will help you to avert the problem of locked knees and/or elbows and the resulting inflammation, tearing, and hypersensitivity that can ensue.

6. *Feel the shoulder blades swinging easily from the spine.* What does your rotator cuff feel like when you are working? You will feel only the front or the back of your shoulders when the shoulder muscles are pinched, depending on whether the shoulders are rotated in or out too far. The subscapularis muscle becomes excessively contracted when the upper extremity rotates in too far in relation to the axial skeleton (spine). The infraspinatus and teres minor are stressed when the arm rotates out too far. Since all of the rotator cuff muscles work together to hold the humerus in relation to the scapula, when one is out of line, other rotator muscles attempt to compensate and tend to be pulled out of line too. When you do not address all of the composite parts of the rotator cuff, rehabilitation takes longer and is more difficult to achieve. (See Chapter 10.)

Exercise 3.4. Visualizing Skeletal Alignment/Structural Relationships in the Body

Sit with your legs crossed and hands resting on the knees, palms upward. Close your eyes and focus on your breathing until you begin to feel relaxed. Allow yourself to feel your skeletal alignment, as you imagine the following.

See the bowl of your pelvis as you sit on the floor (the os coxae, each composed of three fused bones—ilium, ischium, and pubic bone). Visualize the symphysis pubis cartilage, where the pelvis is fused in front, and the acetabulum, where it is fused at the sides. Feel the ischial tuberosities (sits bones) resting on the floor.

Visualize down the thighs and legs. Bring to mind the femur, tibia, and fibula of each leg in turn. See in your mind's eye your tarsals (anklebones), metatarsals, and phalanges (toes) as your foot rests on the floor.

Now imagine a cord at the top of your head at the junction of the coronal and sagittal sutures. Feel the cord lifting up, gently pulling all 26 vertebrae into alignment. Lift your body up and out of your hips and feel the entire spinal column—the coccyx (tailbone) and sacrum touching the floor, and on top of them in order the five lumbar vertebrae, twelve thoracic bones, and the seven cervical spines.

Slightly lift the sternum. Imagine feeling each part of the sternum—the manubrium, the gladiolus (body), and the xiphoid process hanging down. Allow the ribs to expand, including the seven pairs of true ribs directly attached to the sternum and five pairs of false ribs, two of which are floating. Feel all of the ribs as they attach in back to the vertebrae of the spine.

Allow the shoulder girdle to widen. Feel the expansion in the chest, spreading your clavicles (collarbones) and scapulas (shoulder blades). Allow the arms to hang loosely at your sides. Feel each humerus loose and relaxed, and allow the ulna and radius in each forearm to be relaxed. Relax into your carpals (wrists), metacarpals, and phalanges (digits) of both hands as they rest on your knees.

Visualize the bones of your cranium (skull)—the frontal, the two parietals on the sides, and the two temporal bones through which are the ears, the sphenoid in the center of the skull, and the occiput in back. Allow the muscles of the face to relax—around the mandible (jawbone), maxilla (under the nose and upper lip), zygomatics (cheekbones), and vomer (in the center of the nose). The face feels soft, and even the tongue is relaxed; visualize the free-floating hyoid bone supporting the tongue. Reach your hand up under the jaw and palpate the hyoid bone to locate it.

Scan your body again, bringing in a general picture of all the bones. See each joint in the body as open and free. Feel the easy movement of breathing and allow all of your bones to relax with each breath out. When you feel ready, bring your arms overhead and stretch before bringing your attention back into the room.

Exercise 3.5. Examining Dynamic Alignment in the Body

To examine dynamic spinal alignment, begin by getting down on all fours (hands and knees) and focus on the vertebrae. Now arch the back more so that your head and coccyx both rise, then arch the back in the opposite direction so that the head and tailbone both curve toward the earth. Some yogis know this series as the "cat–cow" pose. (See Figure 3.3.)

Continue this examination of dynamic spinal alignment in this next variation. Still kneeling on all fours, place your forehead on the floor and keep head contact with the floor while rolling forward toward the crown of your head. Then roll back to the original contact point at the forehead. (See Figure 3.4.)

Let the head come up. Now feel dynamic spinal alignment on the side, by bringing your head and tailbone closer on the right side, like a dog chasing after his tail. Do the same for the left side. (See Figure 3.5.)

Centering

Being centered means that you have found a center of physical balance. When centered, you feel right at home where you are. When your energy moves from the core of the body, you need less muscle strength to work, move, and massage. When you find your hub, you are more stable, but that does not mean you are more stuck in one position. Actions are also more powerful when they radiate

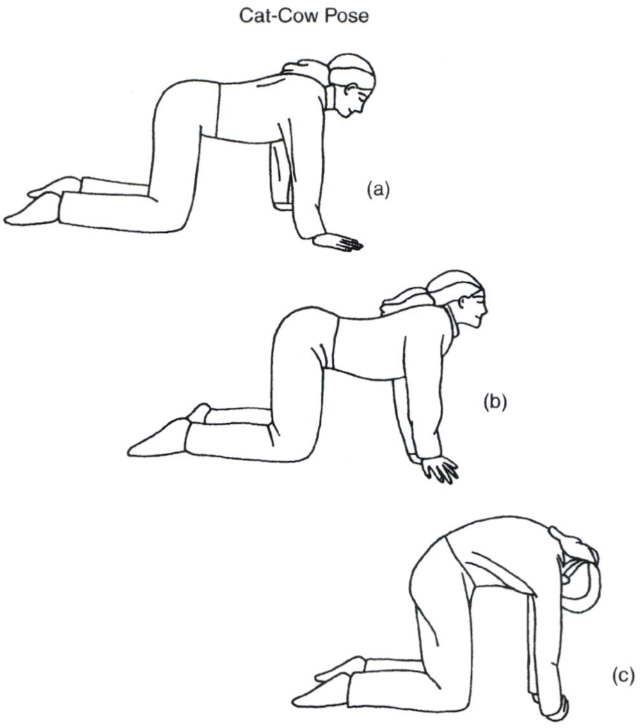

Cat-Cow Pose

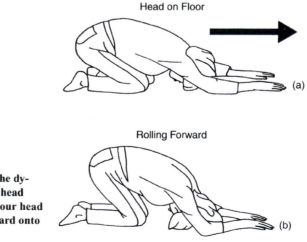

Figure 3.3 (a–c) Arching the back up and down helps you to sense the dynamic alignment of the head and coccyx as you move.

from a strong core. With a solid pivot point, energy can flow freely out through the arms and hands. Being centered entails finding a stable posture and remaining grounded, or aware of your contact with the ground through the legs and feet. (See the section in this chapter on Grounding.) Imagine a tree with roots that go down deep into the earth. When you seek the center, you seek the innermost core, or the heart of the matter. A center is always found within oneself.

The physical midpoint of the human body lies in the belly or abdomen, the

Head on Floor

Rolling Forward

Figure 3.4 (a–b) Sense the dynamic relationship of the head and coccyx as you place your head on the floor and roll forward onto the crown of your head.

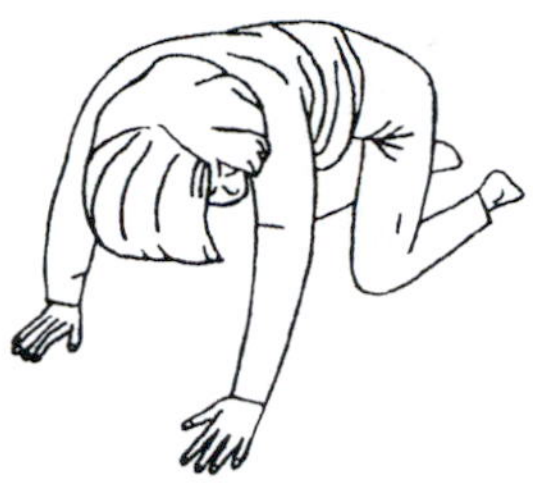

"Dog Chasing Tail"

Figure 3.5   Notice the dynamic alignment of the head and coccyx as you "chase the dog's tail."

soft tissue between the rib cage and pelvic bone. The rib cage is the housing for the lungs, which in turn govern the intake and outtake of breath. Exercise 3.4 demonstrated how attention to the breath can calm the spirit and balance the use of external musculature. The pelvic bowl serves as an attachment for the largest muscle groups in the body. These large and powerful muscles are the gluteals, the quadriceps on the front of the thigh, and the hamstrings, which make up the posterior thigh. Between pelvis and rib cage lies the belly. Most body organs are situated here. All of the body's vital metabolic functions are active here. Geographically, the abdomen is located in the middle of the human gravitational structure. Considering all these contributing factors, we can see how the place residing a few inches below the navel (to be more fully discussed in the Chapter 4, on Eastern influences) can act as a focal point of power, gravity, equilibrium, and stability.

When you begin by physically orienting over your core center of support in deep work, you can still make small adjustments such as shifting wider or more forward. Larger adjustments require a step or other shift, changing the actual center of support. When applying deep pressure, your hands bear the weight of your body. If the client moved away from you at this point, you would fall. The client has become an auxiliary support for your pressure.

When you can rely on core alignment, you will be able to more accurately read the client's musculature and connective tissue. When your body is in line and functioning optimally, you can feel tissue as it softens and opens up underneath your hands (a crucial part of myofascial release, muscle sculpting, Rolfing ®, and structural integration). You can palpate with tougher structures like elbows, because centering creates the clarity to allow you to accurately listen and read very subtle changes in sensations. Moving with a well-established center also allows the client to feel safe as you sink in. If you are muscling into the client, it will feel poky and the client will involuntarily harden to protect against you. The end result is that the client's muscles will contract and push you out.

Staying centered makes for easier passage through inner and outer disturbances. Have you ever seen a potter centering a lump of clay on a potter's wheel, or attempted to throw a pot yourself? If you have, you notice that when the clay is really in the center, it appears motionless on the wheel, no matter how fast it is turning. If the clay is not perfectly centered and the turn of the wheel is accelerated, the imbalance exaggerates into a wobble. If this continues, the clay can actually spin right off the wheel.

Exercise 3.6. Finding the Center of Your Body

Standing or sitting with your feet firmly anchored on the floor, with your eyes closed, gently begin to rock from side to side. Sway from one foot onto the other. Use this pendulum-like motion to help find just the right fulcrum of balance for your body. Allow your head to oscillate until it finds a point of balance on your neck. Gradually slow the motions and make them smaller until the external body becomes still and you are feeling the balance of your head on top of the cervical vertebrae and each vertebra of the spine poised on top of the next. Now concentrate on the pelvis acting as an anchor for the body, with the legs connecting the body to the earth and the entire spine resting on top of this anchor.

Questions for Discussion. Could you feel the center of the oscillations being focused into a geographical middle of the body? If you took a step with your intent starting out from this core, how would it feel? If you took a step originating from your heel, would you be as likely to retain your balance and power? If you moved your arm, would you be as likely to retain your balance and power? If you lifted a weight, would you be as likely to retain your balance and power? If you tried to push a partner off balance (while he or she was trying to do the same to you), would you be as likely to retain your balance and power?

Exercise 3.7. Finding the Centermost Muscle of the Body*

The muscle that is centermost in the body is the iliopsoas muscle. Some bodywork practitioners consider the iliopsoas to be the most important muscle in the body. By connecting two vitally important areas, the lower extremities and the torso, the iliopsoas acts as a powerful lever for transmitting the force of the legs and feet to the upper body. Accessing the power of the lower extremities when pressing and lifting with the arms and hands is crucial in efficient massage.

To feel this muscle, practice the thigh lift, described as follows: Begin by lying down on the floor. Imagine the hip structure as if it were a bowl holding soup. Now tip the pelvic bowl up so that some of the soup might slosh onto your tummy. The back will feel like it is flattening against the floor. Let the pelvis return to neutral. Now repeat this tipping motion of the hip and use that action to lift the leg off the floor. (See Figure 3.6.) While demonstrating this action of the iliopsoas, it may aid the practitioner to put his or her hands between the ribs and pelvis and palpate the muscle during contraction.

Questions for Discussion. Can you see how that movement is very different from powering the leg up by the quadriceps? Try that powering

*Courtesy of *Body Movement: Coping with the Environment* by Irmgard Bartenieff with Dori Lewis (1980). Gordon and Breach Science Publishers: Newark, NJ.

Thigh Lift—Finding the Iliopsoas

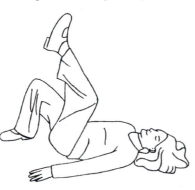

Figure 3.6 To feel the iliopsoas, tilt your pelvis forward to raise your leg, rather than powering it up with quadriceps muscles.

motion and contrast it with moving the thigh by using the centermost muscle of the body—the iliopsoas.

From a psychological standpoint, centering is a process of finding the source of strength, clarity, and peace within. It is a way of focusing, of gathering your energy up into a point so that you can channel it more easily into any activity that you choose. Centering creates higher levels of awareness and enhances your ability to discover what is most important and meaningful to you. When you are mentally and emotionally centered, you feel calm, quiet, strong, secure, balanced, present in the moment, and able to deal with pressures coming in from outside of you. An inner center is a safe haven inside yourself where you can "go" anytime or anywhere. It is a place of special power where you can let go of the tensions and demands of the outside world. Your center or sanctuary is an ideal place for relaxation, tranquillity, and safety. You can create and recreate this inner sanctuary any way that you desire. (See Chapter 4 for further discussion of centering and grounding.)

Exercise 3.8. Mind Centering*

(a) Close your eyes and relax in a comfortable position. Imagine yourself in a beautiful natural scene. Picture any location that holds an attraction for you. Perhaps you will find yourself in a meadow of flowers or a mountaintop stream, in the forest, or beside the ocean. It could even be someplace imaginary, like inside a flower petal or under the sea. Wherever you go, it should be comfortable, safe, and serene. When you imagine yourself in this place, explore the environment, noticing any sights, sounds, smells, tastes, or tactile sensations, along with any other impressions that come to you. Do whatever you like to make the space more homelike and personal. Rearrange things, imagine a light of protection, or create a special ritual to establish this sanctuary as yours. Remember

*Adapted from "Creating Your Sanctuary" in *Creative Visualization* by Shakti Gawain (1995). New World Library: Novato, CA. www.nwlib.com

that this is a place to come to any time that you wish. All you need to do is close your eyes and imagine. If you find yourself wanting an alternate sanctuary, you can start from scratch and create that too.

(b) You can try this variation anywhere, even waiting in a bank line or at a checkout counter. Sit or stand with the weight evenly distributed between both sides of the body. Take some easy breaths, and mentally say to yourself, "Let go." Become aware of the area in the center of your forehead between the two eyes. Hold the attention there for a few seconds. Now draw your attention toward the core of your head to a spot about three inches deep into the skull and brain. Imagine this path intersecting with the line formed by connecting your two ears. After the focus of energy is well established here, drop your awareness down through the middle of the body to the base of the spine. Then move the energy back up the line of the spine. This midline of the body is the stillpoint, the eye of the storm. Allow the energy along this line to build, and then radiate it out to the entire body and beyond.

Questions for Discussion. After you return your awareness to the physical plane, observe how your physical body feels. Are you as tense as you were before the visualization? How do your heart and breathing rates compare? It is difficult to return from your center without retaining some of the qualities of peacefulness and stability.

Breathing

Breathing influences both mind and body. The rhythm and rate of your breathing not only reflect your physical condition, they also help to create it. Notice how breathing can be an accurate indicator of emotional and mental activity. When you are worried or excited, your respiration rate increases and breaths become more shallow and irregular. When you get calm and centered, breathing slows down and becomes fuller and more cyclic.

Voluntary manipulation of the breath can influence and help support more desirable emotional and mental states (Satchidananda, 1972). Do you remember your parents' advice to count to 10 before jumping into a fight? When you count to 10, you are giving your body an opportunity to take 10 deep breaths. Those 10 breaths help relax and free you to see other options. Smoking cessation programs use the same concept to alleviate the compulsion to smoke. Counting to 10 gives deep breathing a chance to calm the body without nicotine. It allows time to elapse, so that you sense that you can let go even without a smoke. These are two ways that observing and deepening your breath can have beneficial consequences for your physical self. Use your breath as a guidepost to remind both you and your client to center, slow down, let go, and relax.

The breath and the way it fills the rib cage also serves as a support to your internal musculature as you stand and move. Expansion is especially important in the thorax as a balance to the external working of the skeletal muscles that move your shoulders, arms, and hands. If you perform a massage stroke with a caved-in chest, what does that do to the rest of your body alignment? How does that differ from following through on a stroke when you have support from the inside out?

When performing massage, there is a need to keep muscle tone in the chest. Observe the rhythmic contracting and relaxing of the primary breathing muscles (i.e., diaphragm and external intercostals contract and internal intercostals relax during inspiration, and vice versa during exhalation). Simply breathe as you normally would, without attempting to change the rhythm or rate. Loss of tone occurs when you hold your breath or forget to breathe. Just concentrate on keeping the flow of breath moving into and out of the lungs. Most people are very toned in the back, and the back takes more than its share of the work. Support for the back comes from the inside. The first rib is under the clavicle, and the lungs are under the ribs. Your breath needs to fill the upper lungs as well as the lower portion. Diaphragmatic (abdominal) breathing by itself is not enough. Filling the thorax is vital to our inner support.

Exercise 3.9. Feeling the Three Dimensions of Breath*

To feel the three-dimensional expansion of the lungs as the air they inspire supports your external rib cage and chest, place your hands in the following three positions/dimensions as you breathe. Try to breathe as normally as possible, without trying to affect the depth or speed of the breath.

To feel for *depth*—Position 1: Cross your hands over your heart. Alternately place one hand in front and the other in back of your chest. Keep the palm facing out on your back hand. This variation is anatomically impossible if the back hand is facing palm in.

To feel for *width*—Position 2: Place your hands on either side of your rib cage.

To feel for *height*—Position 3: Place one hand on the area of your midsection with your thumb on the twelfth (last) rib and your pinkie on your iliac crest (top of your hipbone). (This position also allows you to feel the alignment between your pelvis and your ribs.)

The complete exercise allows you to focus on the thoracic area as you inhale and exhale. This, in turn, tones your intercostal muscles and helps you to breathe easier and more efficiently.

Questions for Discussion. Could you feel the movement of your rib cage in all three directions? Which direction felt least restricted? Which direction felt most restricted? Was the range of movement different in the right side as opposed to the left? How do you think that what you observed could have an effect on your massage work?

Exercise 3.10. The Effect of Filling Your Chest on Skeletal Muscle Movement

Lift your arms. Sense their weight as you lift. Now breathe in to pump up your chest. Lift the arms again and notice any difference in how heavy or light they seem.

*Adapted from Beth McKee, Aston Patterner® personal communication/Body Mechanics Tutorial (1995), Washington, DC.

Questions for Discussion. Did the arms feel heavier or lighter when you lifted them a second time? To what do you attribute this difference? How will this understanding help you when in the midst of giving a massage?

Balance

Balance is more than achieving a stable point that will not tip over. The law of homeostasis requires us to continually juggle the active mix of our lives and to discover "just how much is the right amount" in relation to each. It is a changing flow, a dynamic balance. When our lives are in balance, everything that we do—work, play, relationships—fits in and complements every other part of our lives. Similarly, when we massage with a sense of dynamic balance, the changing flow of passive stretching, compression, effleurage, stillness, and motion creates a dance complete in itself, that is renewing and energizing to both the client and ourselves. On the other hand, when any one component is out of kilter, either in massage or in life (e.g., excessive petrissage is causing the muscles between your metacarpals to be strained), the quality of the whole experience is compromised.

The human body depends on a delicate balance in response to changing stimuli in order to maintain itself. Homeostasis involves active fine-tuning for acceptable amounts of heat and cold, activity and rest, chemicals, hormones, and other substances.

For example, here is an account of how temperature must be regulated in the human body. Human cells and tissues simply cannot function if they get too hot or too cold. Above 105 degrees Fahrenheit, the proteins that make up these building blocks of life literally fry like the protein in an egg. Proteins are the main components of enzymes in the body. Enzymes are the catalysts for chemical reactions in the human body. Reactions that ordinarily keep tissues and organs functioning come to a standstill without proteins to power the change. Neither do cells work well when they get too cold. Many vital chemical reactions, such as the digestion of food, must occur at a certain minimal temperature or they will not take place. All of the body's vital metabolic processes, including breathing and circulation of vital fluids, slow down gradually with decreased temperature until they cease moving entirely.

When you begin to observe the way that you massage and move, you will immediately recognize the need for balance. Consider yourself to be a "massage athlete" when you perform bodywork and reach for the sense of equilibrium. Massage practitioners optimally strive to fine-tune each session to balance in all aspects. They adjust to be neither too slow nor too fast, too weak nor too strong; neither do they lean too far to one side or the other.

Exercise 3.11. Overcompensation*

This exercise can be used to stabilize an "unbalanced" way of moving. For example, if you always tend to throw Frisbees too far to the left, next

*Adapted from "Your Psychophysical Balance" in *Body-Mind Mastery* by Dan Millman (1999). New World Library: Novato, CA. www.nwlib.com

time you play, purposefully aim too far to the right. Dedicate a portion of your attention and effort to consciously maintaining this off-balanced position. By deliberately doing something way out of line, you can observe the action more clearly. This will feel extremely awkward; however, it enables you to see your actions from a new perspective. When you go back to throwing the Frisbee in the old way, it will not feel the same.

Questions for Discussion. How can you use this unsettled feeling to find a more appropriate balance of forces when you perform effleurage? How can you use it to find an appropriate balance of force when you lift a client's leg in a passive stretch for the hamstrings?

Physical and emotional balance go hand in hand. Similarly, an imbalance in one tends to create an imbalance in the other.

Exercise 3.12. The Relationship between Physical and Emotional Balance*

Use this moment to stand and balance yourself on one leg, as shown in Figure 3.7. If this is simple for you, increase the difficulty level by balancing with eyes closed. Make a mental note of how easy it is for you to steady yourself. The next time you are "upset" with too much emotion, be it anger, sadness, or fear, see if you can disengage enough to try the

Tree Pose

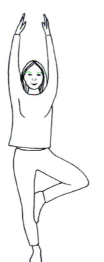

Figure 3.7 Use the tree pose to experience physical balance.

*Adapted from "Your Psychophysical Balance" in *Body-Mind Mastery* by Dan Millman (1999). New World Library: Novato, CA. www.nwlib.com

balancing again. See what effect the physical act of balancing alone has on your emotions.

Questions for Discussion. When you were upset, was it more difficult, easier, or about the same difficulty to balance? On the other hand, when you concentrated on balancing, did you consequently find yourself to be less, more, or about equally involved with the upset feelings?

Grounding

According to Ida Rolf (1989, p. 30), all three-dimensional objects are structured in accordance with gravity or, as she puts it, "the effect of the earth's energy envelope." From this theory, a variety of body mechanics principles emerge.

For easy and efficient bodywork, draw energy from your center of gravity rather than powering away through the use of the hands. Consider the hands as an expression of strength from the lower body. Grounding refers to the way you support yourself, through your feet contacting the earth. You become "ungrounded" or disconnected when the lower body is cut off from the upper part by leaning on the massage table or locking your ankles or knees. Bracing in these ways interrupts energy flow. When you allow yourself to draw support from the earth up through the body, massage strokes and manipulations assume a more continuous flow. In the earth the tree takes root, and from the earth the tree receives nourishment to grow and lift its branches up to the sky.

According to *The American Heritage Dictionary* (1985), one definition of the word *ground* is "an object that makes an electrical connection with the earth . . . used as a return for an electrical circuit and as an arbitrary zero of potential." The physical manifestation of electricity in the body can be measured by physiological tests such as electroencephalograms (EEGs), electrocardiograms (ECGs), and lie detector tests that measure galvanic skin response (GSR). EEGs measure the electrical frequencies of brain waves. ECGs measure the electrical frequencies caused by the contractions of the heart. GSR measures the conductivity of the surface of the skin, increased by perspiration. The living electricity that flows through us can also be observed when we walk across a carpet and then touch a metal object or another person. It sparks! When we touch another being we act as conduits for energy exchange.

The following exercises can help you feel your strong connection with the earth. It is recommended that you try these activities without the restraint of shoes.

Exercise 3.13. The Squat*

Stand with your knees shoulder-width apart. Bend your knees and slowly lower yourself until your buttocks are nearly touching the ground. If you are unable to go all the way down, try moving your feet further apart. If your heels cannot touch the floor in this position, you can remain on your toes or place something under the heels for support. It is also possible to stretch your arms in front of you, holding onto a chair back or doorknob

*Adapted from Amie Rose, personal communication/Hatha Yoga class, 1992.

for support until the soleus and gastrocnemius (calf) muscles and Achilles tendon become more stretched.

Clasp your hands in front of the chest, placing your elbows on the inside of the knees. While in this position, focus on feeling your feet as they contact the ground. You can also focus on feeling the buttocks bouncing up and down, swaying slightly from side to side, or making circular movements. Remember to breathe in this position and imagine as you move that you are gathering in nourishment and energy from the earth. (See Figure 3.8.)

Exercise 3.14. The Mountain*

As shown in Figure 3.9, stand with your big toes pointed in. If possible, have the big toes touching and the heels slightly apart. This creates a stable and supportive triangular base for the exercise. Allow your ankles and knees to be slightly bent. Contract the quadriceps (muscles in front of the thigh) slightly and feel them pulling up on the knee. Let the back be comfortably erect and feel the erector spinae (muscles that hold the back erect) muscles lifting up the spine. Roll your shoulders back and notice how this gentle movement allows your shoulders to relax and your breath to fill and support your upper chest. Allow your arms and hands to hang relaxed from the shoulder blades. Feel your head supported on the cervical vertebrae, easy and light. Imagine yourself strong and still like a mountain. Feel your stable base and secure contact with the earth, and sense your peak reaching upward, through the clouds, toward the sky.

Questions for Discussion.   After you leave either of these positions, how do you feel with respect to your connection with the earth? Do you move any differently? How could you maintain this sense of "groundedness" while moving in a massage? Could you use this as a restorative movement after a massage? How?

The Squat

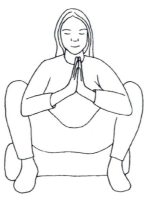

Figure 3.8   Use the squat to feel your relationship with the ground.

*Adapted from Amie Rose, personal communication/Hatha Yoga class, 1992.

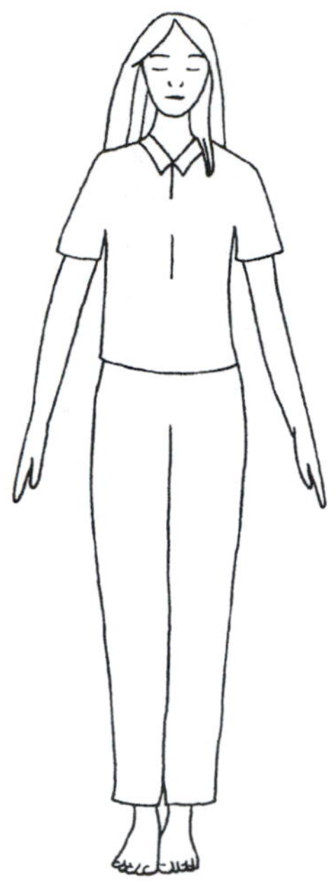

Mountain Pose

Figure 3.9 The mountain pose aids in "grounding."

Weight Shift

Weight shift in massage generally refers to transfering weight from one leg to another. If you are sitting, it refers to shifting in weight between the hips. (See Chapter 10 for more discussion of adapting massage to sitting, kneeling, or other alternative positions.) In Swedish relaxation massage, the weight change occurs *while* doing the stroke. In deeper work, most of the shift occurs *before* putting the hands on the body. When you have a deeper focus, the work is more concentrated in a smaller area and less motion is expended. Thus, the weight needs to be placed where you want to go at the outset. It is as if you are lining up your body to shoot a pool cue.

Use the bones as levers when executing a weight shift. Leverage your weight by bending at the ankle and waist to achieve more downward pressure (McKee, 1995). With most of the weight distributed over the front leg, the back foot becomes like a gas pedal. You can also use weight as a lever by standing on tiptoes, but it will be easier on the calf muscles and more stable to adjust your height by slipping into some clogs or stepping up onto a footstool.

Ideally, when you take a step, the rest of the body follows the ankle movement. A common error when moving the body forward is to lead with the pelvis, rather than the ankle. Similarly, a common error when moving the body back is to lead with the buttocks, rather than stepping back on the foot. Leading with the pelvis is quite different than moving from your center. The first involves jutting your midsection out without the aid of and consideration for the rest of the body, whereas moving from the center requires a sense of connection and support. You can move from the center when you advance a limb or turn your head. You are not moving from the center when you shove your hips forward or back, and the rest of your body stays behind. Another tip is to be careful to initiate weight shifts through the ankle, not the knee. When the ankle dorsiflexes (bends forward) beyond its normal range, the knee takes over. The anterior cruciate ligament can easily become injured when the knee is overstressed in this way. Staying within the normal range of motion will feel like going to a point of mild tension or resistance in the ankle, and not further.

Other common mistakes made during weight shifts include:

1. *Hyperextending the knees.* Instead keep the knees soft and relaxed.
2. *Balancing on one hip or the other (with weight centered over the greater trochanter).* This causes the pelvis to slip to the side and cause back pain. Instead, use the iliopsoas muscle (as practiced in Exercise 3.7.) to lift your leg and keep the weight centered on the center of the thigh bones (over the lesser trochanters) to give central structural bone support.
3. *Rising onto the toes while shifting weight.* This puts stress on the gastrocnemius and soleus (calf) muscles at the back of the leg.

To help you to shift your weight in massage more efficiently, try the following exercise.

Exercise 3.15. Standing Heel Rocks*

Begin to rock back and forth on your heels. Continue this heel rock, except now keep the foot stationary and move the ankle above the foot. This is the same action but in a different plane. Feel the weight transfer from the heel, through the arch, and onto the ball of the foot.

Now practice with your dominant foot in back. To stay aligned on the less favored foot and feel more comfortable, increase the width of your stance a little. This supports your pelvis and keeps your body from twisting and torquing.

Base of Support

McKee (1995) advises that massage therapists should consider their base of support when striving for optimum body mechanics. A general suggestion for finding an optimal base of support *width* is to assume a standing position with the feet hip-width apart. To add a consideration of *length* to your base of support, move one foot slightly in front of the other. You will want some length (i.e., one foot is slightly in front of the other) no matter what stroke you are performing. How much length between the two feet depends on the length of the stroke. When you are gliding over the surface of the skin, you will need a lot of reach. When you want to sink deeper into the muscles or fascia, your movements and foot span will have to be shortened.

The optimal base of support is a direct reflection of what the selected stroke

*Adapted from Beth McKee, Aston Patterner® personal communication/Body Mechanics Tutorial (1995), Washington, DC.

on the targeted muscle looks like. For example, when releasing the rhomboids, you might choose to use longitudinal friction over the length of the muscles. Rhomboids are short, wide, parallelogram-shaped muscles that connect the inside border of the scapula to the spine. Good body mechanics behooves that the legs reflect this intention of the hands and arms. To position yourself efficiently to begin, your legs would be spread wider apart than the distance between the forward and back legs. This position allows you to use forearms (a wide tool) to apply pressure and still line up your body directly behind the stroke. When you change the direction of the stroke, you must readjust and realign your whole body to accommodate the change. This principle becomes more crucial with the deeper work that you do. You cannot "fudge" a comfortable position when you concentrate all your weight as a lever to release a muscle. Because a weight transfer occurs even before you apply your hands, deep work requires you to stand farther away from the table than you would to apply long, relaxing effleurage.

Once you align your body in its optimal position, you can dorsiflex the ankle and flex the trunk to increase pressure or change position to a small degree. More than a slight variation in pressure or alignment requires repositioning the entire body and adjusting your stance.

Exercise 3.16. Feeling the Spinal Curves*

Get onto your hands and knees. The knees are hip-width under the pelvis, and hands are held in a soft fist directly under the shoulder blades. Do some arches like a cat to mobilize the spine. Pay attention to the three curves of the spine (cervical, thoracic, and lumbar). When your middle is curved all the way up or down, the S shape of the spine turns into a C shape. Reduce the range of your motion and find the place where you feel that the S shape is intact; in other words, you can feel all three curves.

Questions for Discussion.   Can you feel the width of your base of support in this position? Is it spread across the chest? Can you feel the support and your weight bearing down through your arms. This is a simplified version of what is happening in your massage work. In bodywork, the idea is to transfer most of the weight through the arms. To do that, the pelvis and ribs are needed to support the shoulders.

TROUBLESHOOTING POOR BODY MECHANICS

From these principles, we can derive a laundry list of symptoms that can be used to troubleshoot poor body mechanics. A mirror or videotape of yourself working will furnish a visual picture to review. You can sense kinesthetically what you feel within your body as you work. Or you can take turns observing with a fellow massage therapist. Remember that observations can be used to help alter nonadaptive patterns only when we truly observe (simply noticing without judging) as we move and massage. The "gremlin" part of us that wants to jump in and crit-

*Adapted from Amie Rose, personal communication/Hatha Yoga class, 1992.

icize or analyze will not be helpful at this point. The task is simply to take note of patterns that are no longer useful, not to beat yourself over the head with what's wrong. Just like pain, these red flags exist to let us know what to focus on and change. Luckily, the red flags often show up much sooner than the experience of pain. Any findings can simply serve to remind you to move easily and more in tune with natural physical and mechanical laws.

Red flags to look for include:

1. *Positions that cause compression (something squished) or compensation (something out of place)* (McKee, personal communication 1995). For example, you may see or feel the shoulders hunching up to the ear.

2. *Bottom half of body (pelvis and lower extremities) moving out of line with the top half (torso and upper extremities)* (McKee, 1995). For example, the body may seem twisted or torqued.

3. *Feet looking or feeling either not wide enough or too wide to support the movement of the body* (McKee, 1995). If feet are too wide apart you will find yourself so connected to the ground that you are stuck in one place. If feet are too close you will find yourself teetering off your center.

4. *Feet looking or feeling either not spread lengthwise enough or too spread out lengthwise to support the movement of the body* (Mckee, 1995). Generally, when performing long, gliding movements (like effleurage), you need a longer base for your stride; when performing most focused and smaller movements (like static pressure or friction), you need a narrower base of support. This is different from how wide the feet are spread.

5. *Excessive or insufficient curvature along the spine, any place from the head to the hips.* If there is extreme cervical (neck) or lumbar (low back) curvature, this is known as hyperlordosis. Extreme lumbar curvature can put a strain on the low back and be the cause of pain. Not enough curvature in one of these areas is called hypolordosis. Lack of an arch in the low back is often a protective response adapted by people who already suffer from low back pain. Too much thoracic (midback) curvature is known as hyperkyphosis; too little is hypokyphosis.

6. *The back foot may be out of line with the rest of the body.* In general, it is helpful to have the "headlights" (the ASISs, bony protrusions on the front of the pelvis) going in the same direction as the rest of your body. Otherwise, with the hips (or one hip) being excessively turned out, muscles that outwardly rotate the leg (piriformis, primarily) put extreme pull on the greater trochanter of the hip. A long-term pattern of outward rotation in the hip can cause pain in the low back and/or pelvic area.

7. *The knees or the elbows may be locked into hyperextension.* When this occurs in either joint, it can cause microscopic tearing of the ligaments, tendons, and muscle filaments around the affected joint with accompanying inflammation (recognized by redness, heat, swelling, and pain).

8. *The therapist is standing fixed in one place.* This becomes even more of a problem when a stroke requires some force to execute it. The force of the stroke, movement, or manipulation should arise from the shift of body weight, like a lever or pulley.

9. *The therapist is using only one or two parts of his or her body as tools for the massage.* Too often, practitioners overly rely on their thumbs and palmar surfaces of their hands and fingers to do all the work.

Summary

This chapter provides an introduction to concepts of physics as they relate to body mechanics and massage. It describes the mechanical laws of inertia, force, and reaction, as expressed in Newtonian physics. Inertia means bodies tend to stay the same unless something acts to change them. Force is shown to be proportional to the mass of a body that delivers the force and the rate of change, including directional change that the force comes from. Every action is said to have an equal and opposite reaction. The law of structural integration says that the form (or structure) of a body is there due to and because of the relationship of the parts. The law of homeostasis says that a human body likes to be organized, whole, and balanced. The chapter establishes guidelines to keep in mind when striving for dynamic alignment along with signals to help you notice when your body is not employing efficient body mechanics. Exercises help you to apply these mechanical concepts to find a kinesthetic perception of your own body mechanics.

References

The American Heritage Dictionary (1985). Boston: Houghton Mifflin.

Bartenieff, Irmgard, with Dori Lewis (1980). *Body Movement: Coping with the Environment.* New York: Gordon and Breach Science Publishers.

Gawain, Shakti, *Creative Visualization* (1995). Novato, CA: New World Library, www.nwlib.com

McKee, Beth (1995). Aston Patterner[R] Body mechanics tutorial. Personal communication. Washington, DC.

Millman, Dan, *The Warrior Athlete* (1999). Novato, CA: New World Library, www.nwlib.com

Newton, Sir Isaac, *Principia* (1686). Cajori Verson (1934). Berkeley: University of California Press.

Rolf, Ida, *Rolfing* (1989). Rochester, VT: Healing Arts Press.

Rose, Amie (1992). Hatha yoga class. Personal communication. Portland, OR.

Satchidananda, Yogiraj Sri Swami, *Integral Yoga Hatha* (1972). New York: Holt, Rinehart, and Winston.

Chapter Four

Eastern Influences on Body Mechanics

CHAPTER OBJECTIVES

The massage student/practitioner who successfully completes this chapter (reading and exercises) will be able to:

- Define important concepts of traditional Chinese medicine, including Chi, yin and yang, meridians, and tsubos.

- Define important concepts of ayurvedic medicine, including doshas and chakras.

- List bodywork techniques that use principles of traditional Chinese medicine.

- List bodywork techniques that use principles of ayurvedic medicine.

- Explain the law of bending the knees.

- Explain the law of maintaining relaxed readiness.

- Explain the law of leaning.

- Explain the law of aligning the fingers, hands, arms, and shoulders.

- Explain the law of grounding.

- Explain the law of maintaining homeostasis.

- Explain the law of using yin and yang.

- Explain the law of using breath to enliven your work.

- List six new signs that your body is not working with efficient body mechanics.

Many Eastern cultures have highly developed massage traditions. Customs from China and Japan and traditions arising out of India comprise two major lines of influence on Oriental bodywork. Eastern massage techniques and the body mechanics guidelines that arise from these techniques are based on a number of concepts that may be unfamiliar to Western massage practitioners. It would be remiss to summarize Eastern guidelines for body mechanics without an introduction into the thought that shapes these influences. Therefore, this chapter begins with a preliminary exposition of Eastern theories about the natural physical world.

TRADITIONAL CHINESE MEDICINE

Ancient Eastern philosophy underlying traditional Chinese medicine is a synthesis of perspectives on the relationship of human beings (microcosms) to their world (macrocosm). The following ideas proceed from this understanding:

1. *Everything is connected.* There is a unity between all that exists. Out of this oneness emerges a duality (described in the next paragraph).

2. *Everything in nature is composed of contrasting forces (yin and yang).* The two opposing forces are known as yin and yang. Yin is the dark, passive, receptive, hidden, negative element in things. Yang is the light, active, creative, open, and positive aspect. Ideas that are said to embody yin traits include the moon, female, nighttime, and the earth. Concepts that are associated with yang characteristics are the sun, male, daytime, and the heavens. The two qualities maintain a dynamic balance that is constantly readjusting and changing. Any prolonged shift excessively toward yin or yang will result in difficulty or disease.

   The relationship between yin and yang can be described as a cycle or a dance. As you can see from Figure 4.1, when the yin (symbolized by the dark area) influence wanes, the yang (or white) influence gets larger. However, even in the part of the diagram with the greatest portion of yin, there is some aspect of yang (the white dot), and even in the most yang area, some element of yin (the black dot) remains.

   The following statements summarize the important characteristics about yin and yang. First, all things in nature have two aspects (yin and yang). Second, any yin or yang object or condition can be further separated into yin and yang aspects. For example, cold (a yin condition) can itself be

Yin Yang Symbol

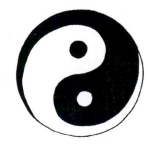

Figure 4.1   The yin yang symbol represents the traditional Chinese medicine principle that everything is composed of contrasting forces. Yin is represented by the dark areas, and yang is represented by the white.

divided into icy cold (yin) and not so cold (yang). Third, the influences of yin and yang cannot be separated. Indeed, they define one another. As an example, cold has no meaning without its definition as a lack of heat. Fourth, yin and yang control each other. When one influence is waxing, the other aspect is waning. In the dead of winter, when the nights are longest, the days are shortest. Finally, the qualities of yin and yang transform each other in a never-ending cycle. One brings on the next. Winter solstice, for example, marks a specific period in the cycle of light and darkness. As the days progress from this time, the length of light (daytime—yang) will gradually increase as periods of darkness (night—yin) lessen. Another example of the cyclical and transformative relationship between yin and yang is demonstrated with each breath. Each time you breathe in (inspiration–expansion—yang), an exhalation (breathing out–contraction—yin) will surely follow. Inhalation brings forth expiration, and exhaling gives birth to a new in-breath.

3. *Chi (also called ki or qi) is the primary energy. This force is the origin of all life.* Chi is, in the broadest sense, spirit or energy, the flow of love and life energy, and the manifestation of harmony. Chi can be either deficient or excessive and it can flow easily or be blocked. You may have experienced these qualities of chi by having too little energy or too much nervous energy, or by being frustrated and unable to access energy when you want it. Rising of energy occurs in anger, fear, or any strong emotional reaction. The sensation corresponds with the physiological release of adrenaline into our bloodstream (Vander et al., 1980). Wilhelm Reich used the term *orgone,* and Gottfried Wilhelm von Leibniz hypothesized about "monads" (or packets of energy) to describe what it is that gives vitality to a corporeal being. Prana is used to refer to the life force too, and this term is often associated with the breath.

Channels along which chi flows in the body are called meridians. These "rivers of energy" have been measured and mapped electronically, thermally, and through radioactivity (Gerber, 1988). With practice, the human hand can palpate meridians, too. Just like rivers in the natural world, rivers of energy can get dammed up and blocked. In areas of the meridian before the obstruction, too much force (called *jitsu*) builds up. In spots that are past the blockage, the chi is deficient (*kyo*). Pressure, needles, electrical stimulation, and moxibustion (stimulation with heat from burning herbs) are used to dissolve blocks in energy channels. They stimulate and move chi through the body. The art of influencing meridians and energy flow with touch is called acupressure. There are a variety of acupressure techniques including amma, shiatsu, tuina, and jin shin do.

Amma (or Anma)

Amma began as a Chinese bodywork system. One translation of the Chinese characters that make up the word is "to calm with the hand." Historically, amma referred to massage given by a blind person. The practice of this form migrated through Korea and Japan and has been influenced by both cultures. Amma involves direct pressure, stroking, stretching, and percussive and kneading touch delivered primarily with the thumbs on special points (tsubos) along the meridians of the body. Practitioners utilize subtle movements of the wrists over each tsubo. Clients are clothed and no lubrication is used. The work involves no diagnosis or specific work on problem areas. Amma is an unvarying protocol that tends to progress away from the heart in order to free the channels of energy (meridians).

Shiatsu

Shiatsu means finger pressure. It is a form of acupressure for manipulating tsubos (points along the meridians where energy flow may become blocked). Shiatsu points are stimulated by pressing with the fingers (most often thumbs) and hands, or by using elbows, knees, and/or feet. There is also stretching, twisting, and tractioning of the client's body and, in the process, of one's own body as well. The client is usually supine, sidelying, or prone on a futon placed on the floor. The therapist is kneeling alongside the client. Often the shiatsu practitioner will begin a session by placing a hand on the hara (abdomen) and palpating the meridians that are represented in this center. This hara diagnosis is known as *ampuku*. The practitioner will tailor the session based on the findings uncovered in the hara palpation, along with the information gleaned through a thorough intake procedure about times of day when the client is most active or fatigued, colors and foods the client prefers, and other questions. The various styles of shiatsu are all performed through clothing and/or a sheet without oil or other lubrication.

Tuina (Chinese Treatment Massage)

Tuina is used to treat a wide range of health problems, from stiff joints to low appetite. In China, all major hospitals have tuina departments, and the technique is taught at all traditional medical schools. Tuina (which literally means "lift and press") is much more treatment and problem solving oriented than other Eastern techniques, with specific protocols for individual diseases. "Rolling" is a major stroke in which the dorsal side of the hand is rotated over the affected area in order to disperse stagnant chi. Pediatric tuina prescribes an entirely different set of gentler protocols for specific childhood diseases, including diarrhea, colic, asthma, and bed-wetting.

Jin Shin Do

Created by Iona Marsaa Teegarden, jin shin do means "way of the compassionate spirit." It is a synthesis of traditional acupressure, Western-style bodywork, Taoist philosophy, and psychology. There are 30 primary acupressure points in jin shin do, derived from approximately 360 tsubos delineated in traditional acupuncture. Therapists place one hand on a point that feels blocked and the other hand on a separate point to release the flow of energy. Each position is held for one to two minutes. As the energy begins to move, the therapist can detect a softening in the muscle tissue, a reported decrease in pain, and/or tingling or pulsing sensations.

Tai Chi Chuan

Tai chi is not a bodywork discipline per se, but it has some strong influences on the way bodywork is performed in Oriental (and now Occidental) cultures. For that reason, it is discussed here. Tai chi chuan, translated into English, means "supreme ultimate martial art exercise" (Dorian Ross, 1992). Chinese have believed for hundreds of years that tai chi is the highest form of martial arts, meditation, and exercise. Tai chi is a series of postures representing martial arts techniques connected by a slow-flowing sequence of transitional movements. When tai chi is performed, you might describe it as kung fu in slow motion and wonder if such slow movement can actually be an exercise. The postures give a dynamic stretch to all the muscles and joints, and the stances generate muscle growth in the legs. The movements are designed to stimulate acupuncture points all along the body and to encourage deep, rhythmic breathing. This oxygenates the blood and fills the body with chi or life-giving energy. Tai chi artists strive to maintain harmony in any situation, never overusing their own force, but rather absorbing, shaping, and balancing the energies present in a conflict until peace and harmony can be restored. As tai chi players move through the routine, they focus complete concentration on the position of the body and the synchronization of their movements. Ideally, all other thoughts and impressions fade until there is nothing left but an active body and an observant mind. This is meditation through movement.

Throughout Asia, tai chi is not regarded as just a martial art, but rather as a part of the therapeutic remedies prescribed by traditional Chinese medicine. According to Oriental medicine theory (and as described above), an intrinsic energy known as chi, the life force, circulates around the body in the same way that the blood circulates through the arteries and veins. The chi travels along the acupuncture meridians, and the obstructions of its flow can lead to sickness, pain, and even death. The movements of tai chi percolate life force from the body's center (hara) and send it circulating around the body. So in a very real sense, every time you practice tai chi, you are more full of life than before.

AYURVEDIC MEDICINE

Indian philosophy has produced ayurvedic medicine, which literally means "the science of life." Ayurvedic medicine proceeds from one question: "How can I be happy in life?" The following principles followed from attempts to answer this question:

1. *Health is the maintenance of homeostasis.* Health means finding a balance between the interplay of vital forces in the body.
2. *Doshas (literally "faults") are the three basic metabolic forces that create the interplay.* Each dosha—*vata, pitta, and kapha*—is recognized in the human form by specific physical and personality traits. Vata, which controls movement, is described as the intelligence of the body. Pitta can be described as metabolism or the transformation of energy as in digestion. Kapha can be thought of as structure and solidity—the physiological tissue and mass of the body. Any imbalance in one of these (too much or too little) creates disease.

Five elements serve to categorize the way in which matter works: earth (solid), water (liquid), fire (power), air (gas), and ether (space). Each dosha is itself composed of two of these influences. Air and ether are the major influences for vata. Water and fire direct pitta. Earth and water conditions impel kapha.

3. *Energy centers (chakras) are an important consideration in ayurvedic health care.* Chakras are vortexes of energy, found along the spine as discrete spheres from the base of the spine to the crown of the head. Each chakra correlates with specific endocrine glands and nerve plexuses (braids of interweaving nerves) that live in the specified section. Colors and sounds (physical expressions of specific frequency variations) reflect the unique vibration of each chakra. Each energy center has a quality (like security and stability in the base or root chakra) that helps describe its influence on the whole person. (See Figure 4.2.)

4. *People are the sum total of all energies and experiences that have affected them up to the present time.* Individual dosha and/or chakra characteristics manifest in each client. Ayurvedic therapies require the massage therapist to consider and work to balance all of these traits as goals for each session.

Chakra Chart

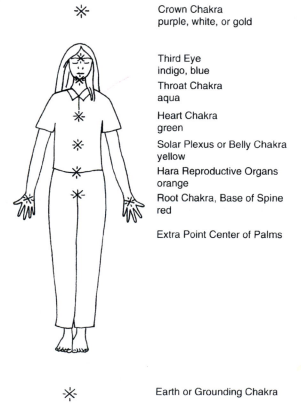

Crown Chakra
purple, white, or gold

Third Eye
indigo, blue

Throat Chakra
aqua

Heart Chakra
green

Solar Plexus or Belly Chakra
yellow

Hara Reproductive Organs
orange

Root Chakra, Base of Spine
red

Extra Point Center of Palms

Earth or Grounding Chakra

Figure 4.2   Chakras are vortexes of energy that extend along the spine. Additional chakras can be found in the center of the palms and the soles of the feet.

Ayurvedic Massage

Ayurvedic prescribes distinct massage oils, powders, and essential oils, depending on which dosha appears to be most dominant in the client at the time of the session. Also, certain colors, sounds, or crystals can be used to enhance desirable qualities for each chakra. Derived from the Sanskrit words, *ayu* (life) and *veda* (knowledge), ayurveda works in harmony with nature and considers mind, body, and spirit as a whole. Balance revolves around the three ayurvedic principles—vata, pitta, and kapha.

Vata constitutions can be described as vivacious, enthusiastic, excitable, or restless. A key word for vata is *changeable,* with mental and physical energies that come in bursts. Vata individuals tend to be on the move, anxious, worried, and quick to tire but slow to sleep. If this describes you, you may want to take time to unwind and balance vata with calming lubricants and strokes.

Pitta individuals tend to be intense and fiery. They are known for a sharp intellect and a low threshold for anger. They have a love of challenge and a tendency to overwork. Under stress, their frustration and irritability can mount. Pittas need to "chill out" and take time to balance pitta with lotions and movements that soothe and cool.

Kapha people are relaxed, easygoing, tranquil, and at times bordering on lethargic. Some are described as fluid and graceful, with great body strength and endurance. Kaphas tend to retain possessions, emotions, and weight when out of balance. Massage for these individuals focuses on warming, stimulating, and rejuvenating the client.

Yoga

The eightfold pathway of yoga is intricately intertwined with ayurvedic medicine. The effect of yoga, specifically hatha yoga, on the efficient execution of Indian massage is as important as the effects of tai chi on the development of body mechanics for shiatsu and other forms of Oriental massage.

Yoga literally means to join together or to yoke. This joining may refer to the union of the self with something higher, like a god. Or it may be joining as in the union of the body with the mind. The union may refer to the merging of the self with other selves (i.e., humans or other living things). Raja yoga, the royal way (also called *asthanaga yoga,* or the eightfold path) includes the teachings of all the paths of yoga. The eight passages are made up of yamas (restraints), niyamas (observances), asanas (postures), pranayama (control of the breath), pratyahara (control of the senses), dharana (concentration), dhyana (meditation), and samadhi (like nirvana, a superconscious state). Hatha yoga emphasizes the postures and breath control as a means to a better life. Asanas (or asans) are specific positions of the body that help to stretch the body and calm the mind. Observing and relaxing into resistance, not forcing past them, perfects these positions. Coordinating the breath with movement into and out of postures is one of the best ways to regulate breathing. Generally speaking, as you breathe in, the body expands. As you breathe out, the body contracts. As you hold a pose, do not restrict the breath. Let it flow, continuing the cycle of energy through the body. Postures are best performed slowly, steadily, and with attention on letting go of unnecessary tensions and bringing in deep, easy breaths. After a series of three or four asanas, practitioners relax in one of the resting poses. Hatha yoga trains the body in relaxation and discipline while it trains the intellect in mindfulness.

THE EASTERN PERSPECTIVE ON BODY MECHANICS AND SELF-CARE

Using logical conclusions from the principles of Oriental and Indian medicine as previously outlined in this chapter can supplement the list of prescriptions for efficient body mechanics. Some suggestions presented here can be considered additional specifications. Some items simply restate guidelines that were profiled in the last chapter. Repeating an ergonomic prescription (like "maintaining homeostasis or balance") in another context acts to reaffirm its usefulness. Remember to confirm or disprove any and all conclusions with kinesthetic observations (without judging) as you move and massage. Check to see what feels good in your body. Note what feels out of line or sync. Use the Eastern guidelines to help you to move more easily and efficiently as you massage.

Bending the Knees

Eastern disciplines make use of specific poses or stances that enable the practitioner to respond quickly, easily, and with maximum power and reach. A good stance keeps the torso balanced over the legs as you work and carries the weight of the body through the legs rather than the back. Three postures that are often used in tai chi and other moving martial arts forms are the *horse stance* (alternately called *sitting stance* in tae kwan do, or *balanced stance*), *bow stance* (alternately called *walking stance*), and *T step* (alternately called *L stance*).

Each stance can be used for different body areas and strokes to achieve maximum leverage. In order to efficiently convert gravity into pressure, your feet must be planted firmly on the ground. (See Figure 4.3.)

Exercise 4.1. Practicing Horse, Bow, and T-Step Stances*

To work in the horse stance, spread your legs approximately a shoulder-width apart or a little more. Keep the feet parallel or slightly turned out. Sink down on bent knees and center your body weight between both legs, as if you were riding a horse. Your weight is distributed evenly over the bottoms of the feet so that you do not feel the weight settling in one particular area. Bend comfortably at the ankle, knee, and hip joints. Relax the belly and entire pelvic floor. Drop the rib cage and float the shoulders back and down. Lower the chin slightly toward the shoulders while gently lifting and opening the cervical vertebrae. The horse stance is a stable place from which movement into standing Swedish bodywork techniques can begin. (There is a danger, however, of settling into a comfortable horse stance and remaining there. With this posture, your feet are not facing the direction of any stroke except those that travel directly across the

*Adapted from David Dorian-Ross, personal communication/Tai Chi class, 1992.

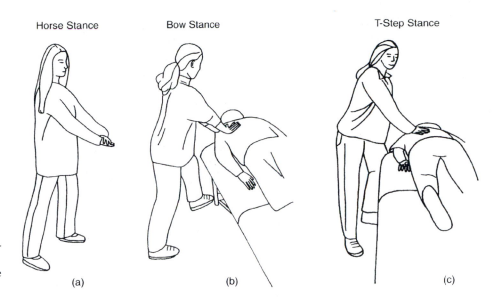

| Horse Stance | Bow Stance | T-Step Stance |

(a)   (b)   (c)

Figure 4.3 (a–c) Use tai chi postures (horse, bow, and T-step) to respond quickly and to maximize power and reach.

body to the spine. I am not aware of any muscle bellies that run strictly transversely into the axial skeleton. Therefore, in order to manually stretch or tone the full length of a tissue, your direction of intent [and your feet] will have to move as you move along the muscle.)

The horse stance allows the axial skeleton to balance over the bowl of the pelvis and the weight of the body to be carried entirely by the legs. (*Note:* You may have to strengthen you leg and thigh muscle to feel comfortable in this posture.) The distance between your feet and the level at which your knees are bent can be varied depending on the area of the client's body you wish to manipulate and the technique you wish to use. Generally, for more strength (depth of pressure), bend the knees deeper or spread the legs farther apart.

To perform the bow stance, begin with feet shoulder-width apart. Your hips and shoulders face forward, pointing straight ahead like an arrow from a bow. Lunge forward and rotate the rear foot outward at a 45-degree angle. For front stance, step forward onto the front foot (about one and a half feet) as though you are taking a step as in walking. Approximately 70 percent of your weight is on the front foot. The back leg is straight, and the front leg is bent at the knee. Both feet remain flat on the floor whenever possible. When increasing strength (depth of pressure), body weight can be further distributed to the front leg. In another variation, the back stance, body weight shifts onto the rear leg. The pelvis remains facing the front, and the forward foot remains pointing straight ahead. The difference is that at least 70 percent of the body weight stays on the rear foot. The more weight you shift to the front foot, the more power becomes available for your massage strokes and manipulations.

To move into the T step from the bow stance, turn the body to the side. Both knees are bent and legs are about a shoulder-width apart. The front foot is pointing forward and slightly turned out, and the back foot is perpendicular to the front, the two feet together making a "T." The body weight is poised on the back leg, readying the practitioner for movement to either side. The T step is used to help the massage practitioner shift his or her weight or change directions. Again, bending the knee will increase the practitioner's reach without sacrificing any strength.

Questions for Discussion. What happens in each stance as you bend your knees? The first rule of body mechanics the martial arts teach us is to use the whole body to generate power. If we use only arm strength to execute a technique, we will only be as strong as our arm muscles alone. If we use our whole body, including our powerful leg, thigh, gluteal, and back muscles, we have the combined strength of all our body weight and muscle.

To access the power of the lower extremities and trunk, we anchor ourselves to the ground in a strong stance and draw strength through our legs and abdominal muscles. These stances also help us use leverage to increase our strokes when applying strokes or pressures. Utilizing leverage makes our weight more effective without having to increase/exert muscle strength. Bending at the waist is said to truncate body strength because it cuts the power of our abdominal muscles in half. Instead of leaning over when working on the extremities, try keeping the head and tail aligned and bending the knees to get to the desired level.

On the other hand, sometimes it may be desirable to trade off maximum body strength in order to maintain flexibility and ease of movement. From your experiences with the horse, bow, and T-step stances, what do you think? How would your massage change if you focused on anchoring and using the legs for power? How would it change if your primary intent were to maintain the flow of energy throughout your body?

Maintain Relaxed Readiness

Another general precept derived from Eastern disciplines is to remain in a state in which body is relaxed and mind is alert and ready. Implementation of tai chi, yoga, and all of the Eastern forms of bodywork requires a balance between the tension that is necessary to move the intended muscles and relaxation of the muscles not being used to execute the technique. In massage, this means shoulders stay relaxed and away from the ears, and hands are tensed only when applying pressure or strokes. This ensures that energy is not wasted and unnecessary tension is not being created in the practitioner. This means releasing tensions and energies externally, but preserving one's chi internally, so that one can adapt more readily to any circumstance. With relaxed alertness, one has the ability to meet any challenge (such as muscle guarding or an emotional outbreak from a client). When practicing the following hatha yoga stretches, let your body feel what tension is needed to achieve the postures and what tension takes away from your ability to maintain the poses in a state of relaxed readiness.

Exercise 4.2. Spinal Twist*

Sit on the floor with knees raised and the soles of the feet touching the floor. Slide the left leg out so that it lies flat on the floor. Lift the right foot and place it outside the left thigh, with the sole resting on the floor. The right knee is close to the chest. Turn your torso so that the left arm passes beyond the right knee and presses against it. Stretch the left arm and take hold of the left leg as it lies on the floor. Now twist the lumbar vertebrae to the right, then the thoracic vertebrae, and finally the cervical spine. Now look as far as you can to the right. Remember to breathe into the ribs, not the abdomen, so as not to hyperventilate as you hold this pose. (See Figure 4.4.) See if you can identify and relax all of the tensions that are not helping to maintain the spinal twist. Repeat on the other side.

Questions for Discussion.   Where did you notice tensions that worked against you as you attempted to feel the spinal twist stretch? Were you holding in your feet, in your calves or thighs, in your hands? Were your shoulders reaching for your ears? Did you remember to let go? Did you remember to let go of tension in your diaphragm by continuing to breathe? Did you find you had more energy to devote to the spinal twist when you let these unneeded tensions go? How could you apply this discovery in a massage session?

Lean or Sink

In shiatsu, practitioners learn to lean or sink into their work, rather than push through muscles with force. Pushing, in contrast, requires a braced and clamped-down body with contracted muscles that exert the force. To sink means to relax completely. All the joints, the whole body, should remain relaxed and loose. One should feel the energy flowing down to the "bubbling well point" (Kidney 1) at the center of the front part of the sole of the foot, at the convergence of the lines

Spinal Twist

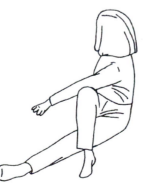

Figure 4.4   As you move into the spinal twist, let your body feel how much tension you require to maintain the pose. Any additional tension is strain that takes away from relaxed readiness.

*Adapted from Amie Rose, personal communication/Hatha Yoga class, 1992.

made when the foot is flexed (Lundberg, 1992). (See Figure 4.7 on page 73.) This means leaning on the client as if you were comfortably resting against a wall or on a table. When leaning, the practitioner's weight is counterbalanced at the point where his or her hands meet the client's body. With equilibrium focused at the contact point, the therapist becomes more sensitive. By leaning into clients, you can be moved or swayed by their subtle movements. In this way, client response directly determines the most suitable pressure and range of motion for evaluation and manipulation purposes.

Moving through healthy tissue is not painful for the client. In contrast, when dysfunctional tissues are palpated, the client's body will automatically respond with a protective movement—either pushing back or moving away. This slight protective movement, in turn, affects the therapist's balance point. What happens is that the therapist is moved slightly off-balance so that changes in the client are reflected in changes in his or her own body. This would not occur if the therapist's body were fixed to apply pressure by pushing from the upper extremity. In this case, postural changes would not be transmitted and no protective movements from the client would be felt.

The same principle applies to stretching. Clients tend to make a protective response when the range of motion is at its maximum. This slight resistance is more easily sensed when the therapist is leaning (and open to sensing change), as opposed to pushing (and benumbed to subtle change), on the client.

Exercise 4.3. Cantilevers

A cantilever is an instrument that projects out beyond a fulcrum (the balance point) and is supported by a balancing object (or downward force). In this activity, two partners become a cantilever by extending limbs to support one another's weight. For example, partner A could reach out an arm while partner B rests a leg on the outstretched arm. Or both partners can sit on a mat with outstretched feet that are touching and holding hands. As one leans back, the other bends forward. (See Figure 4.5.) Instead of two separate objects with distinct centers of mass, the two join to share a single center of support. Experiment with your partner to create several different cantilever poses.

Questions for Discussion. How do the two bodies depend on each other to achieve a joint posture? How does it feel to literally lift, pull, push to the limits, or lean on another? What would happen to your weight if your partner moved? What if they moved even a tiny bit? Do you feel how the body of your partner becomes a support for your own weight rather than an inanimate body to be fixed or molded into a better shape? Does this experience of cantilevers, interrelated balance, and support have an effect on your approach to massage?

Align the Upper Extremities

In the last chapter, we discussed the importance of lining up the trunk and lower extremities of the body to evade wasting energy (having your power split in two

Cantilevers

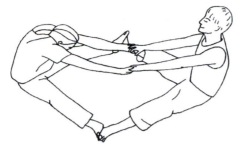

Figure 4.5 Cantilevers give a feeling of joining with a partner to share a single center of support.

or more directions). This will also help to avoid torquing and pulling your body. This concept is reemphasized here with reference to the upper body. In shiatsu, particularly, the use of compressive force requires fingers, hands, arms, and shoulders to be in a straight line so as not to injure the muscles and ligaments that cross a joint. Many shiatsu practitioners aim to keep their force perpendicular to the plane of the client's body. It is as if you are aiming for the core—the bones— of the client. Your focus is deep into the energy meridians. The way to achieve this is to keep your own bones in line (e.g., wrist *not* flexed or extended, abducted, or adducted) with the direction of your effort.

Grounding

Grounding revisits of the notion of "originating from the center for stability and propulsion," discussed in Chapter 3. Centering and grounding involve sinking into the earth in order to relax. All the joints in the body remain relaxed and loose. Eastern traditions of massage and martial arts ask practitioners to sink down to feel a connection with the earth and with their own physicality. Being grounded is an experience of having a relationship to the earth. This translates as being balanced and stable among the forces of the world. Being connected and feeling like an integral part of life are outgrowths of this connection. Having a center from which to operate, a kind of order and harmony emanating from within (as opposed to a chaotic, desperate energy), is a good description of earth dwelling within. It means being at home with one's self, integrated, unobsessed, and at ease wherever we are.

To be "earthy" is to express our rootedness. At any instant, the place where we stand is on the earth. The very solidarity of who we are is determined by the pull of the earth's gravity on our mass. The foods we eat are grown from the earth. Fertility, fecundity, and fullness as well as stability, solidarity, and support are qualities associated with the earth.

The pelvic area has great significance in Eastern cultures, where it is considered to be a key location of a person's feelings. The Japanese call this area the hara; the Chinese call it tan tien; and in ayurvedic traditions and yoga, this is the location of the second chakra or energy center—the seat of self-affirmation. The pelvic base is the heaviest part of the human anatomy—the center of gravity. Franz Veldman (in Noble, 1985) claims that a child who is lifted, supported, and affirmed from the hara develops an expanded sense of self through the body. It is his strong recommendation that babies be held in a "haptonomic circle" (see Figure 4.6) by the caretaker, to provide maximum emotional and physical security. A baby supported through the pelvic base will hold her spine erect even from the moment of birth (Noble, 1985). By analogy, we could reason that holding yourself upon this base of power and working from your strong center could help to sustain an erect spine during massage. By protecting the infant in a crumpled position, caretakers actually limit a baby's postural abilities (Noble, 1985). Similarly, by protecting our adult bodies in a curved fetal slump, we limit our own ability to move and massage.

Shiatsu practitioners typically begin each session with ampuku, which is an assessment of the hara. They focus in on the abdomen first in order to determine which energy meridians need strengthening and which need to be toned down. The vital spirit is also said to reside in the hara. In Japan, "hara" describes the quality of one's energy. The well-known Japanese phrase for killing the self literally translates as killing the hara ("hara-kiri").

Exercise 4.4. Bubbling Well

Take a moment to imagine energy flowing down to the "bubbling well point" (Kidney 1) at the center of the front part of the sole of the foot, at the convergence of the lines made when the foot is flexed (Lundberg, 1992). (See Figure 4.7.) This is the point where the foot connects with the earth. According to Eastern traditions, stimulating this acupressure point at the right time can revive someone who has suffered a

Haptonomic Circle

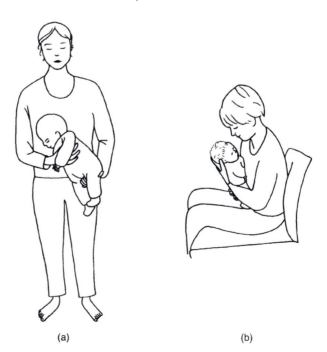

(a)   (b)

Figure 4.6 (a–b)   A baby supported through the pelvic base (haptonomic circle) will hold her head erect.

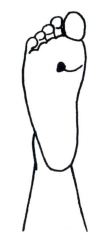

Kidney 1—Bubbling Well Point

Figure 4.7 Bubbling well point (kidney 1) is located at the center of the foot at the convergence of lines made when you plantar flex and point your toes. It "bubbles up" vitality into the body.

life-threatening trauma such as heart attack or stroke. Feel vitality bubbling up from this oft-forgotten source at the base of your feet.

Questions for Discussion.   Can you feel a difference in your body as a result of this guided imagery? How would you describe this? Can you imagine working in a massage session with an awareness of this body feeling? Try the imagery during the session and observe the results.

Traditional shiatsu positioning has the client lying on a futon placed on the floor, and the practitioner on his or her knees leaning into the acupressure points along the energy meridians (although many schools are now teaching shiatsu modified for work on the massage table). A hands-and-knees position can teach students much about their own perception of body mechanics and center of gravity.

Exercise 4.5. Locating Hara from a Kneeling Position

Kneel on all fours. From this position, think about the location of the hara in the area of the abdomen. You can focus on the point which is 2 cun (thumb-widths) below your navel to find the tan tien, and then spread your attention out to the surrounding area. Keeping hands and knees planted on the earth, begin to move and circulate the torso and hips. Rock back and forth, move from side to side, and make revolving movements with the trunk. Exaggerate the movements and see how far you can move and still keep your balance. Keep in mind the sensation of your hara or tan tien throughout the exercise. This is your geographic center and place of greatest balance (Lundberg, 1992).

In the tai chi preparatory stance, sinking down into the abdomen or tan tien is extremely important. The next exercise helps you practice the tai chi stance as preparation for easy action from a standing position while performing massage.

Exercise 4.6. Locating Hara from a Standing Position

In this position, the chest is held in, the back straightened, the shoulders sunk, and the elbows lowered. With the chest held in, the chi or energy of the body will sink into the hara or tan tien. The Chinese say that locating your hara in this way enhances the circulation of blood and energy throughout the entire body. They say when this position is not practiced; the energy collects in the upper body, causing the practitioner to be top-heavy and easily uprooted. The back needs to be straight, so that the energy collected in the spine can influence the body to act as a complete unit. That way, the energy will be very powerful and not dispersed. If the shoulders are raised, chi will immediately rise up into the chest, causing the body to be unbalanced and top-heavy. The elbows and shoulders work together. If the elbows are raised, the shoulders will be raised, too. The end result of raising shoulders or elbows is that the body can be easily uprooted and the movement of energy will be thwarted (Dorian Ross, 1992).

Questions for Discussion. Where is your center when you locate it from a kneeling position? Is it in the same place when you attempt to locate your hara while in a standing position? How does this posture compare to the mountain pose that you practiced in Chapter 3? Where was your center exactly (describe the feeling and placement in as much detail as possible), and what happens to your center when you move?

Maintain Balance

The need for balance when applying massage strokes and stretches was discussed in Chapter 3, and its reappearance here underscores its importance in the field of body mechanics and self-care. An additional yoga exercise to improve your awareness of and facility with balance is provided here.

Exercise 4.7. Adapted Dancer Pose*

Fix your gaze on one spot in the distance. Focusing your eyes in this way will help your whole body to stay balanced as you practice this asana (pose). Now begin to move into the adapted dancer pose by grasping your left foot behind you and pulling the foot up with your right hand. Raise your left arm overhead like a counterweight, pointing your fingers out like an arrow, and rest your upper arm against your ear. Slowly and care-

*Adapted from Amie Rose, personal communication/Hatha Yoga class, 1992.

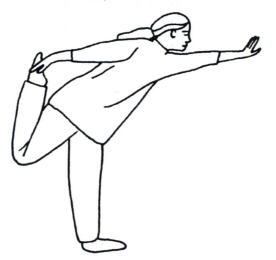

Adapted Dancer Pose

Figure 4.8 **The adapted dancer pose helps you to kinesthetically experience an awareness of and facility with maintaining balance.**

fully lift your left leg up and away from your body. (See Figure 4.8.) If you start to wobble and feel unsteady, stop there and hold the pose where you are more stable. If you really start wobbling and swaying, come out of the pose, rest steady on both feet and start again. Hold the stretch, continuing to breathe easily for several seconds. Relax and repeat on the opposite side.

Questions for Discussion.   What happens to your sense of balance when you move into the position of the adapted dancer pose? How did you feel (physically and emotionally) before you attempted the posture? How did you feel after? Often, you can counterbalance "unsettling" emotional feelings by focusing on physical balance.

Use Yin and Yang

To translate this concept into the language of body mechanics, when the whole body's weight is on the right foot, the right foot is yang. The right foot, because it is holding all the weight, is substantial. The weight is not resting on the left foot at all, so the left foot becomes yin or insubstantial. The idea is that if you can clearly distinguish between which parts of your body hold weight and which do not, your body mechanics become much more efficient. You can see how clearly distinguishing the insubstantial from the substantial—in this case, yin and yang—helps your massage movements to become light and quick, not clumsy and double weighted. If you step forward with your right foot while weight still remains on both feet, your action will waste energy and you will literally be dragging your feet. Your movements become clumsy and heavy. Every part of the body has a substantial (yang) and insubstantial (yin) aspect at any given moment.

Exercise 4.8. Wave Hands Like Clouds*

This exercise is adapted from a tai chi movement demonstrated in class by David Dorian Ross. Begin by standing in the horse stance with arms relaxed and legs comfortably bent. Step your right foot directly to the right and in a continuous motion slowly shift your weight onto that right foot. Now bring your left foot next to the right, again attempting to maintain a continuous flow of movement. Make two or three more shifts (steps) to the side, paying attention to the transfer of weight between the two feet.

Questions for Discussion.   Which foot is yin and which is yang when you first step out with the right foot? Describe how the balance of yin and yang changes as you shift your weight. How can you use this awareness of yin and yang (substantial and insubstantial weight) to improve your massage?

Breathing

In the martial art of karate, breath control is known as ki mastery. The process involves "centralization" (Lundberg, 1992). Centralization means focusing in on the belly (hara) to establish a foundation of strength and stability. Extension is a three-step procedure. First, ki is extended around the body like a magnetic field. From there, ki spreads into a tool (such as a fist, foot, or stick) and projects out from the eye. Eye ki allows one to see clearly with the "eye of God" in order to spot unseen hazards and know an opponent's (or partner's) true motivations. Finally, ki merges with the energy of the adversary, permitting the stronger power to triumph (Tart, 1989).

The word *ki* is also used in aikido. Aikido is literally translated as "the way" (do) "of harmony" (ai) with "the spirit of the universe" (ki). It is a martial art, inspired by Morehei Uyeshiba, in which practitioners work with their partner, rather than seeing themselves as fighting an opponent. This approach seems especially appropriate for the healing arts practitioner.

Chi means energy in tai chi chuan, which literally translated is "supreme ultimate martial art way."

The Indian word for life energy is *prana*. The same word is used to speak of the breath. Swami Sri Satchadananda (1970) calls prana the vital link between and influence over the body and the mind.

Breathing rhythm and rate not only reflect the body's physical condition, but also help create it. Notice how breathing is an excellent indicator of emotional and mental states. When you are worried or excited, the respiration rate speeds up and the breaths become shallower. When you are more calm and centered, breathing rates slow down and become more regular. Taking in life energy becomes haphazard and irregular when we give up, forget, or ignore conscious control of the breath.

Voluntary manipulation of the breath (pranayama) can influence and create

*Adapted from David Dorian-Ross, personal communication/Tai Chi class, 1992.

a more desirable physical, emotional, and mental state (Satchidananda, 1970). Do you remember the advice to count to 10 before you allow yourself to get into a fight? When you count to 10, you give your body an opportunity to take 10 deep breaths. Those breaths help you relax and free you to see other options. Smoking cessation programs use this concept to alleviate the need to smoke. Counting gives the body a chance to relax, so that your need for calming through a cigarette is reduced.

Exercise 4.9. Manipulating Energy Levels via the Breath

(a) Concentrate on the "in" breath as you breathe slowly and fully through the nose. As you inhale, say to yourself the word *energy*. Notice what happens to your own level of energy as you do this.

(b) Now try concentrating on the "out" breath as you exhale slowly and deeply through your nose. Feel the air as it leaves the nostrils. Say to yourself the word *relax* every time you breathe out. Notice what happens to your own energy level when you focus your attention and emphasis on the "out" breath.

Questions for Discussion.   Did you notice a rise or fall in vitality level as you focused on either the inspiration or the expiration stage of your breath? How could you put the effect of conscious breathing to good use during a massage?

The meaning of the word *inspire* suggests lighting a fire, to start the creative juices flowing, to feel more energy rising within. When we expire, we "let go." Indeed, when we take the final breath, we let go of everything in this earthly life, and it is said that we have "expired."

Consciously using these associations can affect the timing of your work. One very practical use of conscious breathing is to be aware of the out-breath during massage. It is well known that compression, stretching, or any significant manipulation of a muscle (including easy range of motion exercises and the return from same) works better when the client is exhaling and letting go (Dixon, 1992). You, as the therapist, can facilitate the "letting go" response in both your client and yourself by making it a point to breathe out (and cueing the client to do so) when focusing in on a soft tissue release.

Expansion and contraction of breath refuels and refreshes every cell in the body. Each time we heighten our capacity to breathe, we facilitate more oxygen delivery and a higher quality of life for every corpuscle. This use and enhancement of breath is the crux of "energy work" (Lauterstein, 1985). Energy work is not some obscure aspect of bodywork accessible only to the "far out" gurus and monks among us. Every breath can open us up to greater life and vitality. Each exhalation lets go of unneeded metabolic and energetic wastes as well as emotional tensions and old patterns of thought, feelings, and behavior.

You might say that breath is a profound source of energy on our planet. Humans inhale an average of 20,000 breaths each day—many times more than we reach for sustenance in the form of food or drink. When we exhale, carbon dioxide is made available to the plant world.

Breath is a fundamental tool in the realm of body mechanics in that it delivers energy to the hands, our structural tools for bodywork. You can use the air that you breathe to influence soft tissue with less effort. To do so, use your hands to shape and direct the chi. Feel that you are shifting the energy, as singers shape each note that flows from their lips, and as dancers mold their bodies into forms that tell a story. When we are consciously in tune with and aware of our breath, bodywork becomes easier and we can allow change to happen, rather than trying to power in and "fix" things. This does not mean that the techniques and tools that we learn are not helpful. They surely are. But breath can be a reminder to let go, or to feel the energy that is already there, inside. Once therapists are conscious of this, their touching is transformed.

Exercise 4.10. The Breath's Influence on Vibration and Percussion

Percussion (or tapotement) can be defined as a series of brisk blows that rapidly follow in sequence. Percussion is used primarily when stimulation and toning is desired (i.e., to psych the athlete for optimal performance before an event).

To limber up before using percussion, the therapist can simply shake the hands freely. Let the wrist, hand, and fingers flip loosely up and down. Bring the palms into position facing one another and continue to feel relaxed. When you alternate the action so that one arm moves up while the other moves down, you are practicing tapotement. Try this movement, holding the breath and continuing the percussive action as long as you can. Now try it again, but let yourself stop the drumming when you feel like taking a break. Take a deep breath while making a smoothing motion, and begin again.

Vibration is a continuous trembling movement. Fingertips are slightly apart, elbows are slightly flexed, and the wrist and finger joints are held stiffly. The stroke can be applied with the whole hand against the client's body surface or with only the fingers, thumbs, or knuckles contacting the client's body. It can be used to relax and soothe (applied lightly), to stimulate (applied vigorously), or to sedate and numb pain impulses (applied at a high frequency—more than 100 cycles per minute—over a long period of time).

For this exercise, first try vibration as long as you can without taking a breath. Then try the stroke with the same modification you just applied to percussion. When your body gets tired, you simply stop and take a breath. Before each new application of vibration, take a new deep breath and breathe out as you are applying the stroke. (See Figure 4.9.)

Questions for Discussion. What difference did it make in your percussion technique when you stopped to take a breath? How did your vibration stroke change? Which was easier? Did you notice any difference in

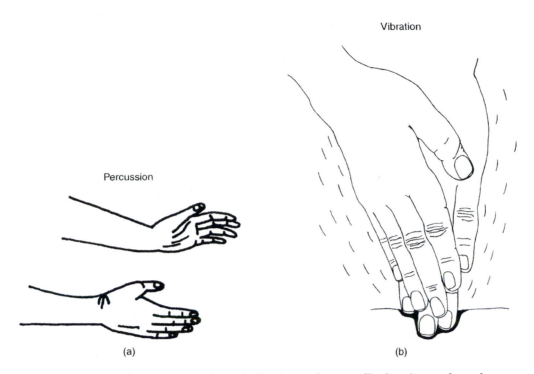

Vibration

Percussion

(a)   (b)

Figure 4.9 (a–b)   Percussion and vibration can be more effective when performed in conjunction with breathing. When you get tired, stop, take a breath, then resume the stroke.

tension levels in the rest of your body—shoulders, head, even back and legs? If you worked with a partner, ask which application felt better—the one that incorporated breath or the one that did not?

TROUBLESHOOTING POOR BODY MECHANICS

Eastern principles add to the list of signs to help spot poor body mechanics. To identify these in your own work, check your observations against symptoms that are red-flagged below. You can use a mirror or videotape to supply a visual picture to critique. You can sense your body kinesthetically as you work. Or you can take turns observing with a colleague. Remember to alter nonadaptive patterns by observing without judging. Take note of patterns that are no longer useful, and do not beat yourself over the head with what's wrong. Allow your findings to remind you to move easily and more in tune with your natural physical inclinations.

Red flags to look for include:

1. *Positions that seem out of balance (so that you are literally falling over) or so much in balance that you cannot shift yourself out of them.* As concluded in Chapter 3, the force of the stroke, movement, or manipulation should arise from the shift of body weight, like a lever or pulley.

2. *Stiffness at the knee joint or, at the extreme, locked knees that are unable to bend.* (Remember the ideals of the horse or sitting stance, bow or walking stance, and T or L step.) When knees are locked into hyperextension, ligaments, tendons, and muscle filaments around the affected joint can tear microscopically with accompanying inflammation (recognized by redness, heat, swelling, and pain).

3. *A feeling of anxiety or unease or, at the other extreme, a feeling of dullness, spaciness, or just not being there.* To counteract these mental states, practice the disciplines of centering and grounding as outlined in this and the previous chapter. This may mean that you consciously need to become aware of your tan tien or hara, the physical space below your abdomen.

4. *The therapist is pushing into the soft tissue, rather than leaning or sinking into the muscles and connective structures.* If you are the therapist and you feel the tissues pushing back at you, wait until they release before going deeper.

5. *Misalignment of the upper extremities.* Especially if the arms and shoulders look or feel as if they are at cross purposes (i.e., shoulders are pointing in one direction and arms reaching in the opposite direction), they probably are.

6. *A sense that you cannot tell which leg is bearing the therapist's weight.*

7. *The therapist is not breathing, or breathing fully and easily.* This demonstrates that the chi or life force is not getting through.

SUMMARY

This chapter provides an introduction to the Eastern perspective and its relationship to body mechanics. Two branches of Eastern thought are examined—traditional Chinese medicine and ayurveda. A number of body mechanics principles can be derived out of major concepts from each branch of Eastern thought. Some of these are new guidelines, including bending the knees, maintaining a state of relaxed readiness, leaning rather than pushing into soft tissue, and being aware of yin and yang. Others restate in a new way body mechanics principles that were adopted in Chapter 3. These precepts include using breath to enrich your work; grounding; aligning the fingers, hands, arms, and shoulders; and maintaining homeostasis.

REFERENCES

Dixon, Marian Wolfe, *Bodylessons* (1992). Portland, OR: Rainbow Press.

Dorian Ross, David, personal communication, Tai chi class (1992). Portland, OR.

Gerber, Richard, *Vibrational Medicine* (1988). Santa Fe, NM: Bear and Company.

Lauterstein, David, *Putting the Soul Back in the Body: A Manual of Imaginative Anatomy for Massage Therapists* (1985). Austin, TX: Lauterstein-Conway Massage School.

Lundberg, Paul, *The Book of Shiatsu* (1992). New York: Simon and Schuster.

Noble, Elizabeth, *Marie Osmond's Exercises for Mothers and Babies* (1985). New York: New American Library.

Rose, Amie, Personal communication hatha yoga class (1992). Portland, OR.

Satchidananda, Yogiraj Sri Swami, *Integral Yoga Hatha* (1970). New York: Holt, Rinehart, and Winston.

Samskrti and Veda, *Hatha Yoga Manual I,* 2nd ed. (1985). Honesdale, PA: The Himalayan Institute.

Tart, Charles, *Open Mind, Discriminating Mind* (1989). New York: Harper & Row.

Vander, A. J., Sherman, J. H., and Luciano, D. S. *Human Physiology: The Mechanisms of Body Function* (1980). New York: McGraw-Hill.

Chapter Five

Movement Reeducation Influences on Body Mechanics

CHAPTER OBJECTIVES

Conceptual Objectives The massage student/practitioner who successfully completes this chapter (reading and exercises) will be able to:

- Define *movement reeducation.*
- Define important concepts of Swedish gymnastics, including active and passive exercise and stretches and variations such as reciprocal inhibition and post-isometric relaxation.
- Define important concepts of Alexander technique.
- Define important concepts of Bartenieff Fundamentals.
- Define important concepts of Meir Schneider's work.
- Define important concepts of Aston Patterning®.
- Define important concepts of Feldenkrais® work.
- Define important concepts of Trager® work.
- Define important concepts of Hanna Somatics®.
- Explain the law of self-observation.
- Explain the law of getting external feedback.
- Explain the law of rest often/take stock of how your body feels right now.
- Explain the law of using baby steps.
- Explain the law of learn to play (as you work).
- Explain the law of recognizing unity in the body.

Practical Objective The massage student/practitioner who successfully completes this chapter (reading and exercises) will be able to:

- List six new signs that your body is not working with efficient body mechanics.

Movement disciplines have always been near to my heart, and I am enthusiastic about synthesizing the wealth of knowledge that they hold for the bodyworker. Movement reeducation therapies are systematic techniques that utilize movement to facilitate healing and body awareness. The original movement therapy was Swedish gymnastics, based on exercise and stretching techniques developed by Per Henrik Ling. A wide variety of movement approaches have become influential during the past 20 years. Founding fathers and mothers, including Milton Trager, Judith Aston, F. M. Alexander, Meir Schneider, and Irmgard Bartenieff, have developed comprehensive movement therapy systems designed to improve posture, self-image, flexibility, and muscle coordination. Some techniques emphasize teaching the client healthier ways of moving with active exercises (e.g., Bartenieff Fundamentals, Alexander technique). Others emphasize table work in which a practitioner induces movement for a "passive" client (e.g., Swedish gymnastics/passive exercise and stretch). Most techniques offer a combination of table work and active exercise and stretch (e.g., Trager, Feldenkrais, Aston, Hanna). Even if movement therapy is not the primary focus of your practice, a familiarity with the techniques can help you loosen, tone, and *learn more about your own body,* thereby improving your natural sense of body mechanics. An added bonus is that the techniques offer fresh alternatives for assisting massage clients.

Swedish Gymnastics

Within the field of Swedish massage, movement therapy refers to what is now called Swedish gymnastics (also known as remedial gymnastics, rehabilitative gymnastics, or just plain gymnastics). Swedish massage, as it was introduced to America in the mid-nineteenth century, was originally part of a larger system of natural therapy called medical gymnastics, developed in Sweden by Per Henrik Ling (1776–1839). In medical gymnastics, a prescription of massage and movement therapy was administered to treat a variety of chronic ailments. Ling described both massage and exercise as "movements," and so the treatment came to be known as the Swedish movement cure (Benjamin, 1996). The movement therapy component of the cure, as it is used in conjunction with basic Swedish massage, is made up of exercise and stretching.

Exercise causes muscles to shorten/contract. In passive exercise (also called range of motion exercise), the client's muscles remain relaxed and the therapist performs the exercise movements. In passive exercise of the biceps brachii, which is an elbow flexor, the therapist flexes the elbow joint without help from the client. This form of exercise can be very helpful to the injured client because it reduces the likelihood that the healing muscles, tendons, and ligaments will adhere and stick to nearby bones and other soft tissues. Since the client's muscles do not contract, range of motion manipulations can be safely performed even when muscles and tendons are injured, because these soft tissues carry no tension with passive exercise. However, passive exercises may be painful if there is a ligament injury, because as the joint moves, it can pull on inflamed ligaments. Remember that pain is a contraindication to any form of movement therapy.

In active exercise, the client contracts the muscles. Active exercise is useful after acute inflammation begins to decrease. It helps the muscles' strength return to baseline after an injury (or increase strength past the customary amount if it is healthy already). There are three types of active exercise. In active assistive exercise, the client moves the joint with the help of the therapist. When muscles are weak, this is the appropriate exercise to use. In free active (or just active) exercise, the client moves through a range of motion without help from the therapist. Active exercise is appropriate when muscle contractions do not cause pain. In active resistive exercise, the client moves a joint through range of motion against resistance. The therapist or a prop such as dumbbells or elastic tubing may offer the needed resistance. Active resistive exercise helps complete the process of rebuilding muscle strength for injured tissue and is the fastest route for building strength when tissue is healthy (Newton, 1998). Healthy massage practitioners can use free weights, elastic tubing, or exercise equipment (e.g., stairsteppers, stationary bicycles, or rowing machines) to build their own strength for massage. (See Figure 5.1.)

Stretching lengthens muscles by increasing the distance from origin to insertion. To stretch a muscle, determine the major action of the muscle over the joint and move the joint in the opposite direction. For example, when stretching the biceps brachii, an elbow flexor, you would extend the client's elbow. The two basic classifications of stretch are passive and active. In passive stretching (sometimes called "placing a muscle in its lengthened position"), the therapist provides all the effort required to stretch a client's muscles. The client remains relaxed and passive and does not assist. Passive stretching relaxes the client and can easily be performed within the context of a full body relaxation massage.

In active stretching, the client elongates the muscle with little or no help from the therapist. There are three types. In active assistive stretching, the therapist provides some assistance as the client moves into the stretch. In active stretching, the client moves through the stretch without any help from the therapist. This form is used when muscle contractions cause no pain to the client. (Therapists can keep their own bodies flexible, free from pain, and ready to perform massage with active stretching.) In active resistive stretching, the client pushes against the therapist's resistance. For soft tissues in which resistance does not cause pain, active resistive stretches provide the fastest and most efficient way of lengthening muscles (Newton, 1998). Practitioners can get the benefits of active assistive or active resistive stretches for self-care, by assisting or resisting, respectively, their major force of effort. For example, to utilize a resistive stretch for the biceps, actively extend the forearm, while your opposite hand presses the back of the forearm in resistance.

Simple guidelines to follow when stretching (any form, for yourself and for clients) include the following (Anderson, 1980):

1. Don't bounce! Any time you pull muscle fibers too quickly, sensory receptors called muscle spindles send a message to the central nervous system (CNS) to engage the "stretch reflex." The CNS responds by sending a signal to the muscles to contract. The stretch reflex is a protective response that will keep muscles from being injured unless they are forced into a lengthened position by another bounce.

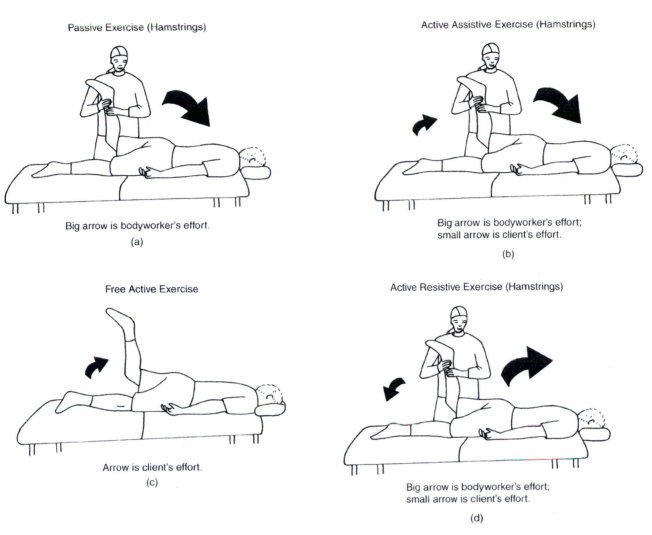

Passive Exercise (Hamstrings)

Big arrow is bodyworker's effort.

(a)

Active Assistive Exercise (Hamstrings)

Big arrow is bodyworker's effort; small arrow is client's effort.

(b)

Free Active Exercise

Arrow is client's effort.

(c)

Active Resistive Exercise (Hamstrings)

Big arrow is bodyworker's effort; small arrow is client's effort.

(d)

Figure 5.1 (a–d) Exercise can be passive, active, active-assistive, free active or active-resistive, depending on who performs the action and whether the client assists or resists the direction of movement.

2. Stretch only to the point of feeling mild tension or resistance. Any time you pull muscle fibers too far, the same nerve reflex tells the muscles to contract. Once again, this keeps the muscles from being injured. Stretching should feel good. Think of reaching effortlessly, like a cat stretching after a nap. Many of us incorrectly learned to associate pain with physical improvement and were taught that the more it hurts, the better. That "no pain, no gain" adage is a myth. Pain is *always* an indication that something is wrong.

3. Always stretch on the exhale. This helps you to let go of the tension.

4. Maintain relaxed continual breathing while holding the stretch. Do not hold your breath!

5. Hold each stretch 8 to 10 seconds to maintain flexibility, 60 seconds or

longer to increase it (Corbin and Lindsay, 1988). (*Note:* The length of time required to encourage flexibility varies widely according to the source. The duration quoted here has always worked well for me, both as a receiver and a giver of the stretch.)

6. Repeat stretches two to three times to achieve a "staircase effect." In muscle contraction, treppe, or the staircase effect, refers to the fact that muscles contract more forcefully after repeated stimuli with brief relaxation periods interspersed with the contractions. The theory is that each contraction raises the availability of calcium for future muscle actions. The muscle effect (treppe) is called the staircase phenomenon for its stairstep appearance on an electromyogram (EMG). Athletes make use of the treppe effect when warming up. Treppe prepares muscles for the best possible effort. I have extrapolated the term *staircase effect* to refer to the phenomenon that repeating a stretch several times with rests in between will be more effective than holding one stretch over a long time period without breaks (Anderson, 1980).

7. Watch for expressions of discomfort (i.e., facial grimaces, unusual smiles, forehead crinkling, toes curling, perspiration, muscles tensing, breathing changes) and release stretch if any are observed. Listen to your body's signals as well. Remember that pain is an indication that something is wrong.

8. Continually monitor for feedback and give clear instructions and/or warnings about what you will be doing next. (See Figures 5.2.)

Swedish gymnastics methods involving combinations of contraction and stretch have also been developed and are used to get even more length into muscles. Two of these resistive techniques commonly used by bodyworkers are post-isometric relaxation (PIR), also called contract–relax or hold–relax, and reciprocal inhibition (RI), also called antagonist contract.

To perform *post-isometric relaxation,* the bodyworker asks the client to isometrically contract a muscle (the agonist) prior to performing that muscle's stretch (Hart, 1998). (See Figure 5.3.) In other words, the client tightens the same muscle that you want to stretch. For example, if I wanted to stretch the biceps brachii, before straightening my elbow, I would first push against the resistance of my other hand, placed on the soft side of my forearm. The biceps flexes against the hand isometrically; hold the contraction for about 8 to 10 seconds, and then stretch. It is a property of muscle that after it contracts ("post-isometric"), it fatigues and can stretch a bit more ("relaxation"). When a muscle relaxes due to fatigue or any reason, it lengthens.

To perform *reciprocal inhibition,* the bodyworker asks the client to contract the antagonist of a muscle prior to performing a stretch on the agonist (Hart, 1998). In other words, you tighten the muscle opposite to the one you intend to stretch. For example, if I wanted to stretch the biceps brachii, before straightening my elbow, I would first push against the back of my forearm. As the triceps muscles tighten in contraction, the biceps muscles relax. When a muscle contracts (in this case, the triceps), the muscles that perform the opposite action (in this case, the biceps) are inhibited from acting ("reciprocal inhibition"). This is quite useful because, otherwise, all the muscles of the body would be fighting with each other

Passive Stretch (Hamstrings)

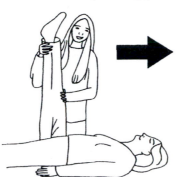

Big arrow is the bodyworker's effort.

(a)

Active Assistive Stretch (Hamstrings)

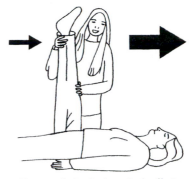

Big arrow is the bodyworker's effort;
small arrow is client effort.

(b)

Free Active Stretch (Hamstrings)

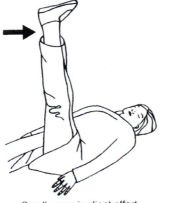

Small arrow is client effort.

(c)

Active Resistive Stretch (Hamstrings)

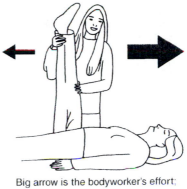

Big arrow is the bodyworker's effort;
small arrow is client effort.

(d)

Figure 5.2 (a–d)   Stretch can be passive, active, active-assistive, free active or active-resistive, depending on who performs the action and whether the client assists or resists the direction of movement.

and the body would be so bound up with conflicting forces that it could not move. When the original muscle relaxes due to this signal from the antagonist muscle on the opposite side, the original muscle lengthens. Reciprocal inhibition can be used when contracting a muscle would cause pain. This would be the case when the muscle that you are targeting for a stretch has been injured (and severely shortened) and cannot contract without pain. (See Figure 5.4.)

Post-isometric relaxation and reciprocal inhibition can be linked in a procedure called "contact–relax, antagonist contract" (CRAC). Using PIR and RI together in this way helps stretch a muscle more effectively than if only one of the resistive methods is utilized. PIR, RI, and CRAC can be adapted for self-care, just like any resistive stretch.

In addition to variations on original Swedish gymnastics exercise and stretch, extensive movement therapy systems have been designed to improve posture, self-image, flexibility, and muscle coordination. Some systems emphasize

Post-Isometric Relaxation (before biceps brachii stretch)

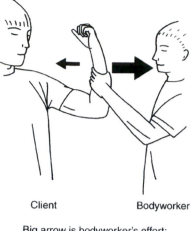

Figure 5.3 In post-isometric relaxation, the bodyworker asks the client to contract a muscle before it is stretched.

Client   Bodyworker

Big arrow is bodyworker's effort;
small arrow is client's effort.

training clients in more ergonomically sound ways of moving (e.g., Bartenieff Fundamentals, Alexander technique). Other methods accent table work in which a practitioner uses massage and manipulation to facilitate motion for a reclining client. Most comprehensive approaches couple table work with client education (e.g., Trager, Feldenkrais, Aston Patterning, Hanna Somatics). Many of these therapies were created when their originator suffered an illness or injury and found traditional medical techniques to be lacking for full recovery. These pioneers used trial and error combined with kinesthetic awareness of their own bodies to develop new ways of being and doing. The new approaches helped cure a

Reciprocal Inhibition (before biceps brachii stretch)

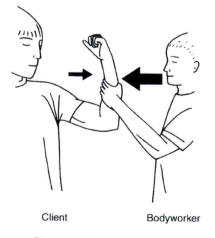

Figure 5.4 In reciprocal inhibition, the bodyworker asks the client to contract the antagonist of a muscle before the muscle is stretched.

Client   Bodyworker

Big arrow is bodyworker's effort;
small arrow is client's effort.

variety of problem symptoms and ailments. "Developing healthier ways of being and doing massage therapy" could almost be the working definition of good self-care and body mechanics. In order to see the influence of individual movement reeducation therapies on body mechanics more clearly, let us begin with a discussion of several acknowledged movement therapies. Whenever practical, sample exercises will supplement the descriptive text.

Alexander Technique

Alexander practitioners help clients to replace unhealthy patterns with healthier ones through positioning the head, neck, and spine and "right use" of the body (Leviton, 1988). They refer to themselves as teachers, as opposed to bodyworkers, to focus on the reeducation aspect of the work. The dynamic relationship between the head and the rest of the body is emphasized. F. Matthias Alexander was originally an actor who lost the use of his voice during performances. With the help of mirrors, he analyzed the position of his body as he spoke and brought his voice back. The culmination of his self-healing efforts is the Alexander work. Alexander work has been applied to help singers, dancers, and musicians make optimum use of their bodies as instruments.

Alexander teachers lead students through ordinary movements but use touch to influence the right head, neck, and torso relationship. Pupils are coached to walk, sit, and stand, with the instructor guiding the student's head to initiate the action of the whole body. (See Figure 5.5.) "If you free the neck and allow your head to move (up and) away from your body . . . it releases contraction . . . and results in better coordination, balance and clarity," says one Alexander practitioner (in Leviton, 1988). The whole body lengthens by following this upward and outward movement of the head. The head, neck, and torso become aligned in this new, less stressful way.

Alexander Work

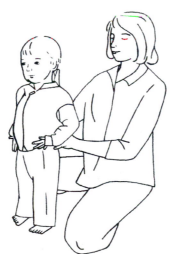

Figure 5.5 Alexander teachers use touch to influence "right use" of the head, neck, and torso.

Bartenieff Fundamentals

Irmgard Bartenieff studied how babies move and applied her knowledge as a physical therapist and student of Laban Movement Analysis to polio patients to help them break down movement into basic "fundamentals" or baby steps. Out of her early experience working with physically handicapped and emotionally disturbed individuals, Irmgard Bartenieff developed several specific exercises which she called *Bartenieff Fundamentals*. Bartenieff Fundamentals are designed to enable individuals to unify their perceptions of three simultaneous activities—breathing, muscular "fluctuation," and feeling (Levy, 1988).

Exercise 5.1. Bartenieff Fundamentals—Rock and Roll*

The purpose of this exercise is to feel the cause-and-effect connection between the heels, spine, and head (Levy, 1988).

Lie flat on the floor, legs and arms extended, the arms resting at the side of the body. Bend your feet down toward the floor (plantar flexion), initiating the movement from the ankle. Reverse the action to bring the feet up into dorsiflexion. Repeat the two actions and feel the movement reverberate into the pelvic area and (ideally) on up through the body to the head. (See Figure 5.6.)

Questions for Discussion.   Where did you feel the movement? Did it travel through the entire body? More importantly, where did you feel the movement stop? The answer to this question will give a clue as to where mobility is most hindered or restricted in your body. Can you put your attention on that stuck, unmoving place and begin your heel rock from there? Originating your movement from a place that does not readily move on its own is a way of unsticking the latch. Do you have places in your body where movement does not happen during a massage? You can use this exercise with clients on the table, or you can apply the exercise to examine how specific strokes, stretches, and manipulations affect your body as you massage.

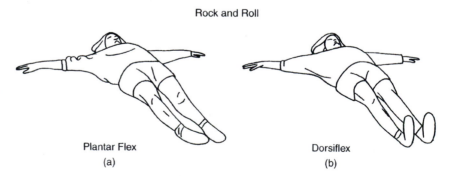

Rock and Roll

Figure 5.6 (a–b)   The rock and roll exercise (heel rocks) helps you to feel connections between heels, spine, and head. Initiate the rocking from the ankle and feel the movement reverberate up the spine.

Plantar Flex
(a)

Dorsiflex
(b)

*Courtesy of *Body Movement: Coping with the Environment* by Irmgard Bartenieff with Dori Lewis (1980). Gordon and Breach Science Publishers: Newark, NJ.

Bartenieff used the heel rock (rock and roll) exercise as a lead-in for all of her other fundamentals of movement. This is the very first of her baby steps. It helps to shape the heel by employing it as a fulcrum through which the foot and leg relate to each other. When babies first start to walk, they often stand on the balls of their feet. Toddlers' heels do not develop until the muscles of the calf extend from use and the anklebones can wedge free. The soft tissue needs to be shaped by use (Schultz and Feitis, 1996). That is the secret behind the Fundamentals—they are not only educational but therapeutic practices. See how working with rock and roll prepares you for this next Bartenieff activity.

Exercise 5.2. Bartenieff Fundamentals—Pelvic Lateral Shift*

The purpose of this exercise is to learn to shift the weight laterally without twist, by using the muscles of the pelvic floor. As a corollary, the pelvic lateral shift trains the muscles of the pelvic floor to aid in rotation and adduction of the hip.

Lie on your back with your knees up. Exhale and hollow out the abdomen. After rocking back and forth in an adapted rock and roll (Exercise 5.1) (i.e., using your ischial tuberosities to initiate the back-and-forth motion), let the back-and-forth action of the pelvis move into a slight lift. Keeping the pelvis lifted, shift it to the right. Then gently lower yourself to the floor. Rest a moment. Now initiate the pelvic lift from the coccyx. To do this, lengthen your low back and feel it flatten against the floor. Try not to tense or clench your gluteal muscles as you do this. Shift the pelvis back to midline and lower yourself down into the starting position. Repeat on the opposite side. (See Figure 5.7.)

Questions for Discussion. Where did you feel the movement? Place your fingers on the greater trochanters on the lateral sides of the hip to track your side-to-side movements. The side-to-side motions should be felt only through the greater trochanters. Avoid initiating the movement from areas above the pelvic rim. The most common error is laterally flex-

Pelvic Lateral Shift

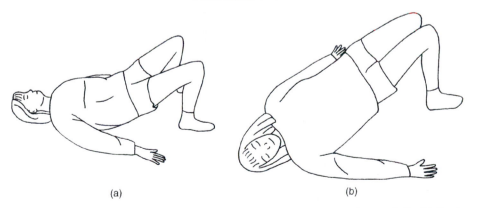

(a)   (b)

Figure 5.7 (a–b) Performing the pelvic lateral tilt can help you shift weight to the side efficiently and without torquing.

*Courtesy of *Body Movement: Coping with the Environment* by Irmgard Bartenieff with Dori Lewis (1980). Gordon and Breach Science Publishers: Newark, NJ.

ing the trunk, which engages the quadratus lumborum and introduces a twist into the pure lateral motion. Also try to avoid all unnecessary upper body and leg tension. When would you use this motion in everyday life? Typically, a pelvic lateral shift is used in normal walking, in sidestepping, and for restorative movements. When would you use it in massage? How can your massage become easier when you practice this movement to ensure a pure lateral shift?

Schneider Self-Healing Techniques

Meir Schneider's self-healing techniques (1994) are practical exercises focusing on breathing, circulation, vision improvement, and neuromusculoskeletal growth. Schneider was born in 1954 in the Ukraine with a variety of vision problems. He underwent five cataract operations without success and at seven was declared legally blind. Years later, by means of eye exercises and movement therapy, he was able to read without glasses and began to work with other physically disabled people. Self-healing exercises have been adapted specifically for populations suffering from muscular dystrophy, multiple sclerosis, polio, back pain, headaches, asthma, arthritis, and vision problems.

Exercise 5.3. Self-Healing Exercise*

Since Meir Schneider is most well known for using movement to improve his own sight, it would seem to be appropriate to include a vision-enhancing experiment here. This exercise is called the "long swing" (Schneider, 1994).

Stand with your legs far apart, and hold one index finger in front of your eyes about two feet in front of your face. Focus on that finger and then move the finger as far to each side as you can, following with your eyes. Move your head so that your finger is always in front of your nose. As you focus on the finger, see in the background all of your surroundings moving in the opposite direction.

Now continue the action while allowing your body to follow the movement of the eyes. As you turn to the left, continue to turn enough to actually bring the right heel off the floor. Do the same on the opposite side. Now increase the swinging of the body to include bending the upper trunk to the side when you are facing forward, and then stretching up at the sides. (See Figure 5.8.)

Questions for Discussion. Did your sense perception of seeing change? How did it feel to look at the world in this new way? How did the rest of your body change? The purpose of this exercise is to increase the sense of movement while you look. Do you let your vision blur during a massage? Next time you do a massage, allow your eyes to track

*Courtesy of *The Handbook of Self Healing* by Meir Schneider (1994). Penguin Books: London, England.

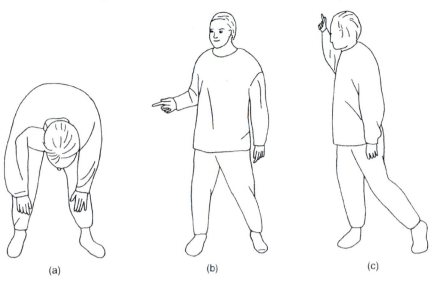

Schneider Exercise—Step 1   Schneider Exercise—Step 2   Schneider Exercise—Step 3

(a)   (b)   (c)

Figure 5.8 (a–c)   Schneider's "long swing" demonstrates one approach to movement reeducation.

your movements. How would it be to massage with easy, open, and clear vision? Would your massage change? What do you think would be the effect on your clients?

Aston Patterning®

This approach originated with deep connective tissue massage (Rolfing) and then integrated movement. Judith Aston invented the method in 1967, after two auto accidents brought her dance career to an end. Unlike the Rolfers, Aston did not believe in a "standard" of one best body posture being applicable to all people. Deep, spiraling massage and movement is the basis for individualized work. The three Aston bodywork techniques are Aston massage®, myokinetics (myofascial mobilization), and arthrokinetics. Although each type of work can be used separately, common themes unite all of Aston's work. First, humans are basically asymmetrical and the concept of traditional "good posture" or exact symmetry is unrealistic and undesirable. Second, the body is an integrated whole, and physical problems are best addressed by treating the whole person, not just an isolated area. Third, natural movements are three-dimensional, with depth, height, and width as factors. Three-dimensional touch takes into consideration the layers, grain, shape, and movement of the tissue (Low, 1988). Aston movement® education is used in conjunction with the bodywork in order to teach the client how to function with the new flexibility that arises from the patterning. Judith Aston believes that if an individual can understand and proprioceptively feel the changes made in a session, then the changes will be more readily integrated into everyday living. The total effect is to encourage bodies to move in an asymmetric spiral, like a feather descending toward earth.

The goal of each Aston Patterning® session is to teach clients how to integrate their newfound body ease into effortless posture and movement. The traditionally accepted model for proper posture is based on the vertical plumb line. With a tuck here and a lift there, we could make our clients' bodies conform to this model. The problem with a standardized plumb line ideal is the constant energy required to maintain verticality. Real people cannot sustain the tension needed to maintain ideal posture and eventually slip back into old habits that cause discomfort and pain (Woods, 1997).

Exercise 5.4. Aston Exercise®*

Consider this experiment to experience the relationship between wholeness, assymetry, and three-dimensionality in the body (Aston, Molnar, and Krier, 1992). Find a chair and sit back in it. Let your spine gently flex and your ribs depress against the back of the chair. Now reach forward while you are lifting a book. Try to feel where the muscles tense to exert this effort. Note the tone of the shoulder muscles in relation to the deeper structure of your upper ribs while lifting. While maintaining the flexed–depressed rib position, lift your left shoulder and check the range of motion in flexion, extension, abduction, and rotation.

Repeat these tests after your shift forward on the chair and assume a more neutral position in the torso. Lean forward slightly by flexing at the hips without hunching over at the shoulders.

Questions for Discussion. What did it feel like to lift the book from the flexed–depressed rib position? What did it feel like to move the arm in circumduction from this position? Range of motion often feels reduced and effort may feel increased. In this alignment, the muscles tend to work excessively to compensate for the compromise in the structure of the upper ribs. How did the feeling of the flexed–depressed rib position contrast with the feeling in the second position? Do you sense that maintaining the integrity of the rib cage decreases the work of the external musculature? Do you notice an increase in the range of motion at the shoulder? Why or why not?

Feldenkrais Work®

Feldenkrais work® engages the body to reeducate the brain through slow, simple movements (Feldenkrais, 1977). Complex movements are synthesized from the simple ones so that your body can create easier ways to move. Feldenkrais work® engages the body to reeducate the brain through slow simple movements (Feldenkrais, 1977). Moshe Feldenkrais, an Israeli physicist and sixth dan black belt in judo, developed the method in the 1940s to heal recurrent knee injuries he was suffering from. The one-on-one table work is known as *functional integration,* and the more familiar group movement classes are called *Awareness through Movement.*

One example of an Awareness through Movement process was given in Ex-

*Courtesy of Judith Aston and Aston-Mechanics®–2000 Personal Communication.

ercise 2.11 (Finding Ease of Motion). The tiny movements that go into the process allow you to find the easiest way to make a larger motion. The intricate detail of the sequence causes you to interrupt patterns that may have been causing pain. Here is a second example of tiny motions that bring about body awareness. Although the steps may look complicated, give it a try. (You may want to read the steps into a tape recorder and play them back as you move.)

Exercise 5.5. Awareness through Moving Tongue and Jaw Muscles*

Lie on your back and begin to sense each segment of your body and the relative tensions that are residing there. Sense how relaxed or tense your feet are, then your legs and thighs and trunk, and so on. You will compare this baseline feeling to how you feel after you have completed the exercise.

Stick your tongue forward to touch your teeth. Then return to a neutral jaw position. Do this a few times. Now draw your tongue back deeper into the mouth and return. Combine the movements. (Remember to perform all the actions in the easiest way possible for you, and if you get tired or if any of the actions feel stressful at any time, rest!) Now jut your jaw forward and return it to neutral. Repeat several times. Jut your jaw back and repeat. Combine the motions to move the jaw forward and back a few times. Now allow the jaw to move to one side and then the other. Make a circle with the jaw. Do this for several rotations. Now allow the tongue to move to one side while the jaw moves to the opposite side. Repeat, then reverse the tongue and jaw movements. Now make circles with the tongue. Do this to one side, then to the other. Rest on one side. Then lie on your back and reassess relative tensions in your head and face.

Questions for Discussion. Did the baseline perception of the whole body change? Did your perception of your tongue and jaw change? How did the rest of your body react? The purpose of this exercise is to increase awareness of all the tiny muscles around the mandible. How would it be to massage with a free and relaxed tongue and jaw? How would the massage be affected? What do you think would be the effect of your relaxed jaw on clients?

Trager® Work

Trager® work uses gentle, rhythmic movements to generate pleasurable sensory input, release tension, and reeducate the nervous system. Dr. Milton Trager first started developing the work when he was an 18-year-old boxer in Miami during the early part of the twentieth century. The story goes that usually his trainer/manager would give him a rubdown after each training session. One day, he decided to return the favor by giving his trainer a massage. The trainer told him he had "hands," meaning that Milton's rubdown was better than any touch therapy he knew how to do. Trager decided to apply these techniques to try to

*Adapted from Maureen McHugh, personal communication/Awareness Through Movement[R] class, 1990.

help his father at home. Trager's father had been suffering from crippling sciatic pains without relief for two years. Within two of Milton's sessions, his father's sciatica was gone (Schwartz, 1997). One component of the Trager® system is the bodywork (known as *Trager Psychophysical Integration®*), which is practiced on a massage table. The other component of Trager work® is movement reeducation instruction (known as *Mentastics®*, literally a fusion of the words "mental" and "gymnastics").

Mentastics relaxes the body, particularly the parasitic tension of the antagonist muscles, so movement becomes easier. Because Mentastics feels good, the body information that arises from the experiences is better accepted. Changes occur gradually, so there is little resistance to improvement. In general, Mentastics improves sensory information about your body and in turn helps you to receive sensory input from others. Knowing how your body moves in time and space helps your functional self breathe, walk, relax, and heal.

Exercise 5.6. Mentastics® Sampler*

The object of Mentastics exercises is to be light, easy, and playful. Work gently and remember that there is nothing that can be done wrong. Ask yourself whenever you feel stuck, "What could be lighter? What could be easier?" Just start the move and let your weight, mass, or momentum do the work. Move without effort. Notice without trying to change. Let in the notion that you deserve to feel good, even though you may not be perfect.

To start, imagine a hook on the crown of your head connecting you to the upper atmospheres. This is your "sky hook." Feel it pulling your entire frame up. At the same time, imagine an "earth hook" attached to your base at the tailbone. Feel your base being drawn toward the earth. Experience the space between your vertebrae opening up as you sense the stretch move up and down simultaneously.

For the upper body: Feel the weight of your right hand with the palm facing up, in front of your body. Do the same with your left. Drop the right hand, as if you were shaking off a water drop. Now make the motion even easier. Drop your hand with larger and larger oscillations, involving more and more of the arm and finally letting the shoulder follow on the outward swing. On the last wave, add a little wobble of the hand (imagine your hand becoming a butterfly), at the end of the motion. (See Figure 5.9.)

For the head: Imagine those little toy figures with their heads on a spring that you often spot in the back windshield of a car. Perhaps you even own one of these nodding creatures with the spring neck. Now try some head bobs. Feel yourself making small light nodding motions, with the head centered on the cervical spine. Now draw shoulders back, while your head keeps nodding "yes." Feel the connections on down the spine.

For the lower extremities: Begin with "foot flips"—kick out one foot at a time, with light flicks. Now do mule kicks to the back. (See Figure 5.10.) Lean on a chair or table and imagine you are throwing away

*Adapted from Joe L. Griffin, PhD, personal communication/Mentastics class®, 1990.

Butterfly Hand

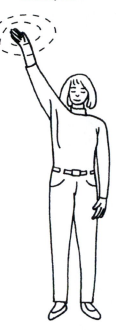

Figure 5.9 Flutter the hand like a butterfly and let it drop. Feel the weight of the hand and ask "How could this movement be easier and lighter?"

your heel to straighten the leg. Try mule kicks to the side, simply by kicking your heel to the side. Feel the lower legs, particularly the calves, as they wobble. Shimmy your legs. Now start walking, incorporating the foot flips before landing. Feel your pelvis drop down and forward slightly as you sense the weight of your leg.

Questions for Discussion. How did it feel to move in this way? How did the part of your body that you focused on change? How did the rest of your body change? How would it feel to move in this light, easy way

Mule Kick

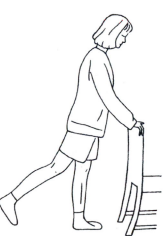

Figure 5.10 Mule kicks dissipate tension in the legs and feet.

all the time? How would it feel to massage with light, easy, and open sensations in your body? How would your massage change? What do you think would be the effect on clients?

Hanna Somatics Education

Hanna Somatics Education (1988) teaches people to take voluntary control of their muscles. This gives a person a conscious input into movement via the cerebral cortex and the ability to bypass patterns and spinal cord reflexes. The idea is to override autonomic responses (reflexes or habits) that may no longer be useful. Thomas Hanna believed that people get sensory motor amnesia (SMA) through repeating unhealthy patterns of movement. This means they lose the ability to sense and control their muscles because of bad habits. Rather than passively giving one's soma over to be repatterned by a therapist, Hanna believes that it is important for clients to take a conscious, active role in the process of resetting their proprioceptors. (*Note:* Proprioceptors are sensory receptors that tell us about the positioning, tension, and length of our muscles, tendons, and joints in space.) The following exercise (Hanna, 1988) on body image training may demonstrate the role of re-"cognition" in Hanna Somatics Education.

Exercise 5.7. Controlling Trunk Flexor Muscles/Body Image Training*

Lie on the back, knees bent, with the soles of your feet planted close to the buttocks. Place your left hand on the pubic bone and your right hand over the lower half of your chest. Now inhale, slowly lifting your lower back as the pelvis rolls down to the tailbone. Exhale, flattening your lower back. Repeat six times. Use your hands to feel how the abdominal muscle contracts when you flatten out the lower back. (*Note:* Emotions of fear and/or apprehension also cause the abdominal muscle to contract in the "red light reflex.")

Place your right hand beneath your head, then inhale, arching back as you did before; exhale, contracting the abdominal muscle to flatten your lower back to the floor as you lift up your head with your right hand. Repeat several times. Use your left hand to notice how the abdominal muscle contracts harder when you lift your head.

Now raise the right knee and hold it in front with your left hand. Continue the same pattern as before, but now, as you exhale, flatten the back and lift the head and also pull the right knee toward the elbow and bring together several times. Notice how the more you lower your back against the floor, the easier it is to bring the elbow to the knee. Stretch out arms and legs and relax, noticing how it feels down the trunk between the right shoulder and hip. Repeat on the opposite side.

On your back with knees bent as before, place your right hand beneath your head. Then lift your left knee and hold it with your left hand. Inhale, slowly lifting the lower back. As you exhale, flatten the back and

*Courtesy of *Somatics* by Thomas Hanna (1988). Perseus Books: New York, NY.

lift the head and right elbow toward the left knee. Simultaneously pull the left knee toward your right elbow and face six times. Sense how the head and elbow must point slightly to the left and feel how the more you round the back down toward the floor, the nearer the elbow comes to the knee. (Hanna says you are now remembering how to regain voluntary control of the muscles of the back.) Repeat on the opposite side.

Interlace both hands and place them beneath the back of the head. Inhale, arching your lower back, then exhale, flattening the back as you lift the head up. Repeat three times.

Keep your hands behind your head and lift up both knees, letting them balance over the stomach. Inhale, arching up the lower back, then exhale, flattening your back as the hands lift the head and both elbows toward the knees. Try to bring the knees toward the elbows. Stretch out your legs with arms alongside the body and rest. Notice how you feel inside your body from the middle of the chest down to the pubic bone and in the area between the legs. As you quietly inhale, allow your lower belly to rise freely with complete relaxation, so that your breathing becomes deep and full. (See Figure 5.11.)

Practice the action of releasing and flattening the back while you are sitting. If you suffer from chronic lower back pain, you may experience swayback with very contracted erector spinae muscles along each side of the spine. Hanna says this is because SMA has caused you to forget what it feels like for the lower back to keep its normal relaxed curve, with weight resting on the vertebrae. Because SMA creates a distorted body image, when your back is relaxed with your head directly over the center of gravity, you feel like you are slumping too far forward. The swayback has come to feel normal. In order to counteract this distorted body image, use a mirror whenever possible. When you do, you may be astonished to find that your back is balanced and the belly is flat. When your internal sense (proprioception) of back position and visual sense adjust to match, you will be able to sit without soreness or fatigue, because your vertebrae are acting as a column of support. It is a matter of adjusting to a new body image. The mirror technique is a simple example of biofeedback training.

Questions for Discussion. How did it feel to move in this way? How did the part of your body that you focused on change? How did your body image change? How would it be to consciously relax the stomach flexors whenever your body tightened up? How would it feel to massage with released stomach flexors? How would your massage change? What do you think would be the effect on clients?

MOVEMENT REEDUCATION GUIDELINES FOR BODY MECHANICS AND SELF-CARE

Logical conclusions from standards explicated in the various movement therapies can supplement our guidelines for efficient body mechanics. Some items on the growing list simply restate suggestions that were explored in the last two

Hanna Somatics Exercise—Step 1

Hanna Somatics Exercise—Step 2

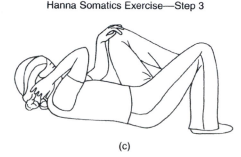

(a)

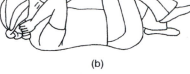

(b)

Hanna Somatics Exercise—Step 3

Hanna Somatics Exercise—Step 4

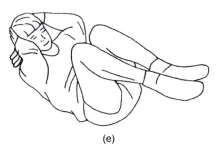

(c)

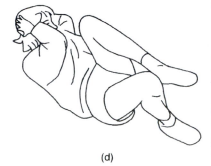

(d)

Hanna Somatics Exercise—Step 5

(e)

Figure 5.11 (a–e) Hanna Somatics focus on replacing unhealthy movement patterns with voluntary and conscious control of muscles.

chapters. Arriving at a body mechanics conclusion (like "maintaining awareness") from a new point of view acts to verify its utility. Remember to confirm or refute any and all data with kinesthetic awareness as you move and massage. What feels good to your body? What feels out of line or out of sync? Your subjective discoveries can prompt body mechanics that are in harmony with your physical world.

Useful conclusions come from probing similarities or peculiarities of method among movement therapies that were outlined in this chapter.

Self-Observation

Sometimes movement therapies are collectively referred to as somatic disciplines. Somatics, derived from the Greek word *soma,* meaning body, is the study of the body as perceived from within. A unifying principle of the somatic disciplines

(Alexander technique, Feldenkrais, Trager, etc.) is that self-awareness is the key to the healthy functioning of the body, mind, and soul. Through self-awareness, we tap into the wisdom of the body and initiate a capacity for self-healing.

Physiologically, the wisdom of the body is in the form of proprioceptors, the afferent neural impulses that give us awareness of posture, movement, and changes in equilibrium. When we take the time to focus on proprioception (what we feel), we access a wealth of somatic information. The information can enable us to equalize the tone of our muscles, use our skeleton for support, and move with more grace and ease. In the movement therapies, self-awareness replaces the dependence on orthodox formulas and rules for body mechanics.

External Feedback

The Hanna Somatics exercise brought out the importance of using an outside tool, such as a mirror, to bring our internal body image into line with the messages we get from the physical world. Alignment of the body by checking with mirrors was also an important principle of the Mensendieck System of Functional Movements, developed by Dr. Bess Mensendieck around the turn of the century. Patterns can be so pervasive that freer ways of moving and massaging can at first seem strange. Sometimes we need an external reality check on those inner perceptions. A mirror is a simple biofeedback device, an easy way of seeing when our bodies are "out of whack" during a massage. It is quite easy to hang a mirror in your office, for the purpose of observing body mechanics. Not only can you use it to prevent injury in yourself, but it could also become incorporated as a tool for showing your clients the difference between less and more proficient ways of propelling themselves. You could incorporate other biofeedback props as instructional aids for yourself and your clients—they also bring an element of fun into your practice. Other devices to use for rudimentary reality checks include:

1. *Biodots.* These are small adhesive dots that you can affix to the webbing between forefinger and thumb. They contain a chemical coating that is temperature sensitive, like the popular "mood rings" of the 1970s. They are used to check stress levels, since peripheral body temperature (in hands and feet) goes up due to increased blood flow when you are more relaxed. This is the same effect achieved for clients by increasing circulation during a massage.

2. *An observer watching as you massage.* This is just what it sounds like. It is easily accomplished within the context of a class. Divide up the class into groups of three students working together. One is the "giver," one is the "receiver," and the third acts as a "silent witness" for the session. Note that this process can feel intimidating unless all participants understand the spirit of "observing without judging."

3. *Videotaping.* Again, this method is easily accomplished in a class setting. Instructors use the camera as the "silent witness/observer" described above. A camera, like a mirror, is truly a witness without judgment. It simply replays the series of steps making up the bodywork session. The advantage here is that the tape can be replayed over and over again to pinpoint areas of

difficulty or "bloopers" in body mechanics. Student givers can evaluate their own performance or receive comments from others.

4. *Use of the Swiss (or Gymnastik, or FitBall) ball.* The Swiss ball is unique in that people associate balls with play and re-"creating." In the United States, the thick, large, vinyl balls were nicknamed "Swiss" because American therapists first saw the balls in use in clinics in Switzerland. The balls were first used in pediatric and neurological settings. Swiss balls have since been integrated into the practice of spinal stabilization exercises, postpartum exercise programs (Elizabeth Noble), and adapted Feldenkrais techniques (Ilana Parker) and exercises to improve golf and other athletic performance. Since 1991, this tool has replaced chairs in school for thousands of European children with the concept of "active sitting." It has been found to calm hyperactive children and improve concentration, handwriting skills, understanding of subject material, and organization (Posner-Mayer, 1995). A variety of repetitive movements can be experimented with using the ball as a counterbalance. It can also be used as a stool by the therapist during a bodywork session for the use of "active sitting," or as a tool for the client after the table work to help integrate and improve range of motion, strength, balance, perceptual retraining (body image), and postural changes. The massage practitioner can utilize the ball between sessions for stretching and renewal with the same benefits that would accrue for a client. Lie over it frontways, sideways, rest your legs on it or sit on it, or be creative. (See Figure 5.12.)

Exercise 5.8. Biofeedback for Body Mechanics

The next time you schedule a client for a bodywork session, try out one of the above-mentioned forms of simple biofeedback. Explain to your clients that you are using this tool for the purposes of improving your body positions and motions during massage, which will ultimately result

Swiss Ball

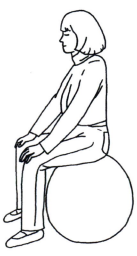

Figure 5.12 Sitting on the Swiss ball gives external feedback about tiny movements in the pelvis, feet, and spine.

in a better massage for them. If you are in a massage class currently, try one of these reality checks during class or during a practice session. Choose the video camera, a mirror, a "silent witness" (meaning an outside observer, or a biodot), whatever is appropriate to your situation. Ask for permission and explain what you want to do to clients. Do not use something that would be intrusive to your clients or a method that would interfere with their comfort in any way.

Rest

This scheme is utilized by several, if not all, of the somatic disciplines. Most notably, rest is a hallmark of Feldenkrais®, Trager®, Hanna Somatics, and Bartenieff work. Think of your massage session as a passage of melody and rhythm in which silences accentuate and highlight the musical flow. Without a pause, the piece has no harmony and the notes incessantly rattle on. Similarly, without pauses, your brain has no time to integrate kinesthetic skills that are learned in a bodywork session. This is true for both givers and receivers of massage. Dr. Henry Holcomb, a research psychiatrist with Johns Hopkins University, found that people who learned a motor skill were more likely to remember the skill later on if they were allowed to do unrelated routines for some time after (Recer, 1997). Test subjects who were trained in a new motor task immediately after learning the first skill lost much of the skill that they had learned first, unlike the group that was allowed a rest. It is thought that immediately introducing a new task tends to erase learning gained from the first task. It is not enough to simply practice something. You have to allow time to pass for the brain to encode the new skill. A shift in brain activities is necessary to render the memory invulnerable and permanent. This time to consolidate memory allows a person to never forget some skills, such as riding a bike or swimming. In the same way, incorporating strategic pauses in our bodywork sessions (when we sense a completion or feel fatigue in ourselves) allows both therapist and client to make the crucial shift in the brain that allows change to happen. Not only is rest important for the therapist who is trying to save his or her hands, but it is also important for the client. This may be different from what was taught in your introductory Swedish massage class. Were you told never to take your hands off the client's body, even when reapplying lubricant or shifting to another segment of the body? I find it annoying when receiving a massage to always be under contact of the therapist. I need time to integrate the work! Test this with your clients and see for yourself whether critical pauses are appreciated as a necessary part of the integration process.

Use "Baby Steps"

For the purposes of improving body mechanics, the "baby steps" guideline translates into two corollary tenets. First, it helps to break difficult strokes and stretches down into their component parts. More basic movements are easier to comprehend in terms of direction of effort and force, positioning of torso and extremities, and postural stance than are complex actions. Second, "babying" means being gentle on yourself and introducing changes gradually. It is generally easier to make smaller adaptations to a routine, rather than abandoning everything you have learned up to this point.

Many movement therapy resources share the concept of breaking overwhelming tasks into smaller steps. We have seen evidence of the belief in Bartenieff's Fundamentals, based on observations of infants' efficient movement. Baby steps are also evident in the tiny movements that make up Feldenkrais Awareness through Movement exercises and also in Hanna Somatics, which builds on Feldenkrais principles. In Trager® work, small movements are used as a way of letting clients feel safe, so that they can open up on their own. Micromovements help the therapist approach their "edge" in order to pinpoint and become more sensitive to resistances in the body. As massage therapists who are learning to protect our bodies from injury, it is also important to cultivate these skills.

Learn to Play

This may well be the most important lesson of the entire book and one in which movement therapists are particularly adept. For example, Milton Trager was a huge proponent of establishing play as part of the bodywork regimen. Mentastics are lighthearted movements, as are the rocking and rolling motions that characterize Trager® "massage." Trager believed that pleasurable sensations were essential for the brain to let go of old hurts.

One of the most wonderful features of humanity is our propensity for play. Children and a few enlightened adults seem to recognize that it is truly all right to play. As individuals enter their "productive" years, they tend to lose sight of play as a worthwhile pursuit. Perhaps we get so caught up in duties and obligations that we fail to see the inherent value in play. Perhaps we have no time or energy left over for play. Perhaps we simply forget how to have fun. Regardless of the reason, what I see is that "grown-ups" (a name that implies that there is no more growing to do) do not play as long or as well as children do. When we suddenly realize that we are not doing anything that we enjoy, we then work too hard trying to have fun. Have you seen joggers with grim and determined faces as they grind out the daily run in sizzling heat or subzero temperatures? What about the aerobics fanatic who suffers recurrent injuries from "going for the burn"? Overly avid "weekend warriors" reveal how working really hard at playing can spoil any amount of fun and can even cause injury and pain. You may recognize some of your regular clients in these stories, or perhaps you may recognize something of yourself as a wounded therapist trying too hard to "fix" your clients' suffering.

Another obstacle that hampers a natural playfulness is the fear of looking foolish. Teens and young adults are particularly prone to forgo happiness in the name of self-image. This age group critiques, criticizes, and downplays their accomplishments, in order to look "cool." Unfortunately for them, the strategy of avoiding anything that might make them look foolish is not sound. If you are unwilling to make mistakes, if you must master a technique on the first try, how can you possibly be open to learning something new? This is especially true for bodyworkers. Typically, we learn new techniques from workshops and seminars in which the instructor has been refining and practicing the technique for years. The instructor has learned to adapt its nuances to his or her own body and has become comfortable with this kind of bodywork, like an old shoe. We learn the technique in a weekend and then are left to practice it on our own. We try to shape our bodies in the way that we remember seeing it demonstrated, but it doesn't feel quite right. How many of us then abandon most, if not all, of the new bodywork technique because it doesn't fit in with our work?

Instead of always turning playtime into work, perhaps it would be better to see if we can turn the massage workday into play. This does not mean we should address bodywork as frivolous and unimportant. It simply means that it might be helpful to bring the energy and joy of play to bear in a bodywork session. But first, we must rediscover how to play. In this regard, movement can be an excellent guide. Moving the body just to see what happens is play. Sensing what strokes feel good as you practice them is enjoyable. Shifting your weight in alternate ways, just to see what happens, can be fun. Using vibration or rocking for the sheer heck of it, because you like to do it, because it feels right—that is the essence of play.

Exercise 5.9. Pretend Play

Animals, like children, seem to be uninhibited in their freedom of movement. It is rare to see a creature with tendinitis or carpal tunnel syndrome. In this exercise, we borrow some playful inspiration from the beasts.

This exercise is best accomplished in a group setting. Appoint one person as the leader. The leader begins by calling out names of animals. All participants in the group act and make sounds like the creature that was named. How would you move if you were a cat, dog, lion, chicken, beetle, snake, deer, or owl?

In the second step, each participant chooses the animal that moves its body most closely to the way you think you move. Write the animal name down on a slip of paper. If you are going on to the third part of this exercise, put that slip of paper away for now. If not, go ahead and propel yourself around the room as if you have become the animal on your piece of paper. Do these movements seem to fit you? Why did you choose this particular animal?

The third stage requires a group of people who have seen each other do physical work. This would be ideal for a massage class or for a support group of people who have taken workshops together and/or done bodywork trades. In this variation, each participant is given as many slips of paper as there are people participating in the exercise minus one. On each tag, write the name of a participant along with the animal that he or she reminds you of. These papers are then distributed to the appropriate partners, lying face down. Now comes the fun part. Read aloud the names of the animals that others have chosen for you, and take turns acting out the parts. Everyone tries to guess the creatures that are being portrayed. As each person finishes his animal repertoire, the others can tell why they selected the animals that they did.

Recognize the Unity of the Body

Somatic disciplines are especially attuned to the body as a whole functioning unit. Although massage therapists need to know individual muscle origins, insertions, and actions for purposes of focusing in on a client's chief complaint, it is important to remember that the human body is a functioning whole. In actuality, no muscle acts alone to move a joint. For every action, other muscles are stabilizing or counteracting each push and pull. Muscles can interweave with each other, as in the case of pectoralis major and the external obliques. Different muscles can share the same attachments of origin or insertion. Sometimes, as in the case of coracobrachialis and pectoralis minor, one muscle begins where another ends. (See Figure 5.13.) That is, the origin of the coracobrachialis is the insertion of the pectoralis minor.

In fact, some bodyworkers claim that there is really no such thing as an individual muscle (Barnes, 1988; Juhan, 1987) since every muscle of the body, every fascicle, and every fibril and microfibril of muscular tissue is surrounded and connected by fascia or connective tissue. These myofascial therapists see the body as covered in a whole body stocking of soft tissue. When there is a pull in this fascial sweater, say at the sleeve, it can affect the material all the way up at the neck and down to the toes. Contraction of muscles pulls the connective tissue tighter. As the muscle fibers relax, the connective tissue recoils, spreading movement throughout the body. When the fibers cannot relax fully due to spasm, the lack of movement can be felt very far from the originating source of pain. I have seen, firsthand, how a localized injury can have system-wide effects on the musculoskeletal complex. I broke my right talus bone and was in a foot cast for about six weeks. I was alarmed to see the amount of muscular atrophy in my right calf in such a short time. Another effect was the overcompensation and subsequent hypertrophy of my left leg. I no longer used my quadriceps muscles on the right side in quite the same way, but instead relied on the left psoas as the main hip flexor when walking. As my psoas spasmed and became sore from overuse, I tended to twist my upper body and neck to compensate. There was a consequent pain and spasm in the scalenes and sternocleidomastoid.

It is important to use both specific mechanical principles *and* a general whole-body perspective for dealing with real live body mechanics issues. How does that translate for the massage practitioner? This double focus is needed to

Muscles with Shared Attachment

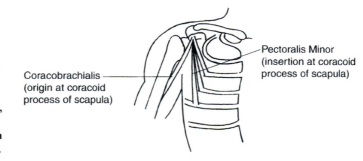

Figure 5.13 The pectoralis minor inserts on the coracoid process of the scapula. The coracobrachialis originates at the coracoid process of the scapula. Where the pectoralis minor ends, the coracobrachialis begins. It is as if the coracobrachialis were an extension of the pectoralis minor.

Coracobrachialis (origin at coracoid process of scapula)

Pectoralis Minor (insertion at coracoid process of scapula)

help us note and deal with all overt signs and symptoms, and then look further for hidden effects. Holding the knees in hyperextension can have repercussions all the way up to the jaw, for example. This open-ended, two-way approach to body mechanics can help save our bodies and our practice.

SUMMARY

This chapter provides an introduction to the movement perspective and its relationship to body mechanics. Introductions to several prominent movement reeducation theories are presented, including the work of Milton Trager, Irmgard Bartenieff, Judith Aston, Moshe Feldenkrais, F. M. Alexander, Meir Schneider, and Thomas Hanna. A number of body mechanics principles can be derived from concepts shared by a movement reeducator's approach to bodywork. Some of these are new guidelines, including getting feedback, taking baby steps, and learning how to play as you massage. Others restate in a new way body mechanics principles that were adopted in the last chapter. These precepts include using self-observation to enrich your work and respecting the unity of the body.

In a typical movement therapy session, the bodyworker will begin by analyzing a client's posture and often-repeated movements. Palpation of the soft tissue follows in order to reveal patterns of musculoskeletal restriction. Bodywork is used to release the most limiting patterns. Last but not least, education is used to help the changes "take." Client involvement leads to personal empowerment, an element missing in the traditional "therapist as fixer" model. Without the educational component, it is likely that the body will slip into old habits and eventually lose its flexibility. Massage practitioners would do well to apply these steps to their own body mechanics as they work.

REFERENCES

Anderson, Bob, *Stretching* (1980). Bolinas, CA: Shelter Publications, Inc.

Aston, Judith, Mary Ann Molnar, and Linda, Krier, "In Your Best Shape with Gravity's Assistance," *Physical Therapy Today* (Fall 1992, Vol. 15, No. 3) pp. 50–59.

Barnes, John, *Myofascial Release Book* (1988). Paoli, PA: MFR Treatment Centers and Seminars.

Bartenieff, Irmgard, with Dori Lewis, *Body Movement: Coping with the Environment* (1980). New York: Gordon and Breach Publishers.

Benjamin, Patricia, "Seeds of a Profession" *Massage Therapy Journal* (Summer 1996), pp. 41–47.

Corbin, Charles, and Ruth Lindsay, *Concepts of Physical Fitness with Laboratories*, 6th ed. (1988). Dubuque, IA: Wm. C. Brown.

Feldenkrais, Moshe, *Awareness Through Movement* (1977). New York: Harper & Row.

Griffin, Joe L. (1990). Personal communication. Washington, D.C.

Hanna, Thomas, *Somatics* (1988). New York: Perseus Books.

Hart, Jon, "Deep Tissue Notes" (1998). Unpublished manuscript.

Juhan, Deane, *Job's Body* (1987). Barrytown, NY: Station Hill Press.

Leviton, Richard, "Better Body Mechanics," *East West Magazine* (September 1998), pp. 92–98.

Levy, Fran J., *Dance/Movement Therapy* (1988). Reston, VA: American Alliance for Health, Physical Education, Recreation and Dance.

Low, Jeffrey, "The Modern Body Therapies," *Massage Magazine* (November, 1988/Issue 16), pp. 48–50, 52, 54–55.

McHugh, Maureen (1990). Personal communication/Awareness Through Movement® class, Arlington, VA.

Newton, Donald, "Pathology Notes" (1998). Portland, OR: Simran Publications.

Posner-Mayer, Joanne, *Swiss Ball Applications for Orthopedic and Sports Medicine* (1995). Ball Dynamics International, Inc: Denver, CO.

Recer, Paul, "Brain Needs a Break for New Skills to Take," (August 1997) *The Oregonian,* Portland, OR, p. A14.

Schneider, Meir, *The Handbook of Self-Healing* (1994). London: Penguin Books.

Schultz, Louis, and Rosemary Feitis, *The Endless Web—Fascial Anatomy and Physical Reality* (1996). Berkeley, CA: North Atlantic Books.

Schwartz, Don, "What Could Be Lighter? The Work of Milton Trager," *Massage Magazine* (May/June 1997), pp. 56–63.

Woods, Jenna, "Forces of Nature in the Aston Paradigm—Key Concepts of Aston-Patterning *Massage and Bodywork* (Spring 1997), pp. 123–125.

Chapter Six

Unpatterning

CHAPTER OBJECTIVES

> **Conceptual Objectives**   The massage student/practitioner who success-
> fully completes this chapter (reading and exercises) will be able to:
>
> - Define the concept of unpatterning.
>
> - Direct specific visual and palpatory questions to determine efficient
>   body mechanics—alignment, weight distribution, tissue quality, joint
>   quality, side-to-side comparisons, motion quality, breath, and patterns.
>
> - List the general steps to unpattern.
>
> - Describe typical patterns in the body that can develop from poor body
>   mechanics.
>
> **Practical Objective**   The massage student/practitioner who successfully
> completes this chapter (reading and exercises) will be able to:
>
> - Devise a strategy for recognizing and altering patterned responses that
>   are no longer adaptive.

Previous chapters have generated hosts of guidelines for applying your body
more efficiently in a bodywork session. These suggestions begin with the meta
principles of the MORE system and are supplemented with prescriptions from
three distinct philosophical perspectives (scientific method, Eastern traditions,
and movement disciplines). As a result, a variety of recommendations exist for
improving therapist positioning and follow-through during a massage. If guidelines and recommendations were all there were to using healthy body mechanics,
the text could end here. Massage therapists need only "just do it" ergonomically,
as the Nike advertisers suggest. Why then are bodyworkers injuring themselves
on the job? Why don't bodyworkers simply make the necessary changes in body
mechanics as they are needed?

Making a shift in body attitude is a necessary precursor to making a shift in
behavior. However, an alteration in body awareness alone is not sufficient to sustain behavioral change. Any health educator can tell you that changing a behavior
(such as quitting smoking or making exercise a regular habit) is the most difficult

kind of transition. Transforming thoughts and attitudes, difficult as that may be, pales in comparison to implementing a lifestyle change. Probably the most significant barriers to implementing ergonomic transformation are the habits, reflexes, and patterns that you hold as you work and move. The guidelines for improving body mechanics have most likely helped you build up an awareness of the discomforts that bad habits can cause, but what good is that if you do not have tools to alter the patterns themselves? This chapter tackles the difficult problem of "unpatterning."

WHAT IS A PATTERN?

For purposes of this exposition, a pattern will be defined as something about yourself that prevents you from living as efficiently, effectively, or enjoyably as you can. In other words, patterns prevent you from massaging in the most optimal way. Patterns are constant or repetitive postures, motions, thoughts, and/or emotions. Patterns arise to help us cope with a certain set of conditions. For example, signing your name and taking the same route when driving to work are examples of adaptive patterns. When conditions change, patterns that used to be helpful may no longer be the best way to respond. Perhaps your writing hand becomes injured or there is a traffic jam on your usual driving route. Then you will need to do a routine task in a new way. Over the years, people can become so used to set ways of moving, thinking, feeling, and standing that they become automatic. Although the familiar behaviors and attitudes were learned at one time, individuals do not think about the set patterns anymore. As a result, habitual ways of behaving unconsciously control parts of us. Physical health, relationships, work performance, eating habits, and posture can all be affected. With reference to body mechanics, patterns are ways of holding the body (or the mindset) that can prevent you from practicing massage in a way that is optimally efficient, effective, and enjoyable. Although a pattern may have been originally developed as a creative solution to a problem, it often becomes generalized to situations in which that answer is not the best response. In essence, patterns can limit you.

Exercise 6.1. Demonstrating a Simple Pattern

This sensorimotor demonstration was inspired by the gentle exercises of Moshe Feldenkrais (1977). To begin, interlace the fingers of both hands. Notice which thumb lands on top. Is it the right thumb or the left? For every individual who winds up with the right thumb on the top, someone else in the world probably prefers the left. Ask yourself which way is correct, that is, which thumb *should* be on top? Of course, the answer is that both options are right. It is okay for either thumb to be on top. Try the procedure again, but this time consciously exchange all your fingers so that the opposite thumb lands on top.

Questions for Discussion. How does it feel to have your nondominant thumb at the top? If it feels awkward, it is probably because you are so used to ending up with the other thumb on top. In short, the dominant thumb on top of interlaced fingers has become a pattern for you. Does that mean that this is the right way? Sure, it is right, but the other way is right too. This pattern limits your options. Consider that probably half of the people you meet prefer to interlace their fingers so that the left thumb comes out on top. Do you feel that these people are misguided and misinformed about the "right way" to interlace their fingers? Continue to hold your hands in this unusual (for you) way. After about 5 minutes, you may notice that what once seemed so awkward and uncomfortable has now become a new position that you have made your own.

Changing a kinesthetic pattern as described in Exercise 6.1 is not always easy. But making the effort to expand your body options can teach two important lessons. First, whatever your way of doing things, there is always someone who can come up with an alternative (and usually equally potent) method. Second, by taking the risk and trying something new, you have more tools available in your bodywork toolbox. After a while, although it seemed awkward and uncomfortable at first, that new way of performing deep friction or stretching the psoas becomes incorporated into your repertoire. The ability to adapt increases, and you can more easily cope with new and unusual situations that arise in your practice. In many life experiences, not just massage, it is only by being willing to be uncomfortable, being willing to take a risk, that you garner the opportunity to grow. Think back to the first time that you rode a bicycle or the first time you kissed. These were awkward moments when you were able to augment your growth exponentially. Why? Because you dared to break a pattern—you dared to try something new.

Patterns can be changed, but it takes conscious input to override the automatic responses that become entrenched from repetition after repetition. Neurologically, patterns are stimulus–response reactions that bypass input from the brain. In a sense, patterns are the information pathways of least resistance and most use. The central nervous system has the very important function of integrating all sensory (stimulus/input) and motor (response/output) information. Integration of data can be expressed as unconscious reflexes (patterns), conscious motor activity, or awareness and thought.

HOW DO REFLEXES WORK?

The spinal cord integrates sensory and motor data through generating spinal cord reflexes. Reflexes usually protect the body from danger (for example, pulling the arm away from a hot flame). Reflex patterns can occur even if the spinal cord's connections with the brain stem are completely severed. The reflex arc acts independently and like a nervous system on a smaller scale. It is a way in which a muscle can respond without conscious influence from our brains (Walker, 1990). In a typical, healthy reflex arc, information from the outside world first activates a sensory receptor somewhere in or on the body. The "outside" information can be a change in temperature on the surface of the skin as in a cool breeze, a shift in blood flow as when you are standing on your head, or a minor trauma as when you cut your finger on a knife. Afferent (sensory) impulses from the periphery approach the spinal cord through the dorsal (posterior) root ganglion. One or more connecting neurons (called interneurons or internuncial neurons) relay the information up to the ventral (anterior) root of the spinal cord. From this point, a motor neuron links the information back out to the appropriate peripheral tissue. An efferent (motor) response will cause you to move a muscle or stimulate a gland. For example, you touch a hot object placed on the stove. A sensory signal goes from your finger to the spinal cord and enters in the back (dorsal root). That message is relayed to the front of the spinal cord by the second neuron. The motor response, in this case to jerk your finger away from the hot stove, is sent back out to the finger via the front neural highway (the ventral root). This simple three-part pathway allows you to remove your finger from the danger even before your brain registers the information that it is dangerous. (See Figure 6.1.)

Reflexes such as these are hardwired into our anatomy in order to let us respond to the environment in healthy ways. Physiologically, reflexes bypass the brain in order to get quicker responses and delegate certain responses to automatic pilot—the autonomic nervous system. This works just fine in many situations, such as the case of withdrawing our finger when we touch a hot stove. It would be nowhere near as adaptive if we had to wait for the information to register in our brains before retracting the finger from danger. In fact, it could be extremely hazardous to our health. However, a problem arises when learned patterns function like automatic reflexes. Patterns can become so intractable that pathological responses are programmed over healthier options. Habits are reflex-like responses that can be so ingrained in our consciousness that we sometimes cannot even see them in ourselves.

One example of such a learned muscular response occurs when we continually hunch our shoulders during a massage. In neurological pathways that are activated over and over again without adequate recovery time, metabolic wastes

The Reflex Arc

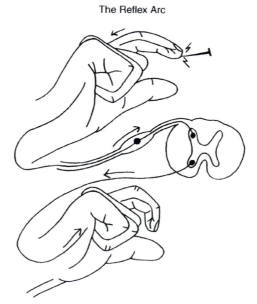

Figure 6.1 The reflex arc consists of a stimulus signal ("pinprick"), a connecting signal, and a motor response ("draw your finger back from the pinprick").

begin to accumulate, including bradykinin, histamine, prostaglandins, acids, acetylcholine, excessive potassium ions, and enzymes that break down proteins. These substances activate pain nerve endings and can even damage them. Nutrients and oxygen are diminished and a vicious reflex cycle of pain–spasm–pain is established (Walker, 1990). Now both mechanical (pressure) and chemical (waste by-products) means are causing the pain. Pain escalates, and the individual contracts his or her muscles even more as a protective device. This causes even more pain and so on and so on (Walker, 1990). This entire reaction process takes place on automatic pilot, to the detriment of the human body.

A further complication that can arise from pathways that are pathologically reactivated over and over is referred pain. More and more ischemia (lack of blood flow—a consequence of tissue held in a continual state of contraction) and resultant waste products build in the tissues. Sensory input into the spinal cord is then significantly increased, both by the mechanoreceptors (for contraction of the muscle) and by chemoreceptors (for the waste by-products). Stimulation can then produce spreading of internuncial messages to other segments up and down the spinal cord. The new impulses tend to take the path of least resistance, that is, a previously activated spinal cord segment. So, if you had an old childhood injury in your right hamstring, holding your lumbar curve in an overarched position during your massage sessions would tend to spread down and activate not only pain in your low back, but also in your right hamstrings.

If left untreated, these distortions can spread to other articulations and create more malfunction and pain. When the stimulation in the spinal cord reaches the brain, the reticular activating system (RAS) activates the whole body as a unit to raise the level of muscle tone body-wide. Sleep patterns are also governed by the RAS, so they may change also, leaving the individual with even less recovery and recuperation time and a general increase in contraction of the entire musculoskeletal system (Walker, 1990). In short, the whole body is "messed up."

PATTERNS OF HABITUAL MOVEMENT

Leon Chaitow (1993) refers to a stockpile of research that indicates that certain muscles of the body tend to shorten in response to stress whereas others tend to elongate and become weak. As a result, the body tends to mold itself more easily into certain postures than others. According to Chaitow, fibers that tend to contract and shorten in response to stress include calf muscles, short adductors of the thigh, hamstrings, psoas and piriformis, tensor fascia latae, quadratus lumborum, erector spinae, lattisimus dorsi, upper trapezius, scalenes, sternocleidomastoid, levator scapulae, pectoralis major, and arm flexors. Muscle fibers that tend to be overstretched and weakened are antagonists to the above muscles. These include the gluteus maximus and medius, abdominal groups, rhomboids, lower and middle trapezius, and serratus anterior. Figure 6.2 provides a clear overall tendency of muscle fibers to impose a fetal curve on the upper body, with the head and feet curled over and the shoulder and chest tucked up and in. The lower body is predisposed to point the toes and shorten the lower back.

This would be the overall pattern if all muscles that tend to contract under stress did so equally and there were no complications arising from other factors. In real life, however, the somatic patterns that develop are a little more complicated.

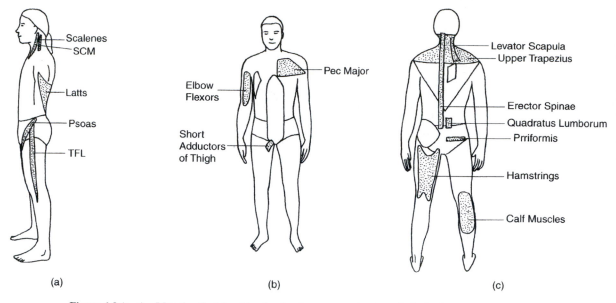

Muscles That Tend to Shorten (Side View)

Muscles That Tend to Shorten (Front View)

Muscles That Tend to Shorten (Rear View)

Scalenes
SCM

Latts

Psoas

TFL

Elbow
Flexors

Pec Major

Short
Adductors
of Thigh

Levator Scapula
Upper Trapezius

Erector Spinae
Quadratus Lumborum
Prriformis

Hamstrings

Calf Muscles

(a)

(b)

(c)

Figure 6.2 (a–c) Muscles that tend to shorten in response to stress include the scalenes, ster-nocleidomastoid, lattissimus dorsi, psoas, tensor fascia latae, elbow flexors, pectoralis major, short adductors of the thigh, levator scapula, upper trapezius, erector spinae, quadratus lumborum, piriformis, hamstrings, and calf muscles.

Generally, a chain reaction evolves in which certain muscle groups shorten and others weaken. Several authors, including Chaitow himself, have begun to ascertain the identity of certain standard imbalances of the body that can be identified and addressed. The goal is to identify the shortened structures and release them, and follow with reeducation in use of the body. Chaitow (1993) quotes Janda as describing an upper crossed syndrome and a lower crossed syndrome, as well as a complicating sagittal instability. He also describes a typical pattern of muscular tightening and weakening for temporomandibular joint (TMJ) dysfunction.

Upper Crossed Syndrome

In the upper crossed syndrome (Figure 6.3), the pectoralis major and minor, upper trapezius muscles, and sternocleidomastoid tighten and shorten, while the rhomboids, lower and middle trapezius, and serratus anterior weaken and get longer. This is a classic example of hyperlordosis of the cervical curve and hyperkyphosis of the thoracic curve of the spine. As these changes occur, they in turn alter the positions of the head, shoulders, and neck so that the head hyperextends and pushes forward, the shoulder blades abduct (move away from each other), and the arm rotates in and becomes more fixed and immobile in its socket.

Lower Crossed Syndrome

In the lower crossed syndrome (Figure 6.4), the hip flexors and erector spinae muscles tighten and shorten while the abdominal and gluteal groups weaken. The

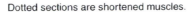

Upper Crossed Syndrome

Deep neck flexors weak

Trapezius and Levator Scapula contracted

Contracted Pectorals

Weak Rhomboids and Serratus Anterior

Dotted sections are shortened muscles.

Figure 6.3 In the upper crossed syndrome, muscles in front of the neck and in the midback weaken and elongate, while muscles in the upper back and chest tighten and contract. The back curves forward in a characteristic slump.

effect on the individual is to tilt the pelvis forward and produce a hyperlordotic lumbar curve with accompanying pain and stress. The stress can be uneven from one side to the other, resulting in a hip hike on one side. In this case, the quadratus lumborum (QL) on the affected side becomes tightened and shortened, and the QL on the opposite side becomes comparatively weak.

It may also be the case that both QLs tighten and the gluteus maximus and medius weaken in response, thereby lifting the entire pelvic girdle and stressing the lumbosacral junction, with accompanying low back pain.

A typical pattern for TMD or TMJ disorder sufferers was also described, with the following muscles showing tendencies to contract: upper trapezius, levators, sternocleidomastoid, suprahyoid, lateral and medial pterygoids, masseter, and temporalis. Scalenes were depicted as a wild-card muscle, which could exhibit the inclination to tighten and shorten, or could instead become weak. Either way, the end result would be spasming and pain in the scalenes.

A postural pattern for a patient could easily involve the entire body (in

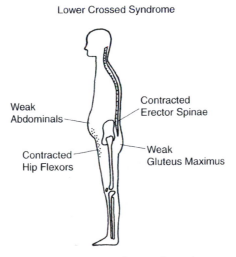

Lower Crossed Syndrome

Weak Abdominals

Contracted Erector Spinae

Contracted Hip Flexors

Weak Gluteus Maximus

Dotted sections are shortened muscles.

Figure 6.4 In the lower crossed syndrome, abdominals and gluteal muscles become weak and elongate, while erector spinae and hip flexors contract and shorten. The tummy bulges and the buttocks sink down.

Chaitow, 1993). For example, hyperextended knees affect the pelvis to increase its anterior tilt. Excessive pelvic tilt causes increased hip flexion and a more pronounced lumbar curve. The shoulders round and wing out to compensate for the hip displacement and that throws the head and neck into forward thrusting and cervical lordosis. The shoulders elevate in an attempt to stabilize the upper body, and this causes even more forward extension of the head, this time with tightening of the jaw (in Chaitow, 1993) and resulting TMJ disorder.

Paul Chek (1995) identifies forward head posture as the most commonly found postural discrepancy in the clinical setting. He notes that when the head is forward only two inches, the neuronal activation of the neck extensors (as measured by an electromyelogram) is tripled. This bears great significance for the massage therapist. Bodyworkers may inadvertently assume a forward head posture due to lack of attention, or due to a desire to "hurry up and get where they are going" or due to the startle response or the misuse syndromes described below. For whatever reason, when a forward head pose is taken, the rest of the body must compensate. Increased tension is generated, and energy, which could be better used on efficient leverage and movement, is wasted. (See Figure 6.5.)

Thomas Hanna (1988) claims postural patterns can commonly end in the loss of ability to sense and control the muscles (what he terms sensory motor amnesia [SMA]). Inability to relax is one example of loss of control. Thus, certain patterns of holding in our bodies can escalate into actually forgetting how to relax.

Conditioning from the environment is said to create a nonvoluntary response (or pattern), as exemplified by the classical conditioning of Pavlov's dogs. Pavlov's dogs were stimulated with a bell and then presented with food. The food sparked salivation as the dogs anticipated their dinner. As the bell was paired with the food, the dogs learned to salivate with the bell. Finally, they were reprogrammed so that they learned to salivate when they heard the bell alone. The particular pathway of neural responses (STIMULUS [bell]—anticipate food—RESPONSE [salivate]) has become so ingrained that the brain loses the capacity

Forward Head Posture

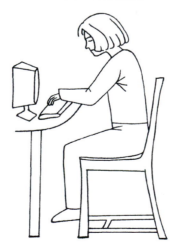

Figure 6.5 The forward head posture increases stress on the back of the neck, and the rest of the body tenses up as a result.

to intervene. The response becomes a conditioned reaction and choice is no longer a part of the equation.

According to Hanna (1988), SMA is caused by specific reflex responses. He lists five recognizable conditioned postural patterns: the *startle* response, the *trauma* response, the *Landau* response, *overuse or misuse* responses, and the kind of response that arises from *disuse and atrophy*. (You may remember Hanna as one of the movement therapists discussed in Chapter 5.)

Startle Response

The startle response (sometimes referred to as the *red light reflex*) is a stress reaction to threatening or worrisome situations. (See Figure 6.6.) It is how our bodies respond to the word "Boo," yelled suddenly and loudly. A turtle retreating back into his shell when frightened can typify the startle response. The body molds itself into a characteristic startled shape, depicted by lordosis of the neck, depression of the chest wall, raised shoulders, and too-forward carriage of the neck. F. M. Alexander also identified the startle response. He believed it begins with a disturbance of the primary head–neck–torso relationship, which causes an individual to raise the shoulders and tense the chest and knees.

Exercise 6.2. Demonstration of the Startle Response

This exercise is derived from a prank that Alexander instructors play with new students (Leviton, 1988). The game goes something like this. There are two partners—one adopts the role of the instructor and one takes on the role of student. The instructor directs the student as follows, "In a minute, I am going to ask you to say hello, but I would like you to do nothing in response." When the teacher makes the request, "Please say hello," what happens?

A general response to the command is for the student to say "hello" or "hel" or "h" or at least to overtense the larynx in preparation for mouthing the word. But when the exercise is repeated often enough, eventually the student learns not to respond at all. This way the power of inhibition, choosing not to respond to some stimuli, is learned kinestheti-

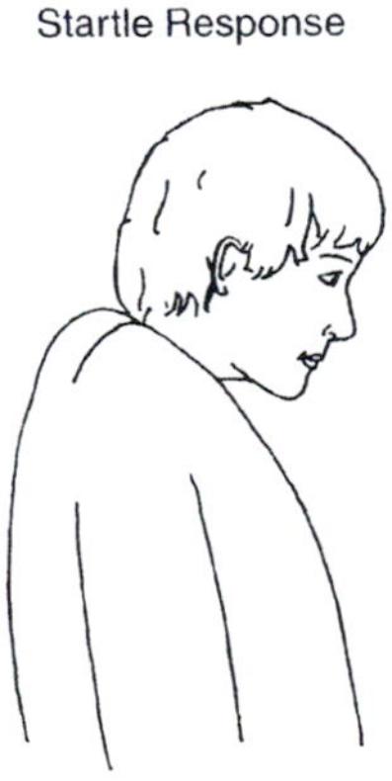

Startle Response

Figure 6.6 The startle response is a reflex that is activated by threatening or worrisome situations.

cally. The student learns to inhibit the entire somatic pattern, rather than just suppressing the intellect alone.

Let me recount another way that massage therapists can begin to somatically, and perhaps unconsciously, teach clients to inhibit a maladaptive pattern. The following scenario may sound familiar. At some point in the massage of a new client, the therapist, placing his or her hands in such a way as to fully support on the client's arms, says something like, "Let me have the weight of your arm. I would like you to let me move the arm without any help from you at all." The client, of course, nods assent. But almost invariably, the client reacts physically by interfering with the movement or manipulation, often at a surprisingly gross level. Once the interference is pointed out, the client can begin to direct his or her powers of attention to prevent or inhibit the unnecessary patterned response, thereby learning more of what it means to relax. Let me stress that the effective way to point out that a client is not relaxing is more subtle than yelling, "You're not relaxing. Just let go." I prefer a more indirect manner, including a short guided imagery directing the attention to the arm or whatever body part is continuing to hold, with suggestions to let that part "feel heavy and supported by my hand or the table underneath."

In this same way, therapists can use positive self-talk (feeling the support, letting go) to help themselves to relax. Perhaps you may even want to record a short guided imagery in your own voice directing your own attention to those areas in your body that tend to guard and hold on. (See Chapter 11 for more in-depth discussion of positive self-talk.)

Trauma Response

The trauma response is a body response to pain—an attempt to avoid the pain or lessen it. It is a protective posture. We can see the response when a person's leg is broken, he or she will avoid using that side of the body and stiffen the opposite side to take all the weight. After surgery for hernia removal, the musculature reveals that the side that was herniated is in constant contraction. The movement of cringing, or flinching, to protect against pain characterizes the trauma response. (See Figure 6.7.) A massage therapist who insists on working even when an injury is causing pain is not just ignoring a problem but actively ingraining the trauma response.

Landau Response

The Landau response (sometimes referred to as the arousal response or the *green light reflex*) is elicited when quick action is required, even demanded from a situation. You can see someone demonstrate the Landau response when they hear a knock on the door or a phone ring, or when they are asked to respond to a request (especially one they might not want or be able to grant). Babies who are over a few months old demonstrate the Landau action when they are placed on their tummies—lifting up their head and neck, pushing up on their arms, and lifting

Trauma Response

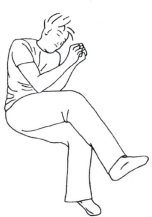

Figure 6.7   The trauma response is a reflex response to pain.

their feet as if they were flying. The adult arousal body response is characterized by the classic military posture, as seen in Figure 6.8. Here, the posterior muscles of the body contract and the back becomes erect in preparation for forward movement. Typically, the erector spinae, rhomboids, gluteus medius, piriformis, and hamstrings tighten in the Landau response.

Misuse or Overuse

Some body carriage patterns arise from habitual misuse and/or overuse. An example of a posture resulting from misuse is one you might spot in the prototypical computer keyboard operator, hunched over a screen, with weak and overextended rhomboids and extremely contracted pectoralis majors. A too-forward head position, as described by Paul Chek (1995), would also be representative of this kind of pattern. (See Figure 6.3.) Repetitive motion injuries, such as carpal tunnel disease and/or false sciatica, can be the end result of overuse syndromes.

Military Posture (Landau Response)

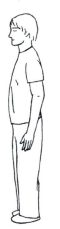

Figure 6.8   The Landau response can be elicited by a phone ringing or a knock on the door. It is also known as the "at attention" pose or military posture.

Disuse or Atrophy

Disuse and atrophy patterns can occur as a repercussion of an injury or illness, where the sufferer is bedridden for a period of time and the muscles waste away from lack of use. A casted limb is emblematic of the predicament, with atrophy of tissues developing underneath the cast. Hanna warns against blaming lack of use on increasing age. It is part of the traditional myth of aging that advancing years correspond with decreasing physical activity. This assumption would be profoundly wrong in our profession and in contrast to the credos put forth in this text. If our bones are not regularly used to bear weight and sustain substantial forces, they become soft, osteoporotic, and prone to break. If our muscles are not regularly challenged in activities and skills, they get smaller, weaker, and less able to contract. If our brain cells are not activated in a wide variety of conscious, voluntary tasks, they deteriorate. Atrophy and weakening of somatic tissue does not take place because of aging per se, but because of aging used as a pretext for inactivity. Wearing down need not be built into the massage therapist's way of life.

ASSESSING SOMATIC PATTERNS

Always ask the next three questions when assessing a somatic pattern. "What can you see?" *This is what you observe.* "What can you feel?" *This is what you palpate.* And do not forget to ask, "what is the story—in terms of the chief complaint, what hurts and what does not hurt, what has been tried in the past (both what worked and what did not work), and are there any prior related or nonrelated injuries." *This is the history.*

Videotape yourself while you work or use a mirror for the critique. You could also ask a fellow practitioner to observe you as you massage. For these visually oriented questions, you need visual feedback. It will not be enough to sense your body kinesthetically. Remember to deal with nonadaptive patterns by observing and not judging.

Then you must consider whether the pattern is a static or dynamic habit. A static pattern will manifest when the client is still. Perhaps you tend to stand with all your weight shifted to one side, and you wonder why you have low back pain only on the right. Perhaps you "rest" against the massage table with knees hyperextended and wonder why they are red and swollen all the time. A dynamic habit does not appear until you execute some massage manipulation. Perhaps you are in the habit of using only your back muscles when you lift and stretch your clients. You wonder why you always feel overworked after a stretching session. Dynamic patterns may be harder to pinpoint; you may have to be more vigilant during your massage.

Finally, in order to fully consider a somatic pattern, frame your inquiries ("What do you see? What do you feel? What have you been told and what do you already know?") in respect to the following attributes. The first five categories are applicable to static or posture patterns. Items 6 and 7 help identify more elusive maladaptive patterns in moving.

1. *Alignment.* What is the placement of body regions or parts in relationship to each other (i.e., foot to leg, pelvis to spine, shoulders to trunk, etc.)?

2. *Weight distribution.* Where is the body bearing weight?

Is grounding sufficient?

    a. Broad and level base—Is the whole foot on the floor? Do you see or feel a release of the hip, knee, and ankle during weight shifts?

    b. Weight close to the base—Are the knees bent or hyperextended? Can you feel a release of tension and a sense of support through the feet into the earth without having to "hold" yourself up?

    c. Line of gravity centered—Where would a plumb line fall if dropped through the center of the body? When a weight shift occurs, how does it affect this plumb line of force?

    d. What is the dynamic alignment of the head and tail? How does the spine align itself, and how does the relationship of vertebrae change as you move?

3. *Muscle or tissue quality.* Where do you see shortening or bunching?

Does the soft tissue look hard and holding or soft and pliable?

Describe the color, texture, and temperature of the tissue.

Which muscle groups have shortened or contracted?

Which have become significantly weaker?

Have any chain reactions occurred? For example, has one muscle group (because of excessive contraction) stretched its antagonists?

4. *Joint quality.* Do the joints appear locked or excessively bent?

5. *Side to side.* Where do you notice imbalances or differences?

Do you see differences between right and left sides?

Do you notice anomalies from upper half to lower half (top to bottom)?

Do you see differences from front to back?

6. *Motion quality.* What is the quantity and quality of each motion?

Is the motion effortless?

Is the motion easily reversible?

Where is the restriction that is pulling you out of the center vertical line of gravity?

As you move through a range, are there glitches or rough spots in the motion?

Do certain motions seem mechanical, as if you were operating on autopilot? (This can indicate lack of awareness and tendency to habituation, reflex, and pattern development.)

Where in the body does the movement originate?

How does the movement sequence through the body?

Where does the flow of movement appear to be blocked? (Blockages can be attributed to tension, muscle imbalance, and disconnection in the kinetic chain.)

Which body parts are active and which are held?

Is the intensity and direction of effort appropriate to the goal?

Is there a balance between exertion and recuperation in the rhythm of the bodywork session?

7. *Breath.* Do you hold your breath? When?

   Does your breathing pattern change during a particular range of motion?

   Does the breathing pattern relate to and support the massage session?

8. Do you recognize any of the patterns discussed in your own habits?

COMPONENTS OF EFFICIENT MOVEMENT

Just as it is easier to identify holding patterns that manifest in the body when it is still, it also takes less effort to change static body attitudes than to alter complex habits of movement. For unhealthy body attitudes, increasing awareness of misalignment or discomfort and then reattuning the body with a shift in posture can do the trick. But a more difficult problem is how to stop and think about altering dynamic body mechanics. That is, how do we effectively change a constantly shifting pattern of motion *while we are moving*?

Perhaps it will help to consider that all movement patterns share a beginning, middle, and end. These three features determine efficient movement, as well as maladaptive habits. Then it may be insightful to examine more thoroughly how and where we start our actions (*initiation*), how the movement proceeds (*sequence*), and where we intend to go (*spatial intent*) (Cox, 1995).

Initiation

Initiation is the biomechanical term that describes how and where we start the actions. Where do our movements begin in space? Where does the movement originate in our bodies? The first question deals with spatial orientation problems that were tackled in previous chapters—how we align ourselves in relationship to the table and to the client. These are general rules for increasing the stability of unstable structures, in other words, principles for grounding. Helpful methods for improving alignment that were generated in the first part of this book include setting the table at a comfortable height, facing the whole body in the direction of the stroke, maintaining the head and tail in line, having the weight centered (e.g., not up on the toes or out away from the center line of the body), and placing the feet wide enough to support the body, but not so wide that you get "stuck."

The second question of initiation has to do with what body part or regions lead specific actions. Where the effort originates can give a stroke a very different feeling and effect, both for clients' and our own bodies. In other words, how you think about leading into a motion will affect the movement itself. For clarity, let us define regions of the body in terms of their proximity to the geographic center. There is the core or the torso (trunk) of the body (the axial spine), and the appendicular skeleton. Limbs can be further categorized into proximal regions (the shoulder and pelvic girdles), middle articulations (elbow and knee), and distal areas (wrist and ankle). To get even more specific, distal extremities can be partitioned into phalanges (fingers and toes). To experiment with initiation, try to step out, thinking of your hip as the source point of the step. Now try the motion again, originating from the knee, and then one more time, allowing the ankle to be the impetus for the step.

Irmgard Bartenieff observed infants turning from a face down (prone) to face up (supine) position. She was astounded by how babies unfailingly instigate the movement from their core (either using the weight of their huge heads or lifting up their buttocks and using that as a counterweight)—a fundamental principle for efficiency in turning. This is unlike what most adults do. Try it for yourself and see.

Exercise 6.3. Initiating Movement from Different Body Regions*

Lie on your tummy with your head to one side. Now turn over so that you end up with your face up to the ceiling and your back on the floor. Rest a moment and think about how you executed that maneuver. Was it easy for you? Most people start to turn themselves over by pushing with their hands or feet. In either of these two methods, a distal region is called upon to leverage the weight all along the entire reach of the spine and outlying appendages of the body. The effort needs to be far greater when it comes from the extremities. Yet adults become so accustomed to pushing themselves up by their hands (and secondarily feet) that they don't even remember how to turn any other way. For comparison, now try turning again from a prone to supine position, but this time initiate the movement from your midsection. This is a "baby step"—how a baby would execute the turn. Surprisingly easier, isn't it? What could have caused us to lose this inherent body wisdom that we all had when we were younger? Could it be that we did not stop to think about what would be the most efficient way to turn, but instead just took on a pattern that our bodies felt familiar with? As previously elucidated, many patterns or reflexes were originally developed as creative adaptations to a challenge, but have come to be employed in more situations than they were initially designed for.

Exercise 6.4. Initiating Massage Strokes from Different Body Regions

Before you begin this exercise, put on some music that you enjoy and allow the sounds to become part of your background perceptions. Allow your arms to move in time with the music. Imagine yourself, if you can, performing various massage strokes, like effleurage (gliding), petrissage (kneading), vibration, friction (focused strokes), and tapotement (tapping or hacking). Now consciously initiate the movement of your whole arm from your pinkie finger. Now try moving from your thumb. Try each finger in turn as the source point of the arm motion. Move now from the wrist. Let the motions that originate from your wrist carry your arm into a variety of expressions. Now try the exercise starting the action from the impetus generated by the elbow. Continue to see what kinds of motions emanate from the elbow area. Do the same with the shoulder, and then fi-

*Adapted from Amie Rose, personal communication/Hatha Yoga class, 1992.

nally have the movement of the arm emanate from the core of the body. Focus on either the point of the tan tien or the broader area of the hara (see Exercise 4.6 or 4.7).

Questions for Discussion.   What did you observe? How does your arm feel now that you have completed the exercise? If you moved only one arm from the various origin points, how does it feel in comparison to the other arm? Can you describe the quality of movement that originates from your pinkie, from your thumb, wrist, elbow, shoulder, and core? Can you describe the differences? Can you describe the similarities? Did you discover some new motions/patterns that you had forgotten you could make? What massage strokes or manipulations would most easily be performed from each of the origin points?

Although you might suspect that the core is the most efficient origin for all bodywork, it is merely the most powerful place to generate motion. Not every massage stroke, stretch, or manipulation is best performed from a core initiation. Sometimes alternate sources of effort are more appropriate and effective. Perhaps you might carry out tapotement beginning with a primary wrist motion. Perhaps you might generate light shaking from a light swing of the shoulder. Can you think of other massage movements that might be more easily inspired from a distal, middle, or proximal extremity as well as movements that proceed most naturally from the center of the body?

Sequence

Sequence refers to how the movement progresses. It is the internal follow-through that unfolds after the initial effort. Sequence refers to the kinetic chains that ripple through as the pattern is made manifest. Hanna (1988) and Alexander (in Leviton, 1998) suggest the importance of experiencing the "means whereby" in order to recover the ability to sense and control the muscles. The theory is that showing the client how to sense and feel the process (or sequence) is just as significant as focusing single-mindedly on a goal. Oliver Sacks, a neurologist renowned for his observations and stories of people with neurological impairments, described sequencing (the means whereby) eloquently in his book *A Leg to Stand On* (1984). Sacks's story begins during a hiking incident when he tore his quadriceps muscles completely off of the bone. He recounts his own healing process and, in particular, the part that sequencing played in recovering function in his leg. After the injury, Sacks literally could not remember how to kick. The ability improved tremendously when his nurses passively moved the knee into extension, so that his body could feel all the intermediate movements. Only after this simple therapy could he achieve the goal—to contract the quads and move the leg. Inasmuch as sequence refers to how the movement proceeds, it also pertains to where the movement stops. The "heel rocks" illustrated in Chapter 5 (Exercise 5.1) can reveal exact locations where sequence breaks down. Another way of locating rifts in the progression of an act, along with a strategy for coping, is portrayed below.

Exercise 6.5. Identifying and Addressing Stops in Sequence

This activity was suggested by Meir Schneider in his workshop "Movement Is Life," presented at the 1996 National American Massage Therapy Association (AMTA) Education Conference. As a baseline for this exercise, stand evenly on your two feet and put hands together in front of your body. Bend your knees, leaning back, and bring your arms over head, as in a yoga sun pose (the yoga sun pose is the first part of the sun salutation sequence as performed in hatha yoga). Focus on your spine as you reach over to touch your toes. Notice where the restrictions occur in your back as you reach over. Now, get yourself into a position on all fours. Begin with the cat–cow movement described in Chapter 3 (Exercise 3.5). As you curve your spine up and down, remember the location of the restriction as you reached over to touch your toes. See if you can amplify the curving movement at the site of the block and reduce the arching elsewhere on the spine. A partner can help you focus on the area of restriction by placing his or her hands over the section (which you pointed out) and pushing back against your arching motions. Do this several times. Then repeat the first part of the exercise, reaching over to touch your toes. Notice the quality of sequencing now.

Questions for Discussion.   Did you feel the same restrictions that you did at the outset of the exercise? Have some eased up? Have you become aware of new blockages further on down the spine? This exercise is an excellent way to identify and loosen up blockages to sequencing in the vertebral line. By focusing attention and movement on the area of most restriction, you can more effectively free the block. How would you use this method to release kinks that arise when performing massage? Is your movement different when the flow is restored?

Spatial Intent

If initiation is where to start from, and sequencing is how to proceed, spatial intent refers to where you want to go. Concentrating on spatial intent helps define a clear pathway in space and in turn gives a basic map for getting there. One of the trickiest parts of getting what you want out of life is learning to focus on what you really want. Attending to spatial intent can provide an "aha!" experience, in which clarity clicks in and an answer to what previously seemed a confusing puzzle appears. Karate masters use a form of spatial intent when they break bricks with their bare hands. They visualize clearly where they want their hand to go, that is, beyond the physical space occupied by the brick. The following exercise that you can try with a willing partner (without risking hurting your hand) also helps demonstrate the power of spatial intent.

Exercise 6.6. Spatially Visualizing a Goal*

Face your partner and place the palms of your hands on his or her palms. Now try to knock your partner back. See how that goes for you. Now try the process again, but this time visualize yourself occupying a place in back of the person you are pushing. Did it work any better for you this time? Spatial intent can be a clear aid to getting where you want to go. (*Hint:* For practical purposes, don't have both partners visualizing their spatial intent at the same time.)

Questions for Discussion. How would you apply kinesthetic understanding of spatial intent to the way you move during a massage session? Try out your strategies and report on the results.

In terms of bodywork, spatial intent helps you be clear about which muscles need attending to or which direction your strokes are heading. A different vector of massage corresponds with a different intent. For example, when you apply deep effleurage or longitudinal friction to a muscle from origin to insertion, this stretches the muscle. When you stroke from insertion to origin of the same muscle, the muscle is being toned (Fritz, 1995). If you are going across the grain of the tissue (as in transverse fiber friction), you will be lining up the fibers (in Tappan and Benjamin, 1998) for greater elasticity.

Once you reach your spatial goal, you may need to reassess and change direction. Sometimes when you get where you initially wanted to go, the next place you need to go comes into sharper focus.

UNPATTERNING

Unpatterning is the process of unlearning patterns and rediscovering alternatives. It dissolves blocks and restores the flow (of matter and energy) to the most efficient paths. In bodywork, unpatterning involves a conscious decision to reroute the paths we are most drawn to take in motor learning.

A pattern was defined earlier as something that prevents you from living/doing/being as effectively, effortlessly, and enjoyably as you can. It is a behavior or attitude that *limits* you in some way. Patterns are like a suit of clothes in three respects. A pattern, like a suit, is something that you put on, but it is not essentially you. When you do wear the suit, however, it seems to have its own personality. The personality is reflected in your body (through its movements and posture), thoughts, and even emotions. And three, the suit has layers, like a sweater over a vest over a shirt over an undergarment. Like the skins on an onion, our patterns are complex. When we uncover one layer, a new twist often appears. This is a new aspect of our personal pattern—an aspect of ourselves that we can meet on a deeper layer.

The goal of "unpatterning" is to live without restrictive patterns. In terms of body mechanics, unpatterning affects learning to move and massage without restrictive patterns. Doing so involves living in the here and now. It means not focus-

*Adapted from David Dorian-Ross, personal communication/Tai Chi class, 1992.

ing on past or future hopes or fears. It means staying grounded in the present and not flying off in imaginings about "what was, what could be, what might have been, what would be, if only I had . . ." Unpatterning gives a sense of freedom that can be experienced in the body, mind, and soul. It is a feeling that one's life is unlimited by habits. The next series of exercises is designed to be performed together to provide you with your own awarenesses about the whole process of unpatterning.

Exercise 6.7. Awakening to New Patterns (Animal Moves)

This exercise requires a group of people. Animal noses are masks that you can buy in toy stores and are a wonderful prop for this exercise. You can, however, either make your own animal noses or do without. You will still reap the kinesthetic benefits.

Each member of the group chooses an animal nose (or an animal) and moves about using the kinds of locomotion that the chosen creature would employ. Now one beast shows his or her actions to the rest and they imitate those movements. Continue on until each participant has shared and all group members have tried on the action patterns of every participating animal.

Questions for Discussion. How did it feel in your physical body to move as the beast you chose? Which animal movement patterns were comfortable, familiar, unusual, uncomfortable, fun, or a surprise? To what do you attribute these qualities? Were there any animal movements that you don't usually make, that seemed "right," restful, or restorative for your body? Were any actions painfully familiar? What does this teach you about alternative patterns for your body?

Exercise 6.8. Steps to Unpattern

(*Caution to participants:* The object of this exercise is to observe, not to psychoanalyze.) On a sheet of paper, note areas of your life that could be better. Then, secondarily, list situations in which you are unable to respond or act effectively. These lists are not limited to uncomfortable body postures or sequences of movements. You are looking for patterns in all aspects of your life that may be amenable to unpatterning. The information that you generate from this exercise is for your eyes only. You will decide what, if anything, you want to share with a partner or with the group.

Questions for Discussion. Choose one item on either of these lists and apply the following steps to unpattern to it. Be aware that these steps are not linear; that is, you could start anywhere in the chain. However, all of the steps are integral to the process of unpatterning.

1. Increase your awareness of the pattern.
2. Find new options for change. You can increase awareness and learn new alternatives through reading books like this one, taking classes, or sharing with a friend, counselor, or support group.

3. Realize the pattern was adopted in order to take care of the self.

4. Ask yourself what you would need to clear the blocks set up by this pattern and what you would need to discharge those blocks. (Answers to these questions that can also surface in a massage session involve laughing, crying, shaking, running, or breathing. These active responses seem to work well as a discharge of energies or emotions.)

5. Ask what else, if anything, you would need to let go of this archetype. Are you willing to do whatever it takes to let the pattern go? If not, consider that the pattern may be the best option for you right now.

Exercise 6.9. Breaking Patterns—Pattern Awareness

(*Caution to participants:* The object of this activity is to listen to your partner, not to psychoanalyze. Remember that the scope of practice and area of expertise for bodyworkers is the body's musculoskeletal system. Like any caring human being, we can listen without straying outside our area of expertise, but counseling is not within the bodyworker's scope of practice. *Caution to facilitators:* Do not force anyone who feels uncomfortable to participate in this or any of the exercises described in this text. If you feel uncomfortable with presenting this kind of work, omit the activity entirely.)

For this activity, work in pairs. One person works at a time. The partner is an open slate—he or she does not offer advice or small talk, but "simply" listens with open attention. The partner is a silent witness, observing without judging. Take 10 minutes for the first person to answer the following questions:

1. Describe the area you want to work on. (Choose something you wrote in response to the previous exercise.)

2. What could be better?

3. Describe the suit of clothes:
   a. What do you do (in this pattern)?
   b. What are your thoughts?
   c. What do you feel?
   d. What happens to your body? How do you move?

Now switch roles. Think about what you learned about yourself and your partner by participating in this exercise. Meet together with other pairs in the group and share what you learned.

Exercise 6.10. Letting Go of the Pattern—Picturing the New You

Consider the pattern awareness activity and what you became aware of as a result of the experience. Think of a movement that would express how you would be, feel, act, and think if you could let go of the pattern. Now pretend and make the motion anyway. If you wish, teach your newly found free expression to the rest of the class.

Alternately (should you prefer a visual medium of expression to the kinesthetic one), draw "YOU" as you would be without your patterns. Hold up your drawing and tell the group what it represents.

Questions for Discussion.   How does the movement or drawing make you feel? Describe yourself now in relation to the issue you have chosen to unpattern. Describe yourself now as you are in relation to everything.

From this series of related exercises, it becomes crystal clear that the process of unpatterning is not to be taken lightly. It can bring up deep-seated issues that in turn must be met and dealt with on new terms. Unpatterning is not just a matter of turning in the toes during a massage or tucking under the gluteal muscles (which, by the way, encourages a posterior pelvic tilt and excessive hypolordosis or "flat back") or straightening the brow. Over the years, I have come to appreciate more and more the strength of massage professionals who have chosen a vocation that continually presents challenges to old habits and patterns. To stay healthy and alive in this field, we simply do not have the option of molding ourselves into old, outdated patterns. We are continually confronted with crossroads where it is no longer feasible to continue on a path of unhealthy habits or reflexive action. Sometimes we do not know what the next step is, only that we must change to survive. It almost feels as if we are falling. Indeed, the next exercise on falling can give us a new kinesthetic awareness of what is involved in the task and what the possible outcomes are.

Exercise 6.11. Letting Go of Patterns—Falling

(*Caution to participants:* Do not attempt this exercise if you have osteoporosis or are otherwise prone to injury or fear of falling. *Caution to facilitators:* Do not proceed with the activity unless you have safeguarded the area and all participants from harm.) Prepare an area by placing futons, mats, or other soft cushioning on the floor. When you are ready, begin to experiment with different ways of falling. For example, try allowing only some parts of the body to fall, varying which parts drop. For example, you could lie on the floor and play with letting your leg drop. Experiment with falling at different rates—in slow motion, double time, in freeze-frame fashion. Try falling in different directions—off to one side, at an angle, straight down, or perhaps exploding up before you go down. Now take your investigations one step further. Continue playing with the action of falling and use the momentum of your body as it accelerates during the fall to carry you into a new movement. For example as your arm swings down, follow through on the motion to let the arm swing back up like a pendulum. Maybe the momentum will even carry your arm all the way around through several revolutions, like a clock.

Questions for Discussion.   How does the action of falling make you feel? Where did the momentum you built up from the kinetic energy of the fall take you? What new position did you find yourself in? How did that feel? This exercise graphically illustrates how the impetus we use to change our patterns can seem to take us into a fall. But if we surrender to the fall (and do not fight it), we may find that the momentum helps propel us to new and unexpected action. In return for the courage to grind through to better ways of being—better ways of expressing ourselves through our bodywork—comes a new freedom. The massage becomes an expression of that freedom, creativity, and uniqueness. This is truly what it means to be a bodyworker.

The next exercise shows how the theory of unpatterning can be put to use while practicing massage. Laura Cox (1995) calls this activity "getting into the client's skin."

Exercise 6.12. Getting into the Client's Skin*

Some preliminary homework needs to be completed prior to this activity. Participants should be prepared to demonstrate for at least two minutes (preferably 5 minutes, although it may be difficult to continue this long) walking, standing, sitting, eating, playing guitar, or other action that they have actually observed in a client or potential client. In essence, the mission is to mimic an individual's locomotive or holding patterns. During class time, each student demonstrates the pattern he or she has brought to share, and the other participants watch. The student who demonstrates can choose to teach the pattern to the rest of the class.

Questions for Discussion. For each pattern, discuss as a group what muscle groups are shortened, which regions are lengthened? Is some aspect out of line? Is there an area where movement is restricted or blocked? Indeed, all of the "questions to ask when assessing a somatic pattern" could apply to the investigation. Based on these observations, what massage strokes, stretches, and manipulations would you want to try with this subject? Based on your experience in the "client's skin," which massage styles do you think the client would be more amenable to? Which techniques do you think might be inappropriate or less than helpful for a person manifesting this pattern? Tell why you would recommend the techniques that you chose. How else would you supplement the process of changing unhealthy somatic patterns? If these questions confound you, try on the pattern (like a suit of clothes) by acting it out. You will literally be embodying the physical complaints of the client. You will achieve an empathy that you may have missed out on before. When you sense how it feels to walk in a certain pattern, kinesthetic awareness can kick in. Then you can put knowledge, conceptual understanding, and practical skills to work. Similarly, in order to make a substantial change in body mechanics, first and foremost you must discover and observe patterns as they manifest in the body. As we have seen, this is no mean feat. I sincerely hope and believe the exercises and insights furnished in this chapter will aid the challenging and substantial life process of unpatterning.

*Adapted from Laura Cox, personal communication, 1995.

SUMMARY

This chapter provides an introduction to the theory and practice of unpatterning. Patterns are defined as an attitude or behavior that prevents you from working as effectively, effortlessly, and enjoyably as you can. Patterns are learned behaviors, unlike simple reflexes. As such, they can be unlearned. They are not essentially you. Several identifiable body patterns are discussed, including the forward head posture (Chek, 1995), upper crossed and lower crossed syndrome (Chaitow, 1993), trauma, startle, and Landau response (Hanna, 1988). In bodywork, unpatterning involves a conscious decision to reroute motor habits and discover alternatives. Steps to unpattern may vary in order, but include the following:

1. Become aware of the pattern.
2. Find new alternatives through reading books, taking classes, or sharing your feelings.
3. Realize that if the pattern was learned, it can be unlearned.
4. Do what you need to clear the blocks set up by this pattern.
5. Check to see if you are really willing to let go of the pattern. Do the benefits outweigh the costs?

Psychological and physical exercises to aid in unpatterning are presented.

REFERENCES

Chaitow, Leon, "Patterns of Dysfunction," *Massage Therapy Journal* (Spring 1993), pp. 77–80.

Chek, Paul, "Corrective Postural Training and the Massage Therapist," *Massage Therapy Journal* (Summer 1995), pp. 83–89.

Cox, Laura (1995). Personal communication. Washington, DC.

Dorian-Ross, David (1992). Personal communication/Tai Chi class. Portland, OR.

Feldenkrais, Moshe, *Awareness Through Movement* (1977). New York: Harper & Row.

Fritz, Sandy, *Mosby's Fundamentals of Therapeutic Massage* (1995). St. Louis: Mosby-Year Book.

Hanna, Thomas, *Somatics* (1988). New York: Perseus Books.

Leviton, Richard, "Better Body Mechanics," *East West Magazine* (September 1998), pp. 92–98.

Rose, Amie (1992). Personal communication/Hatha Yoga class. Portland, OR.

Sacks, Oliver V., *A Leg to Stand On* (1984). New York: Summit Books.

Schneider, Meir, *The Handbook of Self-Healing* (1994). London: Penguin Books.

Tappan, Frances, and Patricia Benjamin, *Healing Massage Techniques: Classic, Holistic and Emerging Methods,* 3rd ed. (1998). Stamford, CT: Appleton & Lange.

Walker, Judith, "The Normal Reflex Arc," in *Neuromuscular Therapy—Care of Soft Tissue Pain and Dysfunction* (1990). International Academy of Neuromuscular Therapies. St. Petersburg, FL: NMT Center.

Chapter Seven

Repetitive Motion and Other Common Injuries

CHAPTER OBJECTIVES

The massage student/practitioner who successfully completes this chapter (reading and exercises) will be able to:

- Define preliminary concepts that relate to common injuries (e.g., ischemia, trigger points, nerve impingement, tensile tissue, contractile tissue).

- Identify and describe symptoms, preventive steps, and treatment options for common musculoskeletal injuries (e.g., spasms, cramps, contracture, tendinitis, strains, sprains, bursitis).

- Define *repetitive motion injuries* (repetitive stress injuries).

- Recognize general steps to avoid injuries that result from incorrect body mechanics.

- Identify and describe symptoms, preventive steps, and treatment options for chronic or repetitive motion injuries (repetitive stress injuries) (e.g., upper extremities [including carpal tunnel and thoracic outlet syndromes], head and neck injuries, mid and low back injuries, lower leg and foot injuries).

(*Disclaimer:* Readers are cautioned against using this information to self-diagnose and treat. Always confirm self-assessments with a qualified health care provider. Neither does this chapter substitute for full courses in pathology or orthopedic assessment skills.)

If you are currently suffering symptoms that suggest a repetitive motion (stress) or other common injury, the information in this chapter will be especially useful. Etiology, contributing factors, and protocols for addressing specific problems are discussed. The information in this chapter can help you recognize early warning signs of repetitive stress and to design strategies to prevent warning symptoms from developing into full-blown syndromes. Repetitive stress injuries are not a "done deal." The more you know about the syndromes, the more equipped you are to ward off debilitating effects.

This chapter covers the most common injuries and repetitive stress complaints throughout the whole body. Most texts focus on upper extremity injuries only. This section includes general and spinal maladies as well as *both* upper and lower extremity ailments. Specific syndromes covered include headaches, cervical strain, torticollis, thoracic outlet syndrome, carpal tunnel syndrome, piriformis entrapment, low back pain, sacroiliac pain, feet problems, and knee difficulties.

Regardless of the specific complaint, rest is a crucial element of the repetitive motion cure. Unfortunately, many injured massage therapists forgo needed rest for fear of immediate loss of income. While it is true that lost workdays are costly, continuing to aggravate the condition can escalate the trauma into permanent disability and loss of livelihood. The good news is that the severe aspects of repetitive stress injuries can often be avoided, if you use early discomforts as warning signals to adapt your body mechanics.

PRELIMINARY CONCEPTS

According to Judith Walker (1990), pain and loss of function in any area can result from six primary factors: ischemia (lack of blood flow to an area), trigger points (areas of hyperirritability with referred phenomena), nerve impingement (pressure on nerves by other body structures), postural distortion, nutrition, and emotional well-being or stress. Walker claims that these factors play a role in determining how the brain and spinal cord and peripheral nerve receptors perceive or relay pain. Postural distortions and alternatives are discussed in almost every chapter in this book. Maintaining emotional well-being and preventing stress is the subject of Chapters 9 and 11. Nutrition is a vast topic that lies beyond the scope of a primer on body mechanics. It is also an area that is deeply fraught with personal beliefs, attitudes, and myths. For all of these reasons, I leave you to research how to create your own optimal nutrition. Books that I have found most helpful in this area are listed in the reference section for the final chapter. The other three contributing factors to the pain and dysfunction of overuse syndromes are clarified below.

Ischemia

Ischemia is the lack of blood and subsequent lack of oxygen in the body tissues. When oxygen and the other needed nutrients cannot get through to cells, the cells starve and begin to die. Blood cannot get through to the tissues because of the spasms or hypertonicity of the muscles. In an overuse syndrome, this is because the muscles are chronically held in one position for such a long time that they begin to spasm. This can set up a pain–spasm–pain cycle (Walker, 1990) that can escalate into trigger points (described below).

Trigger Points

Trigger points are areas of hyperirritability with referred pain or other sensations. Other sensations can include goosebumps, ticklishness, heat, or cold. According to Upledger (1997), increased toxins keep the area in a state of constant irritability. This increased sensitivity to excitation allows normally ineffectual or subliminal stimuli to produce a nerve impulse. This, in turn, causes both skeletal muscles and organs to be maintained in a state of overactivity. By the same token, when massage or some other therapy interrupts the pain–spasm–pain cycle, it removes the source of abnormal stimulation. All tissues affected by that cord segment then have decreased hyperactivity.

Nerve Impingement

When discussing impingement, it is helpful to make the distinction between nerve entrapment and compression. Both result from anatomical pressure on a nerve. Entrapment occurs when soft tissues, such as muscle, tendons, or ligaments, press on nerve fibers. Compression results when tissues such as bones or discs pinch the nerve. Remember that the area of expertise and scope of practice for massage therapists is soft tissue release.

Pressure on a nerve (impingement), no matter what the cause, has the following effects:

1. Inflammation and pain at the site of the entrapment. If left untreated, this pressure can damage the nerve.
2. Numbness and tingling (paresthesia) distal to the site of the pressure.
3. Referred pain in the distal extremity.
4. Reduced electrical impulses innervating the muscles to move. Because of lack of stimulation, muscles distal to the compression site can become atrophied, weak, and prone to injury.
5. Increased likelihood of developing a subsequent injury at a site distal to the original trauma. Headley (1995) refers to this phenomenon as the *double crush syndrome*. For example, pressure on the median nerve at the elbow (proximal) increases the likelihood of subsequently contracting carpal tunnel syndrome (distal). Trauma to the nerve can cause inflammation and scarring around the nerve. Scar tissue adheres the nerve to surrounding structures, causing compression at the new sites.

Impingement often occurs at nerve plexuses (places where the spinal nerves interweave with each other before traveling out to the extremities). The specific nerve that is affected determines what condition will manifest.

If the cervical plexus is affected, you can experience headaches, neck pain, and breathing difficulties. Muscles most likely to press on the cervical plexus are the suboccipital and sternocleidomastoid muscles. (This means these are the muscles you would want to have your therapist focus on in a therapeutic massage.) In addition, the ligaments at the base of the neck can impinge on these nerves (Fritz, 1995). The phrenic nerve, which innervates the diaphragm, also arises from this nerve web.

The brachial plexus gives rise to almost all the nerves that reach out to the upper extremity. It is a complex area situated in both the neck and underarm areas. Muscles most likely to press on the brachial plexus are the scalenes, pectoralis minor, and the subclavius. Thoracic outlet syndrome results from an impingement of these nerves. The median nerve is a branch of the axillary nerve, which itself is a part of the plexus. Impingement of the median nerve is defined as carpal tunnel syndrome. Whiplash may also affect and be affected by the brachial plexus area.

If the lumbar plexus is involved, you may experience low back pain with some pain radiating around the perimeter of the body, like a belt. Primary muscles that squeeze the lumbar plexus are the quadratus lumborum and the psoas. The lumbar fascia covering the low back can also become shortened, creating pressure on the lumbar nerves.

The sacral plexus innervates the lower extremities, as well as the pelvic and gluteal areas. The main branch of this interweaving is the sciatic nerve. The piriformis can press on the sciatic nerve, creating a classic pain syndrome with pain in the glutes, radiating down one leg, and possible accompanying genital or foot pain.

Some physical therapists believe that pain syndromes may be partially the result of neural tension in addition to muscle strain. The greater the tension on a nerve, the less elasticity it has. When you bend your arm or leg, there will be less "give" in the nerve to withstand the stretching. The bending motion tugs on the nerve and causes more irritation, inflammation, and pain.

Tensile versus Contractile Tissue

My beginning massage students see all the "lumps, bumps, and ropy areas" that they palpate in the body as "tightness." What they call tightness can actually manifest from two diametrically opposite sources. First, muscles can feel tight when they are contracted. Contractile fibers are found in muscle that is chronically held in a shortened position. Second, the tightness can emanate from a tensile soft tissue, that is, a muscle that is chronically taut and pulled to its limit. Generally, when one side (agonist) is contractile, the opposite side (antagonist) is tensile, and vice versa. Although both sides will be tight, the contractile side needs lengthening (e.g., stretching) while the tensile side responds best to toning applications (e.g., exercise, short periods of tapotement).

GENERAL CONDITIONS

Spasms

Spasms are abnormal contractions of muscle fibers. The duration of the spasm may be brief or lengthy. Spasms may involve only a few or all of the fibers in a single muscle or they can affect an entire muscle group. The degree of contraction may be mild, moderate, or severe.

Spasms can be caused by postural strain (massaging while standing or sitting in a uncomfortable position for a long time), emotional tension, and fatigue. Strains, sprains, and tendinitis (described later in this chapter) can give rise to secondary spasms in the injured region. Muscles go into spasm as a protective response. They contract to prevent an injured area from moving in a way that would cause pain. Unfortunately, muscle spasms often persist long after the original injury has healed, unless addressed.

Acute spasms occur suddenly and carry a lot of pain. The area feels tender to the touch, hard, and lumpy. When pressure is applied, pain or other symptoms (such as heat, cold, tingly feelings, or ticklishness) may be referred to other body areas. The specific site in the area that produces referrals upon palpation is a classic trigger point (also known as a myofascial trigger point).

Chronic spasms have been present over a long duration and usually are not painful. (However, chronically spasmed areas can contain trigger point sites within the area.) Instead, tissues with chronic spasms are more likely to feel stiff, constantly aching, or fatigued. Someone who suffers from chronic spasms may be unaware of them until they are revealed with pressure. Under pressure, spasms produce pain.

Self-Care. Relieving muscle spasms is what you do every day in your practice. This is indeed good news when we become the clients. Almost all forms of Swedish massage, and especially deep effleurage, longitudinal and cross-fiber friction, and vibration can be effective on spasms. Static pressure on the site is also very useful, especially if referral symptoms are present. You can "map out" a plan of trigger point relief by simply following pain referrals and progressively applying pressure to the next section, until there are no more referrals in the tissue. The more severe and acute a spasm, the gentler the pressure should be. Stretching (as described in Chapters 8 and 10) can help reduce muscle spasms. Remember that what appears to be a muscle spasm may actually be caused by other factors. If a spasm does not seem to be responding to massage, movement, or hydrotherapy, please refer yourself to a health care practitioner who is qualified to diagnose the problem.

Cramps

Cramps are spasms that involve a large area, such as the whole muscle. Muscle cramping has been attributed to a variety of deficiency factors such as not enough salt, potassium, or water in the area of the cramp (Greene, 1995). Cramps are more likely to occur when a muscle has been held in a shortened position for a long period of time without a rest. This is the case when a client lies prone on the massage table without a bolster. The foot is held in plantar flexion, and the cramp develops in one of the calf (gastrocnemius and/or soleus) muscles, which act to plantar flex the foot. Cramping can also occur during strenuous exercise for an extended period of time, such as marathon running or biking.

Self-Care. Treatments for cramping include the following:

1. *Direct pressure* or, as it is colloquially called, "sticking a fist in it." Static pressure applied directly to the belly of shortened muscle groups manually stretches out the fibers.
2. *Reciprocal inhibition (RI).* When you contract the antagonist muscle (the muscle with an opposing action to your targeted muscle), the cramping muscle will let go. If the opposing muscle didn't relax, the body would be stuck in a vector of opposing forces, unable to move anywhere. To release

cramping in the calf muscles, pull toes and ankle toward your head in dorsiflexion. RI also resets the Golgi tendon organs, the nerve receptors in tendons, which are sensitive to how much tension is placed on a muscle.

3. Some authorities recommend *icing*, although it may not be as effective in releasing cramps as other methods (Vaughn, 1995). Ice (and heat) have an analgesic (pain-killing) effect and help interrupt the pain–spasm–pain cycle.

4. *Friction* around the axis of the bone is a method that has been recommended by some massage experts, especially in the case of leg cramps that appear during pregnancy (Stillerman, 1992). To relieve cramps in the lower leg, put your hands on either side of the calf and rotate around the axes of the tibia/fibula.

5. *Origin–insertion approximation (O-I approximation)* means manually bringing the origin and insertion of a cramped muscle together. The theory behind this technique is that if you do the work of a muscle by passively placing it in a shortened position, the muscle itself will not have to contract. O-I approximation resets the muscle spindles (nerve receptors located in the muscles). This stops the reflex from initiating a contraction because the spindles no longer sense that a muscle has been stretched too fast or too far.

Contracture

Sustained spasms can lead to contracture. Contracture is an abnormal decrease in length of a muscle or part of a muscle. Injury or diseases that destroy muscle tissue can begin a process that leads to contracture. Scar tissue or fibrosis replaces the muscle fibers. Scar tissue cannot contract and relax like muscles so that the whole area is shortened. Muscles held in a shortened position for an extended period of time lose their elasticity, producing contractures. Risk factors include ischemia and muscles that cross arthritic joints or injured joints. Hardened, stringy ropy areas can be felt within a muscle with contracture. Range of motion will be reduced because of the shortening of fibers.

Self-Care. Both longitudinal and cross-fiber friction help line up the connective (scar) tissue fibers so that the scar forms a more functional unit. Stretching can manually lengthen the fibers. Heat can increase the efficacy of the manual applications. Note that because muscle tissue cannot regenerate, the muscle does not return to its original state.

Tendinitis

Tendinitis is just what it sounds like—inflammation of a tendon. Direct injury or overstretching or overcontracting the muscle attached to the tendon can give rise to tendinitis. It most often affects tendons crossing the shoulder, hip, knee, or ankle joints (probably because these are areas that suffer the most "wear and tear"). When a tendon sheath is inflamed, the condition is known as *tenosynovitis*. To avoid injuries that give rise to this condition, practice the principles of good body mechanics as laid out in the bulk of this text. Risks for tendinitis increase with whole body inflammation syndromes, such as rheumatoid arthritis, and increased age (Rattray, 1995). Acute tendinitis is red (erythema), hot, swollen (edema), and painful.

Self-Care. According to James Cyriax (Tappan and Benjamin, 1998), cross-friction massage is a good technique for addressing the problem. Make sure to apply friction that does not activate a pain response (if it hurts, there is too much pressure). A good starting protocol would be one to three minutes of light cross-fiber friction. After the area is slightly numbed by the repetitive stroke, use three to five minutes of deeper friction. Follow that with 10 to 20 repetitions of sub-maximal movements (i.e., if the joint flexes, flex and extend it less than it can normally go) and finish with 10 minutes of icing to reduce swelling. Pain at any time is a sign to stop the friction and rest the area. Although it is tempting to apply the massage yourself, it is better to schedule a professional session. Another therapist is less likely to overfriction the area. As the tendon heals, active exercise of muscles connected to the affected tendon can return full strength. Alternating heat and cold is used to speed healing in the subacute phase, and heat is recommended during the chronic phase.

Muscle Strains (Pulled Muscles)

Strains are injuries to a muscle and/or its tendon resulting in partial or total tearing (Rattray, 1995). They can occur anywhere that the muscle or tendon is overused, weak, or contracts suddenly and unexpectedly. Unhealed scar tissue in the muscle, strenuous activity without a warm-up, and habitual postures contribute to the likelihood of developing a muscle strain. Strains occur where the tendon attaches to the bone, within the tendon itself, at the junction of a muscle and its tendon, or within the muscle belly. Redness, heat, swelling, and/or pain is often present. In severe cases, there may have been a snapping sound at the time of injury.

A first-degree (mild) strain is associated with mild inflammation (not much redness, heat, swelling, and pain) and a rapid recovery. A second-degree (moderate) strain involves damage to the soft tissue fibers and moderate inflammation. There is usually some weakness in the injured muscle (i.e., some pain upon use). A third-degree (severe) strain causes tearing of more than half of the soft tissue fibers. It may require surgical repair. There is obvious pain, inflammation, and loss of function.

Strains are also categorized as to how acute or chronic they are. More acute conditions display all the signs of redness, heat, swelling, and pain. The more chronic an injury, the more it feels cooler, harder, and denser because of the laying down of scar tissue and subsequent lack of blood flow. A chronic strain may not be painful at all until pressure is applied to its site.

Self-Care. In acute (and/or severe) strain, rest, ice, compression, and elevation are the best treatments. Light friction and/or ice massage may be performed directly on the site of injury (as long as it does not cause pain) and massage proximal to the area may help reduce swelling.

In subacute (and/or moderate) strain, the goals are to reduce swelling, prevent adhesions, and restore normal range of motion. Edema is reduced through effleurage and petrissage performed proximal to the injury and with pressure toward the heart. Adhesions can be prevented best with cross-fiber frictioning applied directly on site. Range of motion can be restored through passive exercises for the appropriate muscle, as described in Chapter 8. Alternating cold and heat applications bring needed nutrients to the area and flush the site of waste products.

Chronic (and/or mild) strains can benefit from heat applications, deep effleurage, longitudinal or cross-fiber friction, and myofascial release. Stretching (as described in Chapters 8 and 10) may also be helpful, as long as it does not cause pain.

Sprains

Sprains occur when the bones that make up a joint are suddenly taken out of alignment, so that structures such as ligaments, joint capsule, and tendons crossing the joint are torn (Rattray, 1995). For example, if you supinate the ankle joint in a controlled manner, the bones are out of alignment but the likelihood of sprain is minimal. However, if that same action were sudden and weight bearing, a sprain may be more likely to occur.

A first-degree sprain is mild (20 percent or less of the ligament fibers are torn) and usually heals within two weeks. The joint is not loose or unstable. A second-degree sprain involves moderate damage (20 to 75 percent) to the ligament fibers along with noticeable inflammation and pain upon moving the area. There is usually some hypermobility to the injured joint. A third-degree (severe) sprain is a complete rupture (75 percent or greater damage to the fibers) of the ligament. There is significant inflammation and instability in the joint. The damage usually requires surgical repair. There is obvious pain, and movement is not possible (Rattray, 1995).

Pain, heat, swelling, and redness on the injured site identify acute sprains. There also may be some discoloration of the surrounding tissues. This stage usually lasts one to two days. Sprains reach the subacute stage when the above signs begin to disappear. Range of motion will still be limited, and the tissues are very susceptible to reinjury. Chronic sprains occur in ligaments that have experienced incidents of acute inflammation. As a result, scar tissue thickens the ligament fibers and draws them into irregular patterns. The ligament may be permanently lengthened, and the joint may have a tendency to dislocate (Newton, 1998).

Self-Care. Caring for sprains follows the same protocols as for strains (described above). However, sprains generally take longer to heal than strains because ligaments do not have the rich blood supply that muscles have.

Bursitis

Bursitis is the inflammation of a bursa (Rattray, 1995). A bursa is a fluid-filled sac that cushions a tendon from a bone (or other hard structure). It acts like a protective pad to insulate the tendon from wear and tear. Bursitis can be caused by injury, overuse (repetitive motion injuries) of a nearby muscle, an infection, or a systemic inflammatory disease (e.g., gout or rheumatoid arthritis). In many cases, the origin of bursitis is unknown.

In acute bursitis, the area is tender and range of motion is restricted and painful. Chronic bursitis results from repeated local traumas that thicken the bursal wall and attract calcium to reinforce the area. The tissue may feel dense and is easily reinjured. Areas susceptible to bursitis include the Achilles bursa at the back of the ankle, the area of the greater trochanter at the lateral upper thigh, and the subdeltoid (subacromial) bursa at the shoulder.

Self-Care.   Do not receive massage, exercise, or stretch for acute bursitis, because these treatments can reinjure and further inflame the tissue. This is easily accomplished, because massage and movement applied directly to an injured bursa will hurt deep inside. Icing, however, is recommended to reduce the inflammation. If massage or manipulations do not cause pain, your therapist can relax associated muscles that are very close to (but not directly over) the bursa. In chronic bursitis, the caution is not to reactivate the inflammatory process—so, again, do not massage directly over the bursa! Stretching and exercise, along with massage and heat, can be utilized to lengthen muscles surrounding the injury.

SPECIFIC SYNDROMES—UPPER EXTREMITY

Carpal Tunnel Syndrome

Carpal tunnel syndrome (CTS) is the most commonly diagnosed and misdiagnosed repetitive stress condition of the upper extremity. The words *carpal tunnel* are often incorrectly used to describe any repetitive strain injury affecting the hand, wrist, arm, or shoulder.

The bottom of the tunnel is defined by the two rows of carpal bones. The top of the tunnel is formed by the flexor retinaculum (also known as the annular ligament or transverse carpal ligament). The bones and ligament create a limited corridor inside the wrist that cannot expand to make more room. (See Figure 7.1.) The size of the space varies from individual to individual. Nine tendons of the forearm flexor muscles and numerous blood and lymph vessels pass through this fixed space. The median nerve also travels through to innervate the digits of the first three fingers and the half of the palmar side of the fourth finger. Continuous overuse may enlarge the forearm muscles enough to squeeze the median nerve.

CTS is a common injury because so many structures pass through such a small space. If anything happens to decrease the amount of space in the tunnel, pressure on the median nerve increases. Even slight inflammation of a few flexor tendons can generate enough swelling to impinge on the median nerve. Overuse can cause hypertrophy of the forearm tendons or tendon sheaths, with the same outcome.

Signs and Symptoms.   The first noticeable symptom of CTS may be fullness or tightness in the wrists. CTS can affect one or both hands. Classic signs of CTS are pain, paresthesia, and weakness. Shaking the hands may relieve these symp-

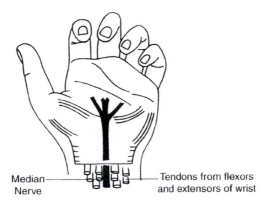

The Carpal Tunnel

Median Nerve — Tendons from flexors and extensors of wrist

Figure 7.1   Carpal tunnel syndrome is an impingement of the median nerve.

toms for a short time. It is common for CTS sufferers to be awakened by night pains and to wake up in the morning with pain.

Pressure on the median nerve reduces the number of nerve impulses traveling to and from the hand. Impingement affects sensations at first, causing tingling and numbness. These complaints surface in the palmar side of the wrist into the palm, first three digits, and adjoining half of the fourth digit. These are the areas innervated by the median nerve. If left untreated, motor problems develop, such as weakness in the hand and/or fingers, lack of coordination, an inability to grip (opposed fingers and thumb), and a tendency to drop things (from impingement of the motor root of the nerves). Continued mechanical pressure acts to damage nerve tissue. Because nerve tissue is made of cells that cannot regenerate, advanced CTS that is not addressed can result in permanent nerve loss. Other symptoms include swelling in the fingers and hands (from lack of venous and lymph return) and cold or pale hands (from lack of blood flow into the area).

Contributing factors include the following:

1. *Incorrect hand positioning* can cause pressure on the median nerve. For example, when the wrist is kept in hyperflexion, over time the median nerve is squeezed against the transverse ligament. Fixing the wrist against an object like the edge of a massage table for long intervals can squash the median nerve against the flexor retinaculum.

2. *Gender.* Women are more prone to CTS than men, probably for the reasons outlined below.

3. *Menstruation, pregnancy, and breast feeding.* Secretion of the hormone relaxin during these times causes ligaments to be more lax and joints to subsequently become less stable. In the cases of menstruation and pregnancy, fluid retention steps up the pressure within the carpal tunnel. With pregnancy, the effects are compounded, as fluid volume increases on the order of 40 percent (Osborne-Sheets, 1998).

4. *Fluid retention or fat absorption.* Other conditions that might cause increased water or fat retention include thyroid disease, diabetes, and taking oral contraceptives.

5. *Lack of vitamin B$_6$ and/or B$_2$.* Vitamin B$_6$ or pyridoxine has been found to relieve symptoms of CTS in clinical trials (Allard and Barnett, 1993). Vitamin B$_2$ (riboflavin) treatments are indicated in severe CTS cases because of its interrelationship with B$_6$ levels (Conner, 1992).

Medical Treatment.   Medical care for CTS often begins with a recommendation for rest and advice to wear a wrist or finger splint. Splints keep the wrist in a neutral position, as well as applying mild compression to the carpal tunnel. If that does not work, diuretics (to reduce water retention) and corticosteroids (to reduce pain) are prescribed. If symptoms persist and worsen, surgery may be recommended. The surgery involves dissecting the transverse carpal ligament and removing scar tissue.

Self-Care.   First, confirm that the problem is true CTS (i.e., there is impingement of the median nerve). Tinel's sign and Phalen's test are the easiest and most reliable home orthopedic tests for median nerve impingement (Conner, 1992).

Exercise 7.1. Tinel's Sign*

Tinel's sign is positive when you experience sharp pain upon light tapping of the affected wrist. (See Figure 7.2.)

Exercise 7.2. Phalen's Test*

Isometrically hyperflex your wrists to increase the pressure on the median nerve. Hold for 30 seconds. Paresthesia in either hand is a positive Phalen's sign. (See Figure 7.3.)

If either sign is positive, the next step is to make an appointment with a medical practitioner to confirm the results. Meanwhile, some self-help to accompany your medical treatment follows.

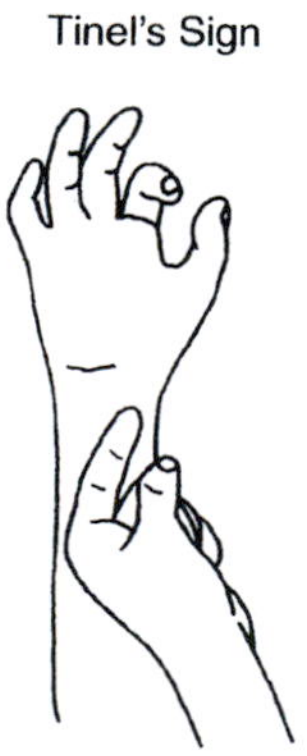

Tinel's Sign

Figure 7.2   Tap the inside of the wrist to test Tinel's sign.

*Courtesy of *Functional Assessment in Massage Therapy,* 3rd ed. by Whitney Lowe (1997). Bend, OR: OMERI.

Phalen's Test

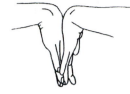

Figure 7.3 Press the backs of your hands together for Phalen's test.

Think about the etiology of carpal tunnel syndrome and you will get many clues as to how to rectify its effects. For example, since pain ensues from overcrowding in the carpal tunnel, anything you do to reduce swelling or inflammation in the area will be helpful. Reducing salt intake will cut down on fluid retention and consequent edema. Rest can quiet inflammation that is due to overuse or misuse. This may mean cutting down on your workload or altering your massage routine to use different body parts (as prescribed in Chapter 2, use the rest of the body, such as elbows, forearms, backs and sides of hands, and knuckles) as tools in your bodywork. It may also mean making a commitment to do restorative or recuperative exercises and stretches in between and after sessions.

Stuart Taws (1999) describes a number of specific stretches based on Aaron Mattes's active isolated stretching for CTS and associated complaints. For CTS itself, have a colleague glide and press from the crease of your elbow down to your wrist. While he or she is gliding, take your hand from full flexion into full extension in a one- to two-second extreme stretch. With the associated complaints, you may be able to manage the self-care without a helper. For tenosynovitis in the abductor and extensor tendons of the thumb (de Quervain's syndrome), he suggests pressing on the tendons in the anatomical snuffbox while taking the thumb in a two-second circuit from extension and abduction to flexion and adduction. For tendinitis pain in the lateral epicondyle (tennis elbow), he suggests compressing the specific site of pain while moving into extreme flexion of the hand and extension at the elbow. For golfer's elbow, use a similar two-second stretch with pressure on the medial epicondyle while moving from flexion of the wrist and elbow into extreme extension.

Daytime splints can allow you to continue massaging while preventing hyperflexion or hyperextension of the wrists. When the area is red, hot, swollen, and painful, use rest, ice, and elevation to offer some relief. Over-the-counter analgesics such as aspirin, acetaminophen, and ibuprofen can also be effective, but consult your health care practitioner about alternatives and proper use. Supplementation with pyridoxine (B_6) and riboflavin (B_2) may be helpful (Conner, 1992). Vitamin B_6 is an essential cofactor in stress hormones and is vital to the production of synovial fluid. The lack of synovial fluid is a factor in severe cases of tenosynovitis, a CTS precursor. Consult with a health care practitioner (MD, ND, NP, PA) to see if B_6 and/or B_2 could help you.

Remember that when you catch CTS in its early warning stages, you can implement changes to help avert the severe nerve pain and functional disability that can arise with the full-blown syndrome.

Thoracic Outlet Syndrome

The thoracic outlet is located between the first two ribs and the clavicle. It is a small, confined area like the carpal tunnel of the wrist. The brachial plexus, composed of an interweaving of nerves C5 to T1, travels through this confined area. Thoracic outlet syndrome (TOS) specifically refers to impingement of nerves C5 to T1. The ulnar, median, and radial nerves all split off from the brachial plexus. Blood and lymph vessels that feed the arm (subclavian artery/brachial artery) also run through the thoracic outlet. Compression of the axillary artery may occur. When blood (and lymph) vessels are compressed, ischemia (lack of blood flow to the area) and decreased venous return (out of the area) result. This can exacerbate the effects of TOS.

Signs and Symptoms. The primary complaint of TOS sufferers is pain in the cervical region and above the scapula. The pain may radiate down the back of the arm to the triceps, then the inner arm, the medial forearm, and the ulnar side of the hand. Diminished nerve impulses can cause paresthesias (unpleasant sensations such as aching, numbness, burning, or tingling) in the shoulder, arm, wrist, hand, and/or fingers. This is a direct outgrowth of the impingement of the sensory root of the nerves.

Reduction in nerve impulses leads to a progressive decrease in strength, dexterity, and fine motor control. In later stages, this can progress to weakening and atrophy of distal muscles along the nerve route because of pressure on the motor root of the nerves. Diminished circulation can deprive the arm of nutrients and oxygen and waste removal needed for healing. The ipsilateral hand may become cold or pale as a result of this reduced blood flow. Sufferers may complain of swelling in the fingers and hands, especially in the morning. This is from lack of venous and lymph return.

In the early stages of TOS, you may notice symptoms only while performing massage in certain positions that aggravate the injury. According to the first rule of body mechanics, this discomfort is a sign to change something! In more advanced cases, discomfort becomes less intermittent and may even be nonstop. Pain is usually worse at night and during activities that provoke the injury. The posterior cervical muscles can go into spasm, creating a chain reaction that spreads to the suboccipital muscles as well. Severe headache pain results from the cervical and suboccipital spasms. Gradual onset is most common in TOS that arises due to overuse and misuse.

The most common cause of TOS is poor posture. Holding your body in positions that bring the clavicle closer to the first rib (i.e., slumping) will decrease the size of the thoracic outlet. This compresses the contents within, including the brachial plexus, and associated blood and lymph vessels. Habitual postures that cause this alteration include holding the arms in a raised position for continual periods of time, or jutting the head forward and rounding the shoulders. Other contributing factors include:

1. *Gender* (women are more prone to TOS than men—the angle of their shoulders decreases the space between the clavicle and first rib)
2. Presence of a *cervical rib* (an extra rib above the first rib)

3. *Hypercontracted scalene muscles* (which pull up on the first rib)
4. *Hypercontracted pectoralis minor muscles* (which pull the ribs forward and up into a rounded position)

There are three common sites of nerve impingement. One is between the clavicle and first rib, where tight scalenes can pull the two bones together or pectoralis minor muscles can tilt the first rib forward to compress the nerves. The second is between the scalenes, where muscular hypertonicity can pinch nerves or spasms can raise the first rib to pinch nerves. Scalene muscles are well known for being the site of many trigger points. Referral patterns can appear in the chest and upper back as well as the shoulder, arm, wrist, hand, and fingers. To address these complaints, apply static pressure or friction at the area of pain and then follow the referrals. If there are pain referrals, go to the next site and repeat the static pressure and/or friction. A third site of TOS compression is within the pectoralis minor, where muscular hypertonicity can compress nerves against the second and third ribs. (See Figure 7.4.) Pectoralis minor entrapment is a condition common to massage therapists, body builders, and large-breasted women. Symptoms include numbness, tingling, and pain in the upper extremity. A mastectomy can cause trauma to the pectoralis minor and diminished venous return, with gradual swelling in the affected arm.

Self-Care.   A first step is to confirm and identify the location of the TOS impingement. Several practitioners (Phaigh, 1995; Aland and King, 1995; Lowe, 1995) advocate and describe orthopedic tests to identify and pinpoint TOS symptoms. These are described and suggested as assessment tools. Remember that any indications should be confirmed by a competent health care professional.

A good test for entrapment of the brachial plexus is the finger curl. If your fingers are swollen from limited venous flow out of an area, the fingertips will not be able to rest on the metacarpal pads at the base of the fingers. This is a common early morning symptom (Aland and King, 1995).

One test for trigger points in the scalenes is the cramp test. If a forceful rotation of the head bringing the chin to the shoulder causes pain in the upper torso or extremities, the test is positive (Aland and King, 1995). A variation on this is to try to tuck the chin behind the clavicle, with pain being a positive sign (Travell and Simons, 1983).

The Thoracic Outlet

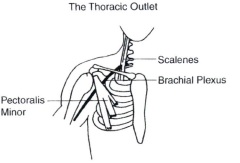

Scalenes

Brachial Plexus

Pectoralis Minor

Figure 7.4   Thoracic outlet syndrome is an impingement of the brachial plexus. Two muscles that can pinch brachial plexus nerves are scalenes and pectoralis minor.

Exercise 7.3. Adson's Test*

Find the radial pulse. Look up and over the shoulder on the affected side and hold the position for several seconds. Palpate for a diminishing pulse as you hold the position. Hold the same wrist and look up and over the opposite shoulder while observing for a diminishing pulse. (See Figure 7.5.) A positive sign indicates either an impingement between the anterior and medial scalene muscles or the presence of a cervical rib. Double check with the traction test, described in Exercise 7.4.

Exercise 7.4. Traction Test*

Find the radial pulse. Have a partner apply firm traction to the arm for several seconds. Palpate for a diminishing pulse as you hold the position. (See Figure 7.6.) A positive sign indicates the presence of a cervical (extra) rib.

Exercise 7.5. Costoclavicular Test*

Find the radial pulse. Pinch the shoulders together, then tuck your chin to your chest. Hold this posture for several seconds. Palpate for a diminishing pulse as you hold the position. (See Figure 7.7.) A positive sign indicates compression between the first rib and the clavicle. Massage of the scalenes and subclavius muscles are indicated.

Exercise 7.6. Wright's Test*

Find the radial pulse. Have a partner raise your affected arm into 120 to 135 degrees of abduction (above shoulder level). Hold this posture for several seconds. Palpate for a diminishing pulse as you hold the position. (See Figure 7.8.) A positive sign indicates compression by the pectoralis

Adson's Test

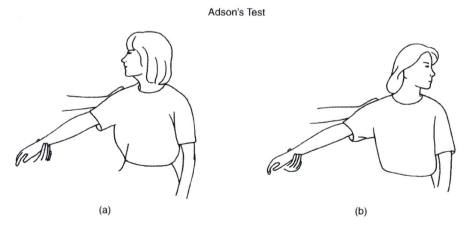

Figure 7.5 (a–b) Look up and over the shoulder on the affected and nonaffected sides while holding the wrist up and palpating the pulse to perform Adson's test.

(a)   (b)

*Courtesy of Rich Phaigh, "Tests for Thoracic Outlet Syndrome" (Spring 1995), *Massage Therapy Journal*, pp. 26–28.

Traction Test

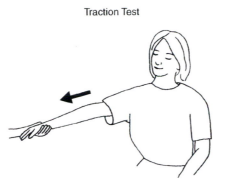

Figure 7.6 Traction the arm while feeling for a diminished pulse for the traction test.

minor muscle or the coracoid process of the scapula. Massage of the pectoralis minor and anterior thoracic fascia are indicated.

Exercise 7.7. Roos's Sign*

Put both arms up with elbows out to the side and palms facing forward like a traffic cop saying "Stop." Keep your arms in this position and open and close your hands rapidly for three minutes. If you feel numbness or tingling in your hands, or if your hands get cold or white during the three minutes, you have a positive test. This suggests that you *may* be suffering from TOS. It is an indication to get your symptoms checked by a medical doctor to confirm or deny the possibility of TOS.

Once you have confirmed TOS, an important step to take is to observe your posture and rectify any tendencies you have toward letting your head fall forward and over the thoracic outlet. Opening up the chest by regularly stretching the pectoralis muscles (see Chapter 8) would also be helpful. Taws (1999) uses another of Mattes's facilitated stretches for TOS. The start position is adduction

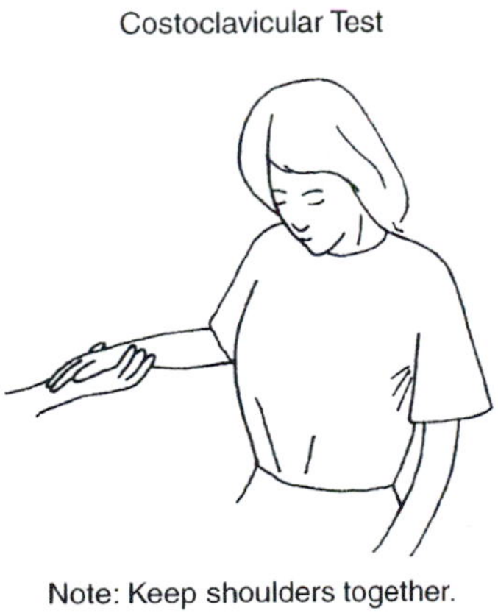

Costoclavicular Test

Figure 7.7 Draw the shoulders together and tuck the chin while palpating for a diminished pulse in the costoclavicular test.

Note: Keep shoulders together.

*Courtesy of Rich Phaigh, "Tests for Thoracic Outlet Syndrome" (Spring 1995), *Massage Therapy Journal*, pp. 26–28.

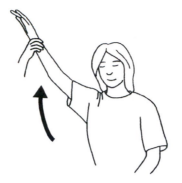

Wright's Test

Figure 7.8 Abduct the affected arm above shoulder height while palpating for a diminished pulse in Wright's test.

and medial rotation of the arm. While a partner applies slight pressure to pectoralis major and/or minor plus attachments, take your arm into full abduction and lateral rotation. Your shoulder should be positioned slightly off the edge of the table to allow for a greater stretch.

Rotator Cuff Injuries

A wide range of pathological conditions fall under the category of rotator cuff tears. A dislocated shoulder often causes associated tearing of the rotator cuff. Because the rotator cuff group is made up of four muscles, a strain to any one of them is considered a rotator cuff tear. Starting superiorly and going posteriorly, the four muscles are the "SITS" muscles—supraspinatus, infraspinatus, teres minor, and subscapularis. All four small muscles also help stabilize the shoulder from pulls by bigger muscles such as the pectoralis major and deltoid muscles. They attach around the neck of the humerus and provide stability and support for arm movement.

For massage therapists, a common overuse injury is to the infraspinatus muscle. This muscle becomes tensile and weak from doing massage with internally rotated shoulders. At the same time, the internal rotator of the cuff, the subscapularis, becomes tight and contractile from having to constantly contract. The subscapularis is often involved in rotator injuries because it is the one muscle stabilizing the front of the arm and shoulder. The supraspinatus is often injured during abduction of the arm. A severe rotator injury that primarily affects the supraspinatus will have a positive sign with the drop arm test (described in Exercise 7.8) (Lowe, 1995).

Exercise 7.8. Drop Arm Test*

Abduct your arm to 90 degrees and then slowly lower it. You could also have a friend tap on the arm just above the wrist. If a severe rotator strain is present, it is likely that you will not be able to lower the arm smoothly.

*Courtesy of *Functional Assessment in Massage Therapy,* 3rd ed. by Whitney Lowe (1997). Bend, OR: OMERI.

It may instead drop suddenly. If this test is positive, seek medical attention immediately.

Shoulder Separation

Along with the four rotator cuff muscles holding the humerus in its socket, a web of ligaments cushions and supports the head of the humerus. A shoulder separation results from a (sprain) tear in these ligaments. Shoulder separation is a displacement of the clavicle from the acromion (Rattray, 1995). The condition frequently occurs from a fall directly on the shoulder. A secondary result is that the humerus is often dislocated or pulled out from the socket as well.

There is likely to be specific tenderness at the acromioclavicular (AC) joint and possible edema. Deformity is another sign. You may be able to see the distal end of the clavicle sticking out in an unusual position. Pain upon movement is likely, particularly as identified with the cross over test (described in Exercise 7.9) (Lowe, 1995).

Exercise 7.9. Cross Over Test*

Sit or stand comfortably. Abduct the arm to 90 degrees and bring it across and over the upper chest. If there is a significant shoulder separation, this movement will cause pain at the acromioclavicular ligament.

Self-Care. Massage can be helpful when applied specifically to muscles that form the rotator cuff. Be sure to address all four of the muscles since they work together to stabilize the joint, and an injury to one may cause weakness or resultant tightness in all. However, severe tears in the rotator cuff may require surgery. A shoulder separation will cause such pain that one will stop all movement in the area. This is adaptive in that it allows the injury time to heal. Inflammation accompanies both rotator cuff and shoulder separation injuries. If unresolved, acute inflammation turns into chronic adhesions that limit range of motion and invite rigidity. Deep transverse friction at the site of the injury and skin rolling help release the adhesions. Joint mobilizations (passive and/or active movements that do not cause pain) help restore movement.

SPECIFIC SYNDROMES—HEAD AND NECK

Temporomandibular Joint Disorders

Temporomandibular joint (TMJ) disorders result from improper alignment of the mandible with the temporal bone. The misalignment can arise from clenching or grinding the teeth in response to stress. TMJ problems often cause headaches and pain in the face and neck. The trigeminal nerve, which controls nerve impulses to and from the temporomandibular joint area, is often irritated in TMJ sufferers.

*Courtesy of *Functional Assessment in Massage Therapy*, 3rd ed. by Whitney Lowe (1997). Bend, OR: OMERI.

Contributing factors include emotional stress, teeth grinding (bruxism), bad posture (especially forward head), trauma, infection or disease of the joint, dental work, long-term gum chewing, and poor TMJ alignment.

Signs and symptoms include clicking, popping, and grinding sounds when moving the jaw, and abrupt or "ratchety" movements and pain in the area that may extend into the head, neck, back, and shoulders. Chronic sufferers may also experience tinnitis (ringing in the ears), dizziness, and drastically reduced range of motion in the jaw.

Self-Care.   Massage can be helpful for TMJ sufferers, if not caused by an underlying malignancy or infection. Suspected TMJ disorder needs to be diagnosed by a medical practitioner. Massage is most helpful when administered in conjunction with other treatments prescribed by a working team. Because some of the acknowledged causes of pain are neuromuscular problems, cranial misalignment, or postural deviations, specially designed massage modalities may be useful in the treatment of pain. Pandiculation (the strong contraction followed by gradual relaxation technique described in Chapter 5 in the section on Hanna Somatics) can be helpful, as well as relaxing the temporal and masseter muscles with Swedish massage. Associated spasms in the sternocleidomastoid, trapezius, head extensor muscles, and suboccipitals may also be relieved by deep pressure (Delany, 1997). Lateral and medial pterygoid muscles are often involved in TMJ disorders and can be addressed by a practitioner who has been trained in intraoral techniques. Extraoral and intraoral craniosacral techniques also address and realign the temporal and mandibular relationship. Make sure that your practitioner wears latex gloves for any intraoral manipulations.

Wryneck and Torticollis

A typical sign of wryneck or a "crick in the neck" is waking up in the morning unable to move the head or neck without pain. Habitual postural patterns, such as holding the telephone with your shoulder or carrying a heavy load, and keeping the head in a forward position can all contribute to wryneck. Massage therapists who habitually look to one side during a session or who carry their tables or chairs to on-site massage sites should be aware of this problem. An easy preventive measure is to shift the carrying shoulder and/or to look to the other side.

Torticollis is a more severe neck spasm that involves primarily the sternocleidomastoid on one side. The head is held locked in a rotated and head forward position where any movement causes pain. This condition can be caused by long-term maintenance of any of the above poor postural patterns and can also be a result of birth trauma (correctable by massage soon after birth) or a by-product of a whiplash.

Self-Care.   Self-stretching for the levator scapula and neck extensors may be helpful (see Chapter 8 for specific stretches).

Whiplash

Whiplash is a neck injury caused by a trauma that rapidly throws the neck into hyperextension (increased backward motion) and hyperflexion (increased forward motion). Although not caused by incorrect body mechanics, whiplash is a problem that can affect any member of the population, including bodyworkers. Different muscles will sustain the most damage, depending on the vector of impact. If the impact is head-on, the posterior cervicals are likely to be the primary site of injury. Trauma coming from the rear is likely to impact the anterior cervicals most severely. A broadside hit will affect both anterior and posterior muscles on the same side. Common whiplash symptoms include stiffness and general achiness; neck, shoulder, and arm pain; dizziness or vertigo; numbness, tingling, and weakness; headaches; chest pain; insomnia; fatigue, anxiety, or irritability; visual disturbances; and digestive distress. These symptoms generally occur one to two days after the injury.

Self-Care. The severity of a whiplash injury can be difficult to detect. For that reason, it is suggested that you wait three days after any accident and until signs of acute inflammation (redness, heat, swelling, and pain) are no longer present before receiving massage (Aland and King, 1995). Always check with a physician to ensure spinal cord integrity and get an x-ray to determine vertebral location and severity of the injury before beginning soft tissue treatment. Watch for any ill symptoms after a massage. The period of one or two days following a massage treatment is a time when tissues are susceptible to reinjury.

Headaches

Structures that are likely to be a site, origin, or contributing factor in head pain are the skin, periosteum, and muscles surrounding the skull; the eyes, nose, and sinuses; the blood vessels of the skull; the trigeminal (V), vagus (X), and glossopharyngeal (IX) cranial nerves; the upper cervical nerves; and the dura mater at the base of the skull (Crawford, 1997). Stimulating one of these structures produces a headache. Thus, for example, when cephalic arteries and veins are irritated and inflamed, the end result is a pain in the head. When cranial nerves are squeezed, the head aches. When sinuses are infected and swollen or when facial muscles are tightened, we can get a headache. Pain can also be referred to the area from trigger points (hypersensitive areas that produce referred phenomena when stimulated) in the head and neck.

Headaches sometimes accompany problems such as caffeine withdrawal; fatigue; constipation; overeating; or ear, eye, and teeth difficulties. The underlying cause of these headaches needs to be addressed by a medical professional. Some headaches occur with serious medical conditions such as brain tumors, meningitis, hematomas, head injuries, infectious diseases, or spinal cord injury. These need to be addressed immediately. Headache symptoms that stem from serious causes include blurred vision; pain behind the eyes; stiff neck and light sensitivity; mental confusion; head pain that attends sudden head turns; persistent throbbing; sudden, severe "bursting" pain; pain that interferes with sleep; and headache that follows coughing, bending, or exercise. In these cases, seek medical care immediately (Crawford, 1997).

Migraine pain is usually found unilaterally (on one side of the head). Migraine phenomena may or may not occur in combination with a headache. Major symptoms of a migraine are pain and nausea. Other possible signs include cold extremities and abdominal pain.

Self-Care. Qualified medical personnel should diagnose suspected migraines. Cool compresses applied to the head and neck in combination with heat packs on the feet may be soothing. Massage strokes that encourage blood flow away from the head may also be welcome. Avoid strong odors, light, and noise. If using aromatherapy in your practice, it may be wise to discontinue its use.

Cluster headache is 10 times more common in men than women. There is usually a rapid onset and the pain is focused on the temple and eye on one side. The pain intensity may be oppressive. The attacks are "clustered" over a period of up to several weeks, with long remission periods that can last for years. Spring is the most likely time that cluster headaches appear. Symptoms require a medical diagnosis.

Sinus headaches are the result of an allergy that inflames mucous membranes that line sinuses in the head. The inflammation causes swelling, pressure, and pain. Signs and symptoms of sinusitis are dull or severe headaches over or behind the eyes and around the cheeks and nose, pain or pressure in one part of the face, discomfort that worsens with damp or cold, fever, and pus in the nasal discharge. Warm, moist heat seems to help diagnosed sinus headaches.

Tension headaches are also known as stress headaches, because tension and stress in the head and neck are the suspected cause. The typical tension headache arises from overuse of the neck muscles, especially in the back of the neck. The upper trapezius, rectus and splenius capitis muscles, sternocleidomastoid, and suboccipitals all can play a role in causing headaches. Trigger points and/or spasms cause referred pain, vision disturbances, and increased pressures inside the skull due to limited blood flow back to the heart. The sternocleidomastoid tends to refer pain to the forehead and behind the eyes (Crawford, 1997).

Self-Care. Standard protocol includes full body relaxation massage with focus on painful muscles. Site-specific cross-fiber friction, followed by 10 to 20 submaximal range-of-motion repetitions, then icing for 10 minutes, is suggested.

SPECIFIC SYNDROMES—MID AND LOW BACK COMPLAINTS

Low Back Pain

Low back pain can result from torn muscle fibers (strain), torn connective tissues (sprains), or slipped intervertebral discs. An exaggerated curve of the lumbar spine (hyperlordosis) increases compression on the posterior side of lower lumbar discs. This is where the gelatinous nucleus pulposus is located. When the disc is squeezed, the cushioning effect of the discs begins to decline.

Anterior pelvic tilt occurs when anterior superior iliac spines (ASISs) tip forward. The hip flexors (psoas, iliacus, tensor fasciae latae, sartorius, and rectus femoris) draw their origins to the insertion rather than bringing insertions toward origins. This draws the posterior pelvis up and pulls the opposing hip extensors (gluteal muscles, hamstrings, and rectus abdominis) taut, into a stretched and weakened position. As the pelvis tilts forward, the curve in the lumbar vertebrae becomes exaggerated (hyperlordosis), which can cause herniation of the discs in the spine.

Posterior pelvic tilt occurs when the pelvis rotates back slightly so that the ASISs tip toward the sky. It is the result of pulling origin to insertion by the hip extensors. The lumbar curve looks "flat."

Not only can pulls on the spine be disproportionate from front to back, but imbalances between the two sides can exist as well. The primary muscle imbalance in the low back is caused by differences in the two quadratus lumborum (QL) muscles, which attach the iliac crest to the lumbar spines and the twelfth rib. Dysfunction is indicated by tenderness in the affected QL and restricted lateral flexion. If you look in the mirror, you are likely to notice an apparently anatomically shorter leg on the affected side, due to the hip-hiking affect of the shortened QL. The ilium on the affected side is also likely to be higher that the unaffected side. Some obvious solutions are postural changes (stop settling in on one leg as you massage), stretching (see Chapter 8 for a good QL stretch), heat applications to soften chronically inflamed tissues, icing for pain, and a trip to your massage therapist to relieve the QL spasms.

Other muscles beyond the QL that can contribute to low back and buttock pain include the erector spinae, multifidi, iliopsoas, abdominal obliques, and gluteals.

Changes in the discs or spaces between the discs are other possible sources of low back dysfunction. Twisting and lifting while bending at the trunk can cause unhealthy changes and/or slippage in the discs. Torquing the back while extending out of the forward bending position is another way to set up discs and paraspinal muscles for injury. Secondary to the disc compression, the gluteals are contracting down hard to stabilize the back. This locking of the gluteals causes ischemia (lack of blood flow) in the area. The resulting pain can refer down the leg to mimic sciatica.

Exercise 7.10. Straight Leg Raising Test (Laseague's Sign)*

The straight leg raising (SLR) test (Lowe, 1995) helps identify lumbar nerve compression below L3. It is used when true sciatica is suspected but not confirmed by a doctor's diagnosis.

Lie down in a supine (face up) position. A partner passively moves your hip into flexion (raises the leg) while holding the leg extended (unbent) at the knee. (See Figure 7.9.) If one of the discs is prolapsed, the movement will compress the nerve against the disc (Lowe, 1995) and cause pain. A positive (pain) response to the SLR suggests impingement of the dural tube. This usually happens within 60 degrees of flexion; if that fails to elicit a response, then passively dorsiflex the foot and flex the neck to provide more traction on the nerve. If no pain ensues, the test is negative for dural tube impingement including disc compression, and massage would most likely be helpful. (See Piriformis Syndrome below.)

*Courtesy of *Functional Assessment in Massage Therapy*, 3rd ed. by Whitney Lowe (1997). Bend, OR: OMERI.

Straight Leg Raising Test

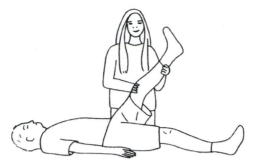

Figure 7.9   Flex the hip and extend the leg in the straight leg raising test.

Piriformis Syndrome (False Sciatica)

Piriformis syndrome is a nerve entrapment syndrome that mimics the symptoms of disc compression. There are six outward rotators of the hip, of which piriformis is one. (The others are obturator internus and externus, gemellus superior and inferior, and quadratus femoris.) The sciatic nerve runs over the other five outward hip rotators. In contrast, the sciatic nerve can run deep to the piriformis or through it, depending on the individual fiber. (See Figure 7.10.) A tight piriformis can constrict the sciatic nerve, causing tingling, numbness, and pain all along the route of the nerve. The piriformis is a primary outward rotator of the hip. Standing with all your weight on one hip while massaging can be a common cause of false sciatica or piriformis syndrome. Adjusting your posture in combination with releasing the piriformis through massage and stretching (see Chapter 8 for stretches for the hip's outward rotators) can ease the discomfort considerably. The gluteus minimus is often a secondary cause of false sciatic pain (Loree, 1995). Since the piriformis and gluteus minimus are deep, the more superficial gluteal maximus and medius muscles must be stretched, massaged, and relaxed before addressing the piriformis and gluteus minimus. (See Chapter 8 for active stretches and Chapter 10 for passive stretches for the gluteals.)

Sciatic Nerve

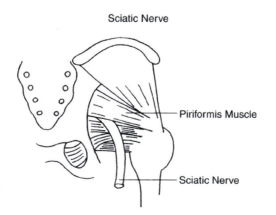

Piriformis Muscle

Sciatic Nerve

Figure 7.10   The sciatic nerve can be compressed by a tight piriformis muscle.

Exercise 7.11. Piriformis Test

Lie down on your massage table close to the edge. Position yourself on your side, with the affected (hurting) side up. Flex the hip and knee of the top side, and let the knee drop down off the table. Have a helper stabilize your hip (do not allow twisting or torquing of the spine) and press down on your knee. (See Figure 7.11.) If this increases pain, the piriformis is probably involved (Lowe, 1995).

Sacroiliac Dysfunction

The sacroiliac (SI) joint (Figure 7.12) is considered relatively immobile. However, it can be twisted or pulled out of alignment. A sudden turning or yanking on the SI joint can cause ongoing dysfunctions. Chronic postural imbalances (such as standing with the weight poised on one foot, or a permanent torque to one side as you massage) are far more likely to create SI problems for the massage therapist.

SI symptoms include pain in the low back or sacral area. Pain may be increased after sitting for long periods or when performing particular activities. Pain and discomfort may also manifest in the gluteal muscles or down the back of the thigh and leg. The sacroiliac ligaments, which attach the sacrum to the ilium, can be assessed for imbalances using the Figure 4 Test, described in Exercise 7.12 (Lowe, 1995).

Exercise 7.12. Figure 4 Test (FABER test) for Flexion, Abduction, and External Rotation*

Lie in a supine position. One leg is straight and the other is *fl*exed, *ab*ducted, and *e*xternally *r*otated, making a figure 4 with the legs. This is

Piriformis Test

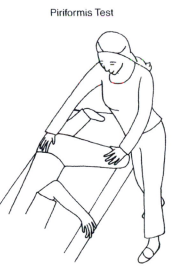

Figure 7.11   While lying on the side with hips and knees flexed, let the top leg drop down in the piriformis test.

*Courtesy of *Functional Assessment in Massage Therapy,* 3rd ed. by Whitney Lowe (1997). Bend, OR: OMERI.

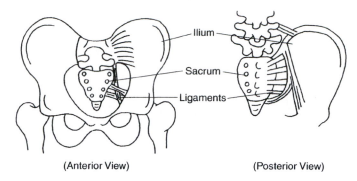

Sacroiliac Joint

Ilium

Sacrum

Ligaments

(Anterior View)   (Posterior View)

Figure 7.12   Although the sacroiliac joint is relatively immobile, it can be pulled out of alignment by postural imbalances or sudden twists and turns.

the origin of the names FABER and Figure 4. (See Figure 7.13.) If you are unable to place the foot on top of the straight leg, position the sole of the foot so that it is touching the medial side of the straight leg. A helper places one hand on your opposite ASIS to stabilize it and the other hand so that it is pressing down on the flexed knee. Pain in the SI region is a positive sign for SI dysfunction.

Self-Care.   After identifying the source of SI pain, stretching and mobilizing the area is often helpful. An easy stretch for the SI joint is to step up with one foot onto your massage table. This can be done as you are waiting for your next client to arrive. Any movement that internally or externally rotates the hip can also help mobilize the joint. (See Chapter 8.) The "gapping" technique, borrowed from craniosacral work, can be helpful. Begin by lying supine on your massage table. Coach a helper to cup one hand under your sacrum (you remain clothed for the technique) and place the forehand of the other arm so that it spans your ASISs. A slight pressure (five grams or less—the weight of a nickel) is exerted medially on both ilia. This pressure frees the joint enough to allow the sacrum to sink into the table and your helper's lower hand (Upledger, 1997).

FABER Test

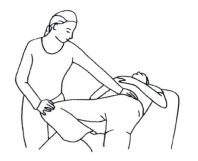

Figure 7.13   The FABER test is an acronym for flexion, abduction, and external rotation at the hip.

Knee Problems

So many problems can occur in the knee joint that it is impossible to cover them thoroughly in the span of one chapter. (See Lowe, 1995, for specifics on categorizing and describing pathologies of the knee.) Most knee problems result from sudden blows to the area that cannot be expected or easily avoided. Chondromalacia patellae or degeneration of the cartilage of the articular surface of the knee can be ruled out with an arthroscopic exam (Rattray, 1995). However, the most common postural imbalance that results in knee problems is knee hyperextension.

Knee hyperextension is commonly known as "locked" knees. The knee is held past full extension and the knees actually go into hyperextension. (See Figure 7.14.) In most cases, the condition exists only in a standing position. When you stand with your knees locked for long periods, the position is likely to affect your low back as well. To evaluate, using a mirror, stand straight with your knees fully extended. The condition is best assessed from a side view. As you look in the mirror, your legs should look vertical. If they move past vertical into hyperextension, it should be quite visible. You may also see a slight concave curvature to the entire lower extremity.

Self-Care. The most effective way to alleviate this condition is through postural awareness and reeducation in the standing position. Keep your knees soft or even bent slightly during massage. Consultation with a practitioner schooled in movement analysis (e.g., Alexander technique, Aston Patterning, Rolfing movement—see Chapter 5 for more ideas) may be helpful. Another recourse is to perform all massages while seated on a height-adjustable, rolling stool.

Knee Hyperextension

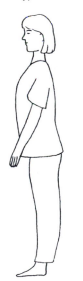

Figure 7.14 Knee hyperextension or locked knees is the most common postural problem contributing to knee pain.

Plantar Fascitis

Plantar fascitis is an overuse syndrome that affects the plantar fascia, the connective tissue that helps maintain the longitudinal arch of the foot. The fascia becomes shortened when the foot is held in a continual arch (i.e., when running for long distances or standing with toes curled under, or when standing for long periods of time). Pain is generally experienced along the plantar surface (sole) of the foot. Discomfort is increased in the morning, or after a period of rest.

Self-Care.   Treatment involves rest and manually stretching the tissues through cross-fiber or longitudinal friction. Be wary of massaging so deeply that you re-inflame the fascia. Also check to see that you are wearing proper footwear during sessions, and perform calf stretches (see Chapter 8) to counteract the effects of plantar flexing the foot.

Tarsal Tunnel Syndrome

Tarsal tunnel syndrome is impingement of the tibial nerve. The condition occurs behind and below the medial malleolus. The actual source of injury is in the tarsal tunnel created by the flexor retinaculum on the top of the foot and the heel (calcaneous) and talus bone on the bottom. The tendons of all the deep posterior compartment muscles of the leg run through this small area. Sharp, shooting pains on the medial side of the ankle while walking are one symptom. The discomfort can radiate onto the sole of the foot.

Self-Care.   Since all five muscles of the posterior compartment of the leg act to plantar flex and invert (supinate) the foot, reducing these actions may relieve some of the hypertrophy, shortening, and inflammation. This, in turn, will reduce crowding in the area and relieve pressure on the tibial nerve. Perform calf stretches (see Chapter 8) to counteract the effects of plantar flexing the foot.

Achilles Tendinitis

Achilles tendinitis is an inflammation of the Achilles tendon, which attaches both the gastrocnemius and soleus muscles to the heel of the foot. Both muscles are used in running and jumping, and both can become chronically shortened when high heels are worn for extended periods of time. Pain is felt upon plantar flexion (pointing your ankle down toward your toes) and is usually experienced closer to the foot than the knee. Pinching the Achilles tendon between your fingers will reproduce the pain.

Self-Care.   Treatment involves rest and reducing the offending activity. (For massage practitioners, this usually means switching to low-heeled shoes. It may mean altering your exercise training, if it involves a lot of running and jumping.) Cross-fiber friction followed by 10 to 20 repetitions of submaximal range-of-motion exercises and ending with ice is recommended. If you can dorsiflex the foot without pain, you can perform calf stretches (see Chapter 8) to counteract the effects of plantar flexing the foot.

Shin Splints

Shin splints refers to two distinct sources of overuse problems affecting the leg. The first type of shin splints arises from repetitive motions made by muscles of the anterior compartment of the leg (tibialis anterior, extensor hallucis longus, and extensor digitorum longus muscles). This happens when these muscles are asked to continually contract while lengthening, as can happen when walking downhill.

The second type of shin splints can arise from overuse of tibialis posterior and other posterior compartment muscles that invert the foot (flexor hallucis longus, flexor digitorum longus). A tendency to massage on tiptoes could duplicate some of the problems.

Self-Care. Both forms of shin splints are treated with rest and cessation or modification of the activity that caused the complaint. Cross-fiber friction followed by submaximal movements (10 to 20 easy circles of the ankle or writing your name in the air with the affected foot) and 10 minutes of ice can reduce adhesions and restore pain-free range of motion. Once you have identified which compartment is affected, you can perform stretches (see Chapter 8) to increase flexibility. Remember that if the stretches cause discomfort, discontinue until the motion can be performed without pain.

SUMMARY

This chapter describes common injuries that can affect the bodyworker as a result of ineffective body mechanics. It includes sections on repetitive stress injuries and common musculoskeletal injuries, including spasms, cramps, contracture, tendinitis, strains, sprains, and bursitis. The chapter can be used as a trail guide to recognize general steps to avoid injuries that result from incorrect body mechanics. Symptoms, preventive steps, and treatment options for chronic or repetitive motion injuries (repetitive stress injuries) are discussed. Carpal tunnel syndrome, thoracic outlet syndrome, headaches, cervical strain, torticollis, piriformis entrapment, low back pain, sacroiliac pain, feet problems, and knee difficulties are covered. Readers are cautioned against using this information to self-diagnose and treat. Always confirm self-assessments with a qualified health care provider.

REFERENCES

Aland, Jeanne, and Donna King, *Deep Tissue Therapy—Theory, Technique and Application* (1995). Heartwood, Institute: Garberville, CA.

Allard, Norman, and Glenn Barnett, "Carpal Tunnel Syndrome," *Massage and Bodywork Quarterly* (Fall 1993), pp. 11–17.

Conner, Robert, "Massage Management of Carpal Tunnel Syndrome," *Massage Magazine,* Issue No. 26 (March/April 1992), pp. 22–28.

Crawford, Dianne Polseno, "The Massage Therapist's Headache Lists—Everything You Need to Know, *Massage Therapy Journal,* Vol. 36, No. 1 (Winter, 1997), pp. 53–64.

Delany, Judith Walker, "Temporomandibular Dysfunction: Neuromuscular Therapy," *Journal of Bodywork and Movement Therapies* (July 1997), pp. 199–203.

Fritz, Sandy, *Mosby's Fundamentals of Therapeutic Massage* (1995). St. Louis, MO: Mosby-Year Book, Inc.

Greene, Lauriann, *Save Your Hands—Injury Prevention for Massage Therapists* (1995). Seattle, WA: Infinity Press.

Headley, Barbara, "Carpal Tunnel Syndrome," *ADVANCE for Nurse Practitioners* (July 1995), pp. 33–35.

Loree, Kins, "Lower Back Pain Syndrome, Part II," *Massage and Bodywork Magazine* (Fall 1995).

Lowe, Whitney, *Functional Assessment in Massage Therapy*, 3rd ed. (1997). Bend, OR: OMERI

Newton, David, "*Pathology Notes*" (1998). Portland, OR: Simran Publications.

Osborne-Sheets, Carole, "Massage and the Pregnant Pelvis," *Massage Therapy Journal*, Vol. 37, No. 2 (Spring 1998) pp. 88–96.

Phaigh, Rich, "Tests for Thoracic Outlet Syndrome," *Massage Therapy Journal* (Spring 1995), pp. 26–28.

Rattray, Fiona S., *Massage Therapy—An Approach to Treatments* (1995). Toronto: Massage Therapy Texts and MAVerick Consultants.

Stillerman, Elaine, *Mother Massage* (1992). New York: Dell Publishing.

Tappan, Frances, and Patricia Benjamin, *Healing Massage Techniques* (1998). Stamford, CT: Appleton & Lange.

Taws, Stuart, "My Hurting Hands," *Massage and Bodywork Journal* (August/September 1999), pp. 62–68.

Travell, Janet, and David Simons, *Myofascial Pain and Dysfunction—The Trigger Point Manual*, Vol. 1 (1983). Baltimore: Williams & Wilkins.

Upledger, John E., *CranioSacral Therapy II—Study Guide* (1997). Palm Springs, FL: The Upledger Institute.

Vaughn, Benny, "Sports Massage," *Massage Therapy Journal* (Winter 1995), pp. 41–43.

Walker, Judith, "How Pain Hurts and Why Massage Helps," *The Australian Massage Therapy Journal* (September 1990), pp. 7–12.

Chapter Eight

Taking Care of Yourself—
Part I (Physiological)

CHAPTER OBJECTIVES

Conceptual Objectives   The massage student/practitioner who success-fully completes this chapter (reading and exercises) will be able to:

- Explain how strength-building exercises can improve one's ability to massage easily and effectively.

- Explain how stretches can help maintain and improve flexibility and the ability to massage easily and effectively.

- Explain how coordination-building activities can improve one's ability to massage easily and effectively.

- Explain how cardiovascular fitness can enhance one's ability to massage easily and effectively.

Practical Objectives   The massage student/practitioner who successfully completes this chapter (reading and exercises) will be able to:

- Demonstrate a variety of strength-building exercises.

- Demonstrate a variety of stretches to enhance flexibility, including a general routine and stretches that target specific areas.

- Demonstrate a variety of coordination-building exercises.

- Choose and enjoy cardiovascular exercises that fit your schedule and in-terests.

Massage therapy is a physically demanding profession. It takes stamina, coordi-nation, and strength to give a good massage. If you cannot physically keep up with the demands of a full schedule, it will be impossible to deliver quality work and to sustain a long-lasting career in bodywork.

Before you take care of any "body" else, you must learn to take care of your own body. Often, massage therapists buy into the myth that they are here solely to help others, and this misconception leads down an ill-fated path. They find themselves giving, giving, and giving until they are depleted and there is nothing left to give. Consider instead that one cannot truly give unless he or she knows what it is to receive. Regular bodywork trades with colleagues can help your body to realize how wonderful it is to receive massage. If you are finding that you do not have the time for exchanges, consider purchasing a massage session for yourself. This is another way of affirming that "bodywork sessions are valuable—I value massage enough to pay for it myself."

On the job, massage therapists systematically observe and palpate how tension accumulates in clients' bodies. In addition to massage, we regularly suggest strengthening exercises, stretching, changes in posture, and coordination-building activities to enhance the table work that we do with our clients. Homework assignments like these help clients integrate the shifts accomplished in a massage session and allow the changes to "take." Stretches, resistance training, and aerobic activities are all practices that we suggest to physiologically support the muscular and fascial releases achieved with massage.

This chapter outlines ways in which massage practitioners can use these same strategies to take care of their physical bodies. Sections are devoted to building the *strength* (stamina and power), *flexibility, coordination,* and *cardiovascular fitness* that you need to sustain a career in massage. A good understanding of these concepts can help you establish a solid foundation for good body mechanics, starting with improved massage posture and alignment.

STRENGTH

Strength is measured by the amount of force you can produce with a single maximal effort (Corbin and Lindsay, 1988). Most of this text has been devoted to showing ways to perform bodywork *without* using maximal effort. However, increasing baseline strength will increase your work capacity, decrease the chance of injury, and prevent low back pain, poor posture, and other sedentary diseases. Taking the steps to increase strength involves work. You will need to walk the fine line between increasing the strength capacity of muscles with more work and sapping your strength by overworking. A little bit of extra work builds and tones muscles; too much extra work injures them.

Note that embarking on a program to increase strength will not effectively enhance cardiovascular fitness, nor will it directly improve flexibility or cause weight loss. (However, secondary effects to an increased caloric expenditure and increase in muscle protein may include reduced overall weight and/or a decreased percentage of fat in muscle tissues.) Muscles will get firmer, and desirable changes may occur in girth, but other aspects of fitness are not directly affected by strength training.

Skeletal muscles (those that move the skeleton) are made up of slow (red), intermediate, and fast (white) twitch fibers. Fast twitch fibers generate more tension than slow twitch fibers, but they fatigue more quickly. These fibers are particularly suited to fast, high-pitched activities such as explosive weight-lifting movements, sprinting, and jumping. The white meat in the breast and wings of a chicken is made of fast twitch fibers. A chicken is relatively heavy and must exert a powerful force to fly up a few feet. This is contrasted with a wild duck that has dark meat (slow twitch fibers) in the flying muscles. A wild duck flies hundreds of miles in its migration path. When the primary consideration is developing the ability to exert a large force with your muscles, then white twitch "strength" must be developed (Tortora, 1994). Strength training requires an overload in the amount of the resistance, whereas endurance requires an overload in the number of repetitions. For bodywork, you need both strength and endurance. When designing a program for strength development, experts generally agree on using a maximum resistance for three to ten repetitions in one to three sets. Practicing this routine three or four times a week will be most effective (Corbin and Lindsay, 1988).

Specific training is known to enhance performance. Thus, massage therapists who want their arms to be stronger in order to lift clients with heavy extremities would focus on specific strength exercises for lifting. On the other hand, if bodyworkers need to have the finger strength to petrissage chronically tough erector spinae fibers, they will practice an entirely different set of strength exercises. Use your arm, back, and leg muscles in the same way that you would to lift a client's leg into a passive hamstring stretch to augment lifting strength. Grip and squeeze a small ball to build petrissaging muscles. Do you understand the concept?

Power is defined as the ability to transfer energy into force at a fast rate (Corbin and Lindsay, 1988). If you are training for a particular technique that requires quick bursts of power, such as Russian massage, strength exercises should be modified into movements with less resistance and greater speed.

On the other hand, if you are planning to train for eight to nine hours of back-to-back Swedish massage, you would do best to concentrate on increasing *endurance* or stamina. Building stamina entails using less weight and more repetitions. Muscular endurance is defined as the ability of the muscles to repeatedly exert an effort (Corbin and Lindsay, 1988). A fit bodyworker can repeat movements (wrist extension) over a long period of time (even eight-hour shifts) without undue fatigue.

What you use to provide the resistance to build muscles is up to you. You can lift free weights (e.g., barbells), pull elastic tubing, squeeze tennis balls, or push against the resistance of your own body. Probably the best way to increase the overall ability to massage is to massage more. Increasing the duration of your massage time means treading a fine line between hypertrophy of the muscle to build up size and strength and working so hard that you tear or otherwise injure the muscle fibers. This is the danger in relying solely on massage as a strength training regimen. If one muscle group is being strained due to overload in massage, more massage will not build strength, it will only injure tissue. If one muscle group is being neglected as you work, more of the same work will build other muscles but the lazy muscles will not get stronger.

Muscle fibers adapt only to the load placed on them; therefore, in order to continue increasing strength, you must progressively increase the stress on fibers as they adapt to each new load. Weight training is considered the fastest and best method of improving strength. Isotonic exercises refer to activities in which the muscles alternately shorten (concentric contraction) and lengthen (eccentric contraction) (Newton, 1996).

There does not seem to be any difference between eccentric and concentric exercise in terms of effectiveness for developing strength (Clarkson, 1997). Eccentric exercises, such as walking downhill as opposed to uphill, may be more comfortable to do. However, there is a tendency for eccentric exercises to cause more muscle soreness afterward (Clarkson, 1997). The stress on a muscle will vary with the speed, joint position, and muscle length in isotonic exercise.

Isometric exercises (when the muscle contracts but does not move) are effective for developing strength. They require no equipment and only minimal space. Research has shown that isotonic training can be enhanced by adding isometrics at the glitches or sticking points during the range of motion. However, isometric exercises work the muscle only at the angle of joint used in the isometric exercise. Isometrics may be more dangerous for those with high blood pressure or cardiovascular disease, because they cause a marked rise in blood pressure and may produce irregular heartbeats. Isometrics are also questionable as a method for adolescents because their bones have not matured. It is thought that normal growth may be stunted in teens who rely on isometrics (Corbin and Lindsay, 1988).

Isokinetic exercises are isotonic concentric muscle contractions performed on special machines. These machines match their tension to the effort and provide maximal resistance throughout the range of motion. They are typically expensive, however, and usually available only in a health spa or gym setting.

The following are guidelines for safe and effective strength training according to Corbin and Lindsay (1988).

1. When beginning a strength program, *start* with weights or resistances that are too *light* so that you can avoid soreness and injury.
2. *Progress gradually.* For example, use one set of three repetitions with a light weight to begin, add repetitions when it gets too easy. Repeat until you get to a maximum of ten repetitions for three sets. After this has been achieved, then you can increase weight resistance.
3. *Body workers should train muscles in the way they will be used in their skill.* Employ similar patterns, range of motion, and speed.
4. *Choose an exercise sequence that alternates muscle groups* so that muscles have a rest period before being involved in another exercise.
5. *Isometric exercises should be performed at several joint angles.*
6. *Use motivating techniques* such as music, partners, competition, and variation in routine.
7. To prevent injury:
    a. Warm up before the workout and stay warm during the session. Warm-up exercise refers to light to moderate activity, including stretching, done prior to serious exercise (Corbin and Lindsay, 1988).
    b. Do not hold your breath while exerting force. This can cause blackout or hernia.
    c. Wear shoes with good traction.
    d. Keep the weight close to the body.
    e. Keep a definite rhythm and avoid pauses between repetitions.
    f. Remember that the expression "no pain, no gain" is a fallacy. If it hurts, you are probably harming yourself.

Mental influences on human strength were tested on a group of undergraduates from George Williams College. Arm strength was measured under four experimental conditions—normal conditions, immediately after a loud noise or while the subject screamed loudly at the time of exertion, under the influence of recreational drugs, and under hypnosis. The hypnotic suggestion was that the subject would be considerably stronger than usual and should have no fear of injury. All of the additional stimuli augmented strength, but the greatest increment in strength occurred when subjects were under hypnosis (McArdle et al. 1986).

The investigators speculated that strength improvements were due to a temporary modification in central nervous system function. The theory is that most people normally function at a level of nerve inhibition that prevents them from expressing their full strength capacity. During the excitement of competition, under the influence of certain drugs, or under hypnotic suggestion, the inhibition is removed. The result is an apparent superoptimal performance. This notion may also explain the feats of strength attainable in emergency situations. Athletes can create a similar self-induced hypnotic state by "psyching themselves up" prior to competition. These studies suggest the importance of mental factors in developing strength. The first two exercises help the bodyworker explore some of the psychological aspects of strength.

Exercise 8.1. How Much Is Enough Strength?

This easy hatha yoga warm-up helps you to gauge how much strength is enough. Your task is to kinesthetically find the balance between too little effort and too much.

To begin, stand with your arms at your sides and exhale. Now start to inhale, abducting the arms slightly (bringing them up to the side) and rising up on tiptoes. Fix your gaze on a spot on the wall in front of you. (Do not look down at the floor, because your body will follow and you will topple.) As you rise, let your hands form themselves into fists that settle under the rib cage to help support the lifting motion. Hold the balance and the breath for eight to ten seconds. Return to the starting position as you exhale and relax. Repeat two or three times.

Notice your energy/strength/effort level as you rise. If you bring too much force to the rising, you will topple. If the strength you manage to muster is not equal to the task, you will fail to rise at all.

Exercises 8.2. How Do You Use Excess Strength?

For this inquiry, you will observe how you respond in times when your experience creates a great deal of inner energy and strength. You are most likely to catch yourself in this state during moments of excitement (e.g., your favorite sports team has just won the championship or you have just received a promotion at work). You may become more aware of the coursing of the blood and the pumping of the heart. What happens after this initial burst of strength? Where does the energy go?

Most of us do not have a strategy for dealing with a burst of strength. We do not know how to save our power for future times when we may be feeling lackluster and dull. All too often, we waste the accumulated energy by picking a fight or getting angry over a matter of little consequence. Wouldn't it be helpful to harness the excess for constructive purposes. Make a list of things that you like to do when you have extraordinary amounts of energy and strength (exercising to burn off steam or finishing an unpleasant physical chore like vacuuming).

Although learning or other psychological factors can enhance one's ability to express muscular strength, the ultimate limit for strength is determined by anatomical conditions within the muscle. The physical state of the body can be augmented with appropriate training exercises. Exercises designed to target and strengthen muscles used most often by massage therapists are outlined in Exercises 8.3 through 8.7.

Exercise 8.3. Abdominal Strengthener A—Crunches

The abdominal muscles are important to maintain because they help support the back. Without abdominal strength, the muscles of your back get overloaded as you massage or lift and become primed for injury and chronic pain.

To do crunches, lie down on a mat or futon with knees bent and the soles of your feet resting on the floor. Interlace your fingers behind your head at ear level to support your head. Now, contract the abdominal muscles to slowly pull yourself forward and up toward your knees. Do not use your arms to pull up your body and head! (*Note:* The very beginning of the abdominal effort is the most effective for building strength. Do not feel that you have to sit up completely.) Hold for eight to ten seconds. Return to the starting position. Repeat two or three times. (See Figure 8.1.)

Exercise 8.4. Abdominal Strengthener B—Pelvic Tilt

Pelvic tilts will strengthen both the gluteal and abdominal muscles (especially the psoas), so that you are able to sit and stand with good posture. You can practice a variation of this drill to control tension when sitting or standing anywhere.

Lie down on a mat or futon with knees bent and the soles of your

Crunches

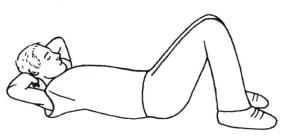

Figure 8.1   Abdominal crunches strengthen the back.

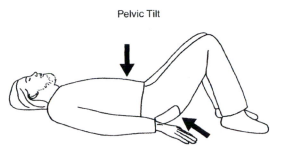

Pelvic Tilt

Arrows show muscles to tighten (gluteals and abdominals).

Figure 8.2   Pelvic tilts strengthen the abdomen and the gluteal muscles.

feet resting on the floor. Tighten your gluteus muscles (buttocks) and, at the same time, flatten your lower back by tightening your abdominal muscles. When you tighten, concentrate on maintaining constant muscle contraction. Hold this feeling of tension for eight to ten seconds, then relax. Use the breath in the following way. As you tighten your muscles, breathe in. When you hold the tension, breathe little, easy breaths. When you release the tension, breathe out. Repeat two or three times. (See Figure 8.2.)

Exercise 8.5. Inchworm

This is one of the most important exercises that you can practice for the health of your feet. The "inchworm" strengthens your metatarsal arch and toe muscles. This exercise gives your toes the strength they need to press down every time you support or shift your weight during massage. With this strength, you will be able to balance, stand, walk, and change levels with more power, control, and stability. You can practice this whenever you find an empty moment.

The exercise can be practiced sitting or standing, and seems to work best if performed while barefoot. You will be working with one foot at a time. If you are standing, unlock the supporting leg, while you exercise the opposite foot. Point your feet straight ahead. If sitting, make sure that both feet are squarely on the floor.

Press the bottoms of all five of your toes down on the floor and lift up the entire ball of your foot. Imagine that you are pressing your feet into clay or sand to make an imprint. Press your toes down firmly and pull your heel toward your toes. Hold this feeling of tension for eight to ten seconds, then relax. Now raise your toes forward (not up) and rest your toes and the ball of your foot back down on the floor for a count of eight to ten seconds. Repeat this inching forward two or three times. Repeat on the opposite side. (*Note:* To prevent cramping, finish by dorsiflexing the ankle and manually spreading the plantar fascia on the soles of the feet out to all directions.) (See Figure 8.3.)

Inchworm

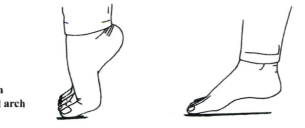

Figure 8.3   The inchworm strengthens the metatarsal arch and toe muscles.

Exercise 8.6. Toe Open and Close

The purpose of this exercise is to stretch and strengthen the toe muscles. It may help your toe muscles to respond more efficiently to motor signals from the brain, and may help them increase mobility and dexterity.

Sit where your feet can rest and your ankle can be relaxed. If your legs are extended, place a bolster or small pillow underneath your knees. Let the rest of your body be aligned.

Extend your toes and, at the same time, spread them apart as far as you can make them go. Hold this feeling of tension for eight to ten seconds, then relax. Close your toes together and still try to keep them extended. Repeat this open and close, spread and squeeze sequence as long as it is comfortable. At first, exercising your toes may be frustrating because you are not accustomed to coordinating that area of the body. Be patient with yourself and keep practicing to achieve maximum benefit. (See Figure 8.4.)

Exercises 8.7. Wrist, Hand, and Finger Strengtheners

Increasing strength in the hands can be accomplished while accomplishing everyday tasks such as typing, weeding, or playing a musical instrument. Other, more structured exercises are provided here. These easy activities can be practiced anytime—before, during, or after massages. They focus on the wrists and hands, the bodyworker's basic tools. These

Toe Open and Close

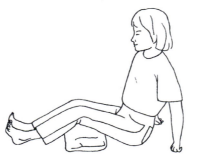

Figure 8.4   The alternate toe open and close both stretches and strengthens the toes.

are the anatomical tools most often overused during the practice of massage.

1. Squeeze a firm ball (e.g., a tennis ball, a balloon filled with sand, or silly putty works well) for 10 counts. Repeat two or three times.

2. Making "steeples." This exercise derives from the old childhood rhyme: "Here's the church and here's the steeple. Open the doors and see all the people." Put your hands together as if you are praying. Then press the fingers together eight to ten times. You can press all the fingers simultaneously or move from little finger through thumb, sequentially.

3. Press your fist into the palm of your opposite hand. Repeat two or three times on each side.

4. (This one is my personal favorite.) Fill a pail full of sand, or just use sand straight from the beach. (This may necessitate a relaxing trip to the ocean.) The pail must be big enough so that you can slip your hands comfortably into it. Open and close your hands so that you are extending your fingers against the resistance of the sand. This exercise most closely imitates the action of pressing against the resistance of the client's body. The sand yields to your movement, though, and builds up your arm/hand strength in a delightful way. *Note:* If sand is not available, you can substitute a thick rubber band (thick enough so that it doesn't cut into your skin) wrapped around the fingers. In my mind, although the action of extending the fingers remains the same, this is a poor substitute for the soothing action of the sand.

In all of these exercises, both left and right sides of the body need to be manipulated so that one hand will not be weaker than the other.

FLEXIBILITY

Flexibility can be defined as the range of motion available in a joint (Corbin and Lindsay, 1988). When we say that someone is physically flexible, we generally mean that he or she is able to adapt easily to new physical positions without too much stress and strain. I believe that developing flexibility or fluidity in your body also has an effect on your psyche. It helps a therapist become more able to "roll with the punches." A flexible mind can adapt more readily to new situations without psychological stress or emotional strain. I also believe that fluidity, as reflected in a massage therapist's body, has a strong influence on the client. When you express more ease and range of motion in your movements, you can more successfully transmit and inspire those qualities in those you touch.

For bodyworkers, target areas for stretching include the small muscles in the hands and feet, the repeatedly used muscles in the arms and thighs, and the fibers that accumulate tension in the neck, shoulders, and back.

Active stretching requires sensitivity to your pain level. Do not go past a point where you feel a comfortable tension. This is the point of mild resistance, and it is the place where stretching has the most impact on lengthening muscles. When stretching correctly, after about 10 seconds have elapsed, the tension of the stretch should start to fade. If the feeling does not subside and/or grows in intensity, you are overstretching (Anderson, 1980). Your muscles are protected by an internal mechanism called the *stretch reflex*. As described in Chapter 7, any time you pull muscle fibers too far or too fast (e.g., by bouncing or overextending), the stretch reflex is activated. A signal is sent to the muscles involved telling them to contract. This prevents injury to the muscles. It is similar to the involuntary reaction that occurs when you accidentally touch a hot stove; without thinking your body pulls away from the heat. When you stretch too far, the end result is a tightening of the very muscles you are attempting to lengthen.

Pushing a stretch as far as you can past the point where it hurts, or bouncing up and down (ballistic stretching), will strain muscles and activate the stretch reflex. These harmful procedures cause pain and physical damage due to microscopic tearing of muscle fibers. Tearing leads to the formation of scar tissue in the muscles, with a gradual loss of elasticity. Torn and scarred muscles become even more tight and sore.

Over time, bodies tend to contract and become tight unless they are challenged. Before the age of 18, we do not need to stretch to maintain suppleness. After that age, practitioners must sustain a pose for at least eight to ten seconds just to maintain what flexibility is already there. To increase range of motion, a posture must be sustained for at least one full minute (Corbin and Lindsay, 1988).

The following guidelines can help coax your body into a more flexible state (Anderson, 1980):

1. *You are the expert when it comes to determining your stretching needs.* You know better than anyone does exactly when, where, and just how much your muscles need to loosen, in order to accomplish what you are asking it to do. No one else can feel this as well as you.

2. *Relax into the stretches.* Whenever you feel tight, first sense and feel the breath move into the places where you are tense (e.g., neck, low back, or behind the knees). Then consciously let go of the tensions by breathing out and imagining the tight area likewise loosening and letting go.

3. *Stretching should feel good, like a cat stretching after a nap.* Many of us incorrectly learned to associate pain with physical improvement and were taught that the more it hurts the better. That "no pain, no gain" adage is a myth. Pain is an indication that something is wrong. Listen to your body's signals. A sharp, acute pain is a warning to immediately stop what your are doing. Any pain that does not go away after four or five days is a cue to seek medical attention.

4. *Stretch when the body is warm.* It is easier to do, it feels better, and it is better for your body. Cold stretching hurts more and creates a greater opportunity to tear muscles.

5. *Stretch only a little each time you stretch, but stretch often.* The effects are cumulative. Five minutes of relaxed stretching twice a day is more effective than an hour spent grinding and groaning on the weekends.

6. *Don't bounce*!!!!

For massage practitioners, the whole body can benefit from increased suppleness and resiliency, but some regions tend to accumulate tightness more than others do. Stretches for these special areas are presented here.

The first activity provides basic stretches to help relax the muscles of the upper body, focusing on neck, upper back, shoulder girdle and joint, and arms and hands.

Exercise 8.8. Basic Stretch Routine

This is a basic routine for all-around shaking, stretching, loosening, and relaxation. It is arranged so that the movements can be practiced as a whole routine, from standing to sitting to lying down. Following this preliminary are muscle-specific active stretching exercises.

While standing, take three deep breaths. On the first, say to yourself, "I am relaxing my mind—letting all thoughts go." On the second breath, say, "I am relaxing my body—allowing tension to flow out." On the third, think, "I am relaxing completely—letting go of anything else that is not needed right now."

Now shake the right arm. Start with the fingers, hand, and wrist. Then include the forearm and then the upper arm in the shaking. Repeat with the left arm. Be aware of your joints as you shake.

Shake your right leg. Begin with your toes, foot, and ankle. Then continue to include your lower leg and thigh. Repeat on the other side and keep an awareness of the joints as you move.

Stand with your feet shoulder-width apart and with the knees relaxed and slightly bent. Drop your chin to your chest. Allow the weight of your head to lengthen and relax the muscles in the back of your neck. Continue to curl down, one vertebra at a time until you have curled over as far as you comfortably can. Allow the weight of your upper body to just hang down and let gravity do the work of stretching and relaxing your lower back. Hang like a rag doll, allowing your arms to dangle. Sway slightly from side to side. (*Note:* If you feel like your back is overstretching at some point, stop and rest your hands or forearms on your thighs to give your back some support.) Slowly curl up again, vertebra by vertebra, until you are standing again.

Exercises 8.9–18. Upper Body Stretches

8.9. Warm-up. Breathe in as you interlace your fingers and press them out in front of you for 10 seconds and then above your head for the same amount of time. Breathe out as you feel the stretch in your arms, shoulders, and upper back. You can repeat this several times.

8.10. Head Extensor Stretch. Lie down on a mat or futon with your knees bent and the soles of your feet resting on the floor. Interlace your fingers behind your head and rest your arms on the mat. Using the arms to initiate the effort, lift your head forward until you feel mild tension. Hold the position for eight to ten seconds. Breathe in as you move into

Head Extensor Stretch

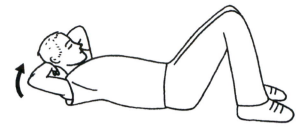

Figure 8.5 Support your head in your hands as you pull up to stretch the neck extensors.

the stretch and breathe out as you imagine the neck muscles lengthening and letting go. Repeat two or three times. (See Figure 8.5.)

8.11. Sidebends. Sit, stand, or lie with your head in a comfortable, aligned position. Breathe in as you slowly tilt your head to the left side to stretch the muscles on the right side of your neck. Hold this feeling of tension for eight to ten seconds. Breathe out and feel a good, even stretch without overstretching. Repeat two or three times on each side. (See Figure 8.6.)

8.12. Deltoid and Triceps Stretch. Stand and hold your right elbow with your left hand behind your head and give yourself a pat on the back. Do this slowly. As with all of the stretches, breathe in as you move into position, and breathe out as you hold the position and feel the muscles letting go. Repeat, reversing the positions of your arms. Notice if one side feels tighter than the other. (See Figure 8.7.)

8.13. Lattisimus Dorsi Stretch. From a standing position, reach up behind your head and take hold of your right elbow with your left hand. Keep your knees slightly bent, and gently pull your right elbow overhead as you laterally flex your trunk to the left. As with all of the stretches, breathe in as you move into position, and breathe out as you hold the position and feel the muscles letting go. Repeat on the other side. (See Figure 8.8.)

Because massage can be so taxing on the thoracic body, several stretches are suggested for the pectoralis muscles. Depending on the exercises you emphasize, you can also have secondary effects to tone the rhomboids, stretch the upper abdominals, or focus on the shoulders.

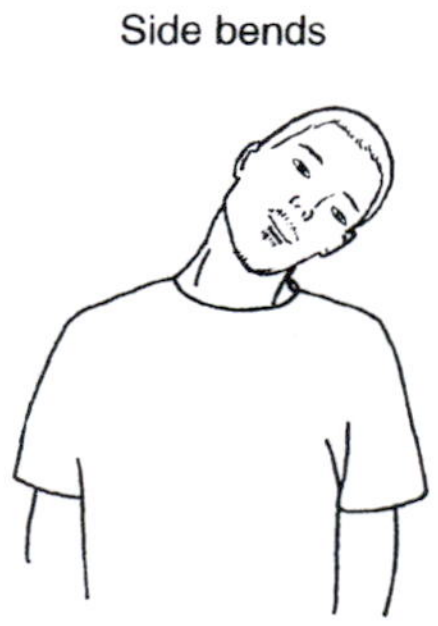

Side bends

Figure 8.6 Tilt your head to the side to stretch the lateral flexors of the neck.

Anterior Deltoid and Triceps Stretch

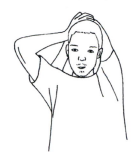

Figure 8.7   A supported pat on your own back stretches anterior deltoids and triceps.

8.14. Pec Stretch A. To stretch your chest and shoulders, clasp your hands behind your back. Straighten your elbows and pull your shoulders down from your ears. Open your chest and lift, pretending to squeeze an imaginary grapefruit between your shoulder blades. This will bring your arms up behind you. Turn your elbows medially while straightening your arms. Do not tilt your torso forward. Rest your hands on the back of a chair for support. Take a few steps away from the support object and straighten your arms to increase the stretch. Do not overstretch. This is great for rounded shoulders and gives an immediate feeling of energy. Breathe in as you walk into position. Breathe out as you imagine the muscles lengthening and getting more relaxed. Hold for eight to ten seconds as you continue to breathe easily. Repeat two or three times. (See Figure 8.9.)

8.15. Rectus Abdominis and Pec Stretch. Standing with your knees slightly bent, place your palms on your lower back just above your hips with your fingers pointing down. Now breathe in as you lean back nice and easy. This is an especially good stretch to do when you find yourself

Lattisimus Dorsi Stretch

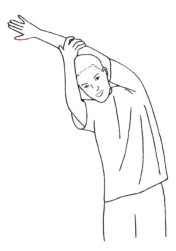

Figure 8.8   Bend to the side to stretch lattisimus dorsi.

Pec Stretch A

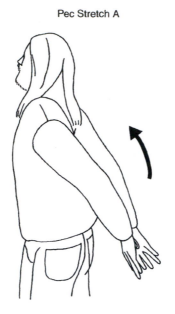

Figure 8.9   Clasp hands behind your back and pull them up for a pectoralis stretch.

sitting for extended periods of time. Breathe out as you hold for eight to ten seconds. Repeat two or three times. (See Figure 8.10.)

8.16. Rhomboid Toning and Pec Stretch. To begin, lie down with your knees bent and the soles of your feet planted on the floor. Breathe in as you pull your shoulder blades together. Feel the tension in between the shoulder blades as you contract the rhomboid muscles. These muscles often get overstretched and painful when performing massage in a chroni-

Rectus Abdominus and Pec Stretch

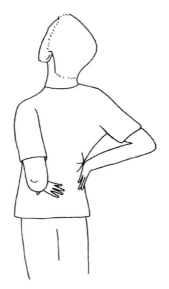

Figure 8.10   Support your low back with your hands and bend back for a rectus abdominis and pectoralis stretch.

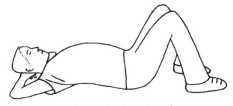

Note: bring shoulders together.

Figure 8.11   Draw your shoulder blades together to tone the rhomboids and stretch the pectorals.

cally hunched position. Notice that as you contract the rhomboids, your chest moves upward. Breathe out as you hold for eight to ten seconds, and then pull your head forward with your hands cupped behind your head, to release the tension. Repeat two or three times. (See Figure 8.11.)

8.17. Deltoid and Pec Stretch. Hold a towel at the two ends (folding it diagonally gives the most width). Breathe in as you move it behind you with your arms straight. Move it up, over your head, and down behind your back. Do not strain or force. Your hands should be far enough apart to allow for a smooth movement up, over, and down. To isolate and add further stretch to any particular area, hold the stretch for eight to ten seconds at the area(s) where you feel resistance. Breathe out and imagine the area loosening and letting go. As you move into the next area of resistance, breathe in again and breathe out as you hold the stretch and feel the muscles letting go. Repeat two or three times. (See Figure 8.12.)

8.18. Shoulder Shrugs and Shoulder Rolls. Shoulder shrugs are just what they sound like. Breathe in as you bring the shoulders up close to the ears and hold them there. Breathe out as you feel the shrug squeezing out the tension. Hold this feeling for eight to ten seconds and then relax your shoulders down into their normal position. Repeat several times and them move into slow shoulder rolls forward, up, back, and down. End by reversing the direction of the circles so that the shoulders are moving back first, then up, back, and down. (See Figure 8.13.)

Exercises 8.19–27. Lower Body Stretches

The lower body acts as a mainstay for all the reaching and pressure delivered by the shoulders and arms during massage. Without regular stretching, the muscles of these areas will tighten up and be unable to deliver support when it is required. This series is especially beneficial because each position targets a body area, which is generally hard to relax.

8.19. Adductor Stretch.

(a) Sit on a mat or futon and begin with knees bent and the soles of your feet touching. Breathe in as you allow your hips to rotate out (the knees will move away from each other to the sides) and completely relax as you exhale. This comfortable position will stretch the groin muscles. Let the pull of gravity do the stretching. Maintain the position for eight to ten seconds. Repeat two or three times. (See Figure 8.14.)

Deltoid and Pec Stretch

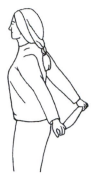

Figure 8.12   Pull a towel behind your back for a deltoid and pectoralis stretch.

(b) Sit on a mat or futon with your legs extended out to the sides. Inhale as you allow your hips to rotate out (your legs will extend out to the sides) and lean forward slightly. This position focuses on stretching the long adductor muscles. Exhale as you hold the stretch for eight to ten seconds. Repeat two or three times. You may feel the tendons stretching at their origins on the pubic ramus or at the insertions at the distal end of the medial femur. If you wish, massage these attachments while stretching to get even more release.

You can do a variation of this stretch with a partner, by facing one another and holding hands. As one partner leans back (leading with the back of the spine), the other is pulled forward into the stretch. Come out of the position into a straight-up resting pose after eight to ten seconds. Repeat with the opposite partner leaning back. (See Figure 8.15.)

8.20. Reclining Abdominal Stretch. Lie down on a mat or futon with your legs extended and your arms extended overhead. Inhale as you point your fingers and toes, and exhale while you reach as far as is comfortable in opposite directions with your arms and legs. To also stretch the abdominal obliques, let your arms and legs extend out from the center of your body in an X shape. Alternate your reach, so that you are reaching first the left arm and left leg, then the right arm and right leg, then the diagonal through the left arm and right leg and the diagonal through the right arm and left leg. Now stretch in all four directions at once. Breathe

Shoulder Shrugs

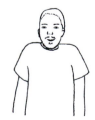

Figure 8.13   Bring your shoulders toward your ears in a shoulder shrug.

Adductor Stretch A

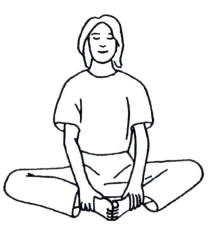

Figure 8.14   Adductor stretch A focuses on stretching the short adductors of the thigh.

in as you reach and breathe out as you hold the position for eight to ten seconds. Repeat each variation two or three times. (See Figure 8.16.)

8.21. Quad Stretch. *Caution:* When stretching the quadriceps muscles, you must take care not to stress the knee joint. If you feel more than a mild tension, relax. Pain is a sign that something is wrong.

Lie down on your side on a mat or futon, with your knees bent into the fetal position. Extend the lower leg so it is lying long. With the lower hip extended, bend the knee and reach behind you to the ankle of the upper leg. You may wish to hold a towel in both hands and hook it across the foot if you cannot reach the ankle. Inhale as you reach, and exhale as you feel the stretch in the front of the thigh. To isolate the rectus femoris muscle, which is the only quadriceps muscle to cross the hip joint, also extend and lift the whole upper leg back.

To focus your stretch on the lateral or medial side, simply rotate your leg at the hip joint and hold the stretch where you feel the most tension. Hold each position for eight to ten seconds. Repeat all variations two or three times. Anderson (1990) suggests that it may be easier to

Adductor Stretch B

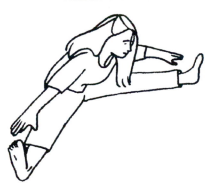

Figure 8.15   Adductor stretch B focuses on stretching the long adductors of the thigh.

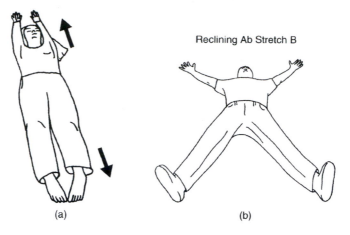

Figure 8.16 (a–b)   Extend your arms overhead, feel your back on the floor, and reach with arms and legs for the reclining abdominal stretch.

(a)   (b)

stretch the hamstrings after the quads have already been stretched, although he provides only anecdotal experience to support the theory. Experiment for yourself and see. (See Figure 8.17.)

8.22. Hamstring Stretch. Lie down on a mat or futon, with one leg extended and the other knee bent and sole of the foot standing on the floor. Lift the long leg up to a vertical position (or past vertical, if that feels good to you). Place your hands behind the thigh or the lower leg. (*Note:* Avoid putting pressure just behind the knee.) You may wish to hold a towel in both hands and hook it across the foot if you cannot reach behind your leg. Make sure that your lower back muscles remain flat on the floor. Breathe in as you extend the leg, and breathe out as you feel the stretch in the back of the thigh. Pay attention to whether the tension is focused on or near the tendon attachments at the hip or at the knee. If you wish, massage these attachments during the stretch to achieve more release. Remember to keep the straight leg straight. Sacrifice elevation for straightness. Proper position is important to target the muscles that you want to be stretching.

Flex the knee and the ankle, and let the leg relax toward your chest. Now straighten the leg and allow it to stretch farther this time. Release and flex again, then stretch even farther.

Quad Stretch

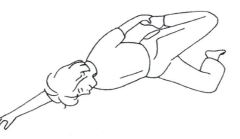

Figure 8.17   Pull your leg toward you to stretch your quadriceps. Stop if you feel pain at the knee.

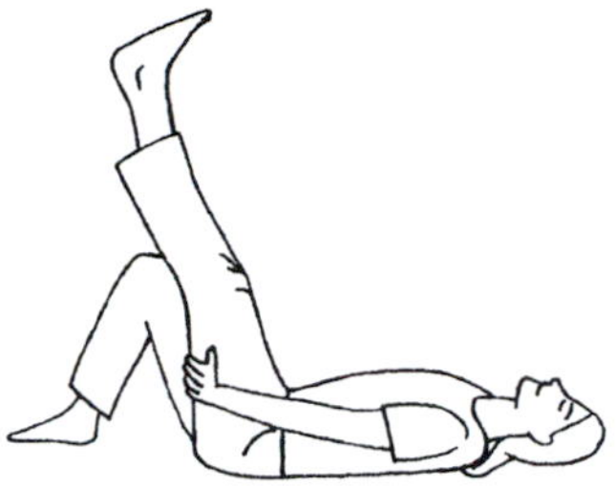

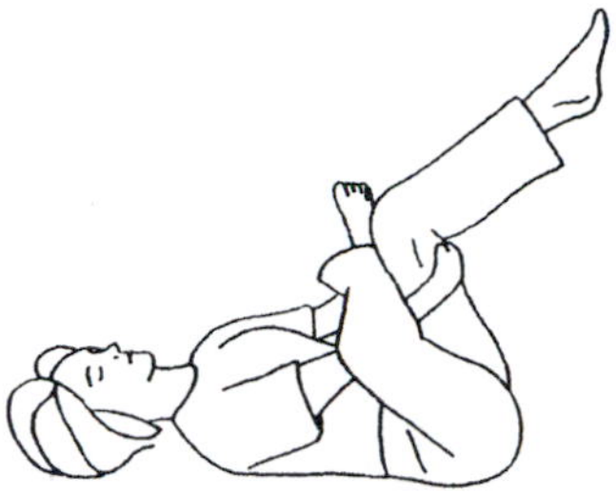

Hamstring Stretch

Hamstring Stretch—Figure Four Position

Figure 8.18 (a–b) To stretch hamstring attachments at the knee, pull a straight leg toward your nose. Use the figure 4 stretch to lengthen the hamstring attachment at the hip.

(a)

(b)

To focus on the attachments at the ischial tuberosity, cross your bent leg over the extended one. This brings your legs into a figure 4 position. Then reach behind the thigh of the posterior leg and pull toward you. Hold each position for eight to ten seconds. Repeat both variations two or three times. (See Figure 8.18.)

8.23. Gluteal Stretch. Sit on a mat, with one leg extended and the other knee bent and sole of that foot standing on the floor. Inhale as you reach down to the bent leg and pull the knee toward the opposite shoulder. Make small circles with the bent knee to find areas of resistance. To isolate and add further stretch to any particular area, exhale as you hold the stretch for eight to ten seconds at the area(s) where you feel resistance. Release any tension that is not needed to hold the pose. Hold for eight to ten seconds. Repeat two or three times. (See Figure 8.19.)

8.24. Psoas Stretch. From a standing position, inhale as you lunge forward on one foot. Exhale and feel the stretch in the groin area of the leg that is in back. Hold for eight to ten seconds. Repeat on the other side. (See Figure 8.20.)

8.25. Quadratus Lumborum Stretch. Lie down on a mat or futon, with both knees bent and the soles of the feet standing on the floor. Cross the right leg over the left. Inhale and use the weight of the top leg (right) to pull your bottom leg (left) toward the floor. Stretch until you feel mild tension along the side of your left hip and lower back. Exhale and let the tension go. Keep the upper back, shoulders, and elbows flat on the mat. To feel the stretch further up the back, turn your head away from the knee (to the left). Hold for eight to ten seconds. Repeat on the opposite side. (See Figure 8.21.)

8.26. Piriformis Stretch.

(a) The piriformis is the muscle that overlies or runs around the sciatic nerve. Releasing this muscle with a stretch can be very helpful in alleviating what can be known as "false sciatica," or pain running in the direction of the sciatic nerve.

Since the piriformis becomes an internal rotator when the thigh is flexed and crosses the midline, you can use the figure 4 position as described in the hamstring stretch (see Figure 8.18).

Gluteal Stretch

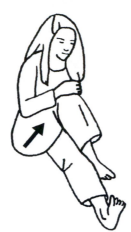

Figure 8.19 From a seated position, cradle your leg and pull it toward your opposite shoulder for a gluteal stretch.

(b) Lie down on a mat or futon, and extend your right arm straight out from the shoulder. Bend the right knee at a 90-degree angle. With your left hand, pull the bent leg up and over the left leg as shown in Figure 8.22. Turn your head to look toward the right hand (away from the direction of stretch). Breathe in and, using the left hand that is resting on your thigh, pull your bent leg down toward the floor until you feel mild tension along the side of your right hip and lower back. Make sure to keep your "sits" bone on the floor throughout the stretch. Breathe out and let the tension go. Keep the head, upper back, shoulders, and elbows from lifting off of the mat. Hold for eight to ten seconds. Repeat on the opposite side for the left hip.

8.27. Calf Stretches. Face one of the walls of the room or something else (like a beam) that you can lean on for support. Step back and rest your forearms on the wall and let your head rest on the back of your forearms. Now bend one knee and bring it toward the support. To stretch the superficial gastrocnemius muscle, let the back leg be straight. The front leg is

Psoas Stretch

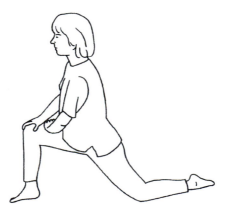

Figure 8.20 Lunge forward in a psoas stretch. Make sure the front hip and leg are at a 90-degree angle or more to avoid stressing the knee.

Quadratus Lumborum (QL) Stretch

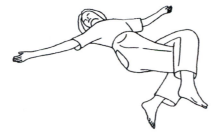

Figure 8.21   Use the weight of the crossed over leg to pull the bottom leg toward the floor.

bent, and the wall supports your arms and head. Breathe in as you imagine your ankle reaching for the floor. Breathe out and feel the stretch in the back of the calf. To isolate the deeper soleus muscle (which unlike the gastrocnemius, does not cross the knee joint), bend the back knee slightly. Once again, breathe in and reach with your ankle toward the floor. Exhale and feel the pull in your calf move down and a little to the side. You are now feeling the soleus muscle. Hold each position for eight to ten seconds. Repeat on the opposite side. (See Figure 8.23.)

COORDINATION

Coordination (or dexterity) is the ability to combine the senses with the body parts to perform motor tasks smoothly and accurately. Juggling is an example of an activity demanding good coordination. Fluid massage transitions and smooth execution of strokes also require dexterity.

Small muscles of the spine, foot, and hand are called intrinsic muscles. We also have very small muscles around the ankle, knee, shoulder, and elbow. These muscles have limited range of motion and very little overall strength. Their importance is in fine movement control. Quite interestingly, much of the reason why we have back pain, are clumsy, or fall is because we lack control of the smaller muscles. Why do these smaller muscles not get enough exercise to help us out? When large muscles (such as the gluteals or quadriceps groups) contract, they overpower the ability of the small muscles to affect the movement. Over the course of our lives, we have kinesthetically "learned" to rely on the strength of the large muscle groups and neglect the development of these intrinsic muscles. Thus, our coordination suffers.

Piriformis Stretch

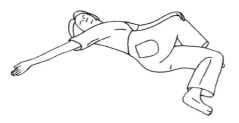

Figure 8.22   Pull your top leg over and down to the floor with your hand.

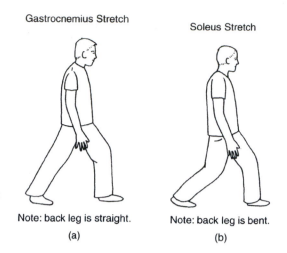

Gastrocnemius Stretch

Soleus Stretch

Figure 8.23 (a–b) Keep the back leg straight for a gastrocnemius stretch and bend it for the soleus stretch.

Note: back leg is straight.

(a)

Note: back leg is bent.

(b)

One way to test your coordination is the "paper ball bounce," described as follows: Wad up a piece of paper into a ball. Bounce the "ball" back and forth between the right and left hands. Keep the hands open and the palms up. Bounce the ball three times with each hand (for a total of six bounces) to demonstrate good coordination. Alternate hands for each bounce.

A stretching program utilizing the Gymnastic or Swiss ball (introduced in Chapter 5) can help lengthen and relax the large muscle groups so that smaller muscles can get to work. The ball necessitates response by each and every muscle in the body. You must remember that many years were spent learning the dysfunctional skill of ignoring the intrinsic muscles of the spine, so learning the replacement skill will take some time. Swiss ball exercises provide a coordination program for life. Additional exercises on the Swiss ball follow (Posner-Mayer, 1995).

Exercise 8.28. Pelvic Rock

Sit on the Swiss ball. Keep your shoulders relaxed while keeping them from hunching over. Allow the upper body to be still while you rotate the hips in four directions—north, south, east, and west. Go only as far as you can while maintaining pain-free motion. Always return to the center before proceeding to the next direction. This exercise will help you to locate pain-free lumbar spinal motion and to support the large muscles of the lumbar spine (erector spinae, quadratus lumborum) while freeing and rotating the small intrinsic ones (rotatores, multifidi).

Exercise 8.29. Trunk Twist

Position yourself on your knees with the ball in front of you. Use a mat or pillow to cushion your knees. Rest your hands on the ball. Keeping your back straight, walk the ball with your hands from the center to the side and back again. Repeat on the other side. This exercise will help you to support the large muscles of the thoracic spine (erector spinae) while freeing and rotating the small intrinsic ones (rotatores, multifidi). It is good for the upper back, lower back, sides of the hips, and rib cage. Spinal twists are also beneficial for internal organs and will help to keep your waistline trim by stretching and toning the external and internal obliques. Trunk twists aid in your ability to turn to the side or look behind you without having to turn your entire body.

The next exercise helps you to improve toe coordination at the same time that you stretch and lengthen the toes.

Exercise 8.30. Toe Curls

Sit on a mat on the floor and extend your legs. Place a bolster under your knees if you wish. Sit up tall or rest back on your arms extended behind you. Make sure your elbows are not locked. Align your head with your chin tucked in.

Curl the toes on both feet at the same time. Do the action gently and slowly so that you will not cramp your feet. Take five counts to curl your toes. Now point your feet by extending your ankles, while keeping your toes curled. This is hard to do, they will want to uncurl. Now flex your ankles in five counts with the toes still curled. When your feet are as curled as they can go, change direction and extend, uncurling your toes and flexing them as much as you can. When your feet are as extended as they can be, curl your toes; repeat the exercise two to three times. (See Figure 8.24.)

Freeing the small muscles around the eyes can keep the eyes soft and free from tension. In the following exercise, it is important to allow your eyes to move and blink between the movements so that your gaze does not become fixed.

Toe Curls

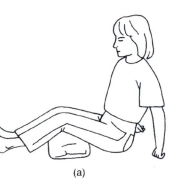 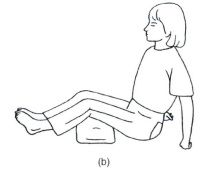

Figure 8.24 (a–b) Curl the toes while flexing and extending at the ankles to improve toe coordination.

(a)

(b)

Exercise 8.31. Improving Eye Coordination

This activity can be practiced as a group. Everyone participating sits in a circle on the floor. Each member takes a turn (one at a time) looking at every other person in the group, allowing the eyes to make contact for a moment and then move on. Do not move the head, just the eyes.

Questions for Discussion. Did your ability to focus change after the exercise? Do you see any more clearly? Did you feel contact between your eyes and the eyes of others? Was there a flash of recognition? Did you glance at others or stare? Did you blink your eyes?

The group can perform the next two variations in unison.

(a) Without moving heads, everyone looks to the right as far as possible. Blink and then glance up, then down. Repeat to the left, and then complete the entire sequence two or three more times.

(b) Again without moving heads, everyone makes a full circle with the eyes. First look to the right, then roll your eyes upward and around to the left. Then move the eyes downward, around and back up to the extreme right. Make two or three circles in this direction and then repeat the sequence to the left.

Questions for Discussion. Were you breathing during the exercise? Did you find it difficult to blink or move your eyes? Did you feel dizzy or get a slight headache? Was there any tension in the muscles of the eye or the back of the neck at the base of the skull?

Other ways to evaluate and at the same time improve hand–eye coordination include the following (Dixon, 1994):

1. Pretend to type or play the piano. Any movement like this that moves the fingers individually will improve your fine motor skills.
2. Use Chinese exercise (also called Baoding or health) balls to increase hand–eye coordination. Exercise balls are small metallic or enamel-covered balls that fit in your hand two at a time. They have a nice bell sound that tinkles as they move. The object is to move them around in your hand using your fingers and to avoid clanging them together. Rhythmically rolling two or three marbles or large steel ball bearings in the palms will mimic the action of the Baoding. Practicing this skill allows each finger to work independently of each other. This dexterity is transferred (hopefully) to other activities where you use you hands, such as playing a musical instrument or performing massage.
3. Increase circulation to the hands before and during a massage by shaking the hands out for 10 counts at high speed.
4. Increase circulation to the wrists before and during a massage by rotating your fists forward 10 times and then backward 10 times.

5. Make a fist with your hand and rhythmically squeeze it tighter, moving from little finger to ring finger to middle finger to index finger to thumb.

CARDIOVASCULAR FITNESS

Cardiovascular fitness is a significant aspect of taking care of your physical self, because those who exercise regularly have a lower incidence of heart disease. The massage therapist should consider doing aerobic exercise for stress reduction and renewed feelings of energy. Walking, swimming, and cycling are all exercise choices that will keep you in good cardiovascular shape. Massage therapy is a physically demanding profession. It takes stamina, concentration, and sensitivity to give a good massage. If you cannot physically keep up with the demands of a full schedule, it will be impossible to deliver quality work.

The heart is a muscle, and just like any other muscle tissue, it must be exercised to become stronger. If the heart is not exercised, it becomes weaker. The heart muscle will expand in size and power when called upon to do more work (Starling's Law). The increase in size and power allows the heart to pump a greater volume of blood with fewer strokes per minute.

Both aerobic and anaerobic exercises can build cardiovascular strength. Aerobic exercises are activities that can be sustained for relatively long periods of time. When practiced continuously over at least 30-minute intervals, they can result in considerable calorie expenditure and are good for reducing body weight. Aerobic activities must also be performed continuously to improve the health of the heart and blood vessels. Aerobics are also valuable in developing muscular endurance, particularly in the quadriceps and calf muscles. These thigh and leg muscles need endurance in order to support the massage therapist throughout the session. Not all aerobic exercise translates into cardiovascular fitness. Bowling and golf are aerobic activities that do little to stimulate circulation. Popular types of aerobics include bicycling, dancing, running, cross-country skiing, swimming, rope jumping, and walking.

Anaerobic exercise requires the use of the body's high-energy fuel. Because it is so intense, this type of activity can be sustained for only short periods of time without rest. You must alternate vigorous anaerobic exercise with frequent rest periods. It does not depend on the body's ability to supply oxygen. Examples of anaerobic exercise include "speed play" (jogging interspersed with brisk calisthenics and walking) and interval training (sprint running or swimming interspersed with slow recovery jogging or swimming). These kinds of workouts should use maximum speed with rest intervals lasting from ten seconds to two minutes, and the series should be repeated eight to thirty times (Corbin and Lindsay, 1988).

General guidelines for cardiovascular activity include the following (Corbin and Lindsay, 1988):

1. *Wear proper shoes* and exercise on a surface that "gives" rather than on a very hard floor (i.e., concrete).
2. Take time to *warm up* before and *cool down* after the workout.
3. *Consider exercising with a partner* or group to help motivate you.

4. *Start "too easy"* rather than "too hard." You can always increase intensity after you determine your reaction to the exercise.

5. It is recommended that you not perform the activity seven days a week. *Rest* at least one and preferably two days a week to lessen the risk of injury.

6. If an injury does occur, *take time to rehabilitate* up to preinjury activity levels.

7. *Vary the exercise routine* daily but make sure all body regions are exercised.

POSTURE REVISITED

As described in Chapter 6, the most common posture problems in the massage therapist are rounded shoulders (hyperkyphosis), a forward head (chin jutting forward), a protruding abdomen, and an exaggerated lower back curve (hyperlordosis). It is not uncommon for several of these inefficient holding patterns to manifest together as a syndrome in a suffering bodyworker. For example, when a practitioner has an exaggerated posterior tilt of the pelvis, he or she is likely to display rounded shoulders and a forward jutting head. In the case of a bodyworker with an anterior pelvic tilt, the outward signs include both a protruding abdomen and hyperlordosis.

Using the physiological components of fitness (stretching, strength, coordination, and cardiovascular health) previously discussed, we can create a concrete plan to positively affect our posture. Indeed, these elements provide us with a practical strategy for building an ergonomically sound carriage.

For example, we know that extra weight in the abdominal area puts additional strain on the lumbar spine. Both pregnancy and paunch can be a source of physical stress. As discussed in Chapter 10, the best strategy to use when pregnant is understanding how to accommodate our changed form. However, when excess weight is not desired, cardiovascular exercise can be used to combat the paunch.

Vertebrae lose bone mass, and intervertebral discs dehydrate as we age. This causes a flattening of the discs and compression of these structures downward. In turn, this can cause loss of height and a more pronounced thoracic curve (hyperkyphosis or dowager's hump). Such skeletal changes lead to muscle tightness and stiffness, and the cycle can degenerate from there. Maintaining healthy bones is important for a healthy back as we age. Again, regular practice of weight-bearing anaerobic and aerobic activities, such as jogging, cycling, and interval weight training, will be most helpful.

Deficiencies in strength and flexibility of key postural muscle groups (abdominals, back muscles, and hip flexors/extensors) contribute to back discomfort and pain (Corbin and Lindsay, 1988). Inadequate abdominal muscle strength allows the pelvis to tilt forward, creating an exaggerated lumbar curve (hyperlordosis or swayback). Exercises like sit-ups and crunches (described earlier in this chapter) work to strengthen the abdominals.

Back muscles need to be both strong and flexible, so both stretching and strengthening is important. Upper back muscles like the trapezius extend into the shoulders and neck, so attention must be given to the physiological fitness of these areas as well. Coordination of the small muscles of the back allows our strength, flexibility, and stamina to be fine-tuned into the supple motions of a healthy and happy bodyworker.

Both the hip flexors (which pull the leg up to your chest, i.e., psoas, quadriceps group) and the hamstrings are important for a balanced posture. Inflexibility in either of these groups can pull the pelvis out of balance. Strength in both groups is important for support against gravity when standing, shifting from a seated to a standing position, and lifting.

Cardiovascular fitness allows blood in every cell in the body. Moving nutrients in and toxins out of an area provides optimal conditions for all of the muscles and muscle groups. Thereby, cardiovascular fitness enhances the effects of all strength, flexibility, and coordination training for improved posture.

Maintaining strength, flexibility, coordination, and cardiovascular fitness is imperative for maintaining good body mechanics. This example (of posture) shows how taking care of yourself physiologically ties directly into establishing good alignment for massage. Body mechanics also involves finding and maintaining alignment while moving. Stringing together a variety of gestures into a session that flows is an athletic feat that requires even more preparation. Because massage is such a physical activity, the importance of maintaining physical health cannot be denied.

SUMMARY

This chapter discusses the physical preparation that can help bodyworkers maintain optimal fitness, needed to sustain a career in massage. Components of physiological health that are discussed here include *strength* (stamina and power), *flexibility, coordination,* and *cardiovascular fitness.* Understanding these aspects of bodyworker fitness can help you identify and use a personal workout that will support your body mechanics.

Strength is the amount of force produced by a single maximal effort. Increasing strength increases your ability to work and reduces the likelihood of acute and chronic injury. Power and endurance are components of strength. Power is the ability to transfer energy into force quickly. Lifting a lot of weight with few repetitions builds power. Russian or pre-event sports massage techniques may be easier when you increase your power. Muscular endurance is the ability of the muscles to repeatedly exert an effort. If you need to perform eight to nine hours of back-to-back Swedish massage, concentrate on increasing endurance or stamina. Building stamina entails using less weight and more repetitions.

Flexibility is the range of motion available in a joint. Flexible bodyworkers are better able to adapt to new physical positions without stress and strain. Stretching enhances flexibility.

Coordination (or dexterity) is the ability to perform motor tasks smoothly and accurately. Massage transitions and even delivery of strokes require coordination.

(continued)

Cardiovascular fitness enhances the effects of strength, flexibility, and coordination. Improving blood flow provides optimal functioning for the therapist's muscles. Aerobics are valuable in developing cardiovascular fitness and muscular endurance.

Massage is a physical activity that requires sustaining physical health through engaging in the appropriate fitness-building activities. Maintaining strength, flexibility, coordination, and cardiovascular fitness is imperative for maintaining good body mechanics. Good posture reflects all of these aspects of physiological preparation.

REFERENCES

Anderson, Bob, *Stretching* (1980). Bolinas, CA: Shelter Publications.

Clarkson, Priscilla, "Oh Those Aching Muscles—Causes and Consequences of Delayed Onset Muscle Soreness," *ASCM's Health and Fitness Journal,* Vol. 1, No. 3 (May/June 1997), pp. 12–17.

Corbin, Charles, and Ruth Lindsay, *Concepts of Physical Fitness with Laboratories,* 6th ed. (1988). Dubuque, IA: Wm. C. Brown Publishers.

Dixon, Marian Wolfe, "Massage I Class Notes" (1994). Portland, OR: Simran Publications.

McArdle, William, Frank Katch, and Victor Katch, "How Muscles Adapt," in *Exercise Physiology: Energy, Nutrition and Human Performance* (1986). Philadelphia: Lea & Febiger.

Newton, Donald, "Massage II Notes" (1996). Portland, OR: Simran Publications.

Posner-Mayer, Joanne, *Swiss Ball Applications for Orthopedic and Sports Medicine* (1995). Denver, CO: Ball Dynamics International, Inc.

Tortora, Gerard, *Introduction to the Human Body: The Essentials of Anatomy and Physiology,* 3rd ed. (1994). New York: HarperCollins College Publishers.

Chapter Nine

Taking Care of Yourself— Part II (Psychological)

CHAPTER OBJECTIVES

Conceptual Objectives   The massage student/practitioner who successfully completes this chapter (reading and exercises) will be able to:

- Define *personal space.*

- List and define important communications skills for the massage therapist (including asking and receiving permission, equalizing, and assertiveness).

- Describe methods for improving assertiveness (including consistent body language, DESC [describe, express, specify, consequences], broken record approach, escalation, delaying, compromise, clarification, deciding not to assert).

Practical Objectives   The massage student/practitioner who successfully completes this chapter (reading and exercises) will be able to:

- Role play three situations in which boundary issues could create problems for a massage therapist.

- Identify and articulate professional boundaries.

- Identify ways to take time out from massage.

- Identify sources of support for massage therapists.

- Identify referral options.

Ask any good bodyworker and they will acknowledge that clients are not simply a jumble of sore muscles and injured anatomical parts. People need nurturing for their whole selves, not just for their bodies (although the medium of touch interfaces with the physical skin). Clients have hearts and minds and souls as well as flesh. Likewise, it is true that massage practitioners are more than physical bodies. Perhaps you are questioning how mental and emotional states can affect body mechanics. If you doubt the effect of psychological factors on body mechanics, consider the following experience.

Exercise 9.1. Exploring the Effect of Emotions on Physical Balance

Pause, now, to stand up and balance on one leg. If this is easy for you, stand up and balance on one leg with your eyes closed. Make a mental note of this baseline—how easy or difficult the task is to do. The next time you are emotionally upset, see if you can detach enough to repeat the one-legged balancing act. I will hazard a guess that the emotional upset will affect the control and awareness of your body. First, it will probably be difficult to separate from your feelings enough to stop to balance on one leg. Second, the upset feelings are likely to make you wobblier on your feet.

When we are feeling uneasy, we lose the mental edge that allows us to observe small difficulties in moving and massage. We are more likely to injure ourselves from not paying attention. We are also more likely to injure ourselves because we no longer care. It becomes "too difficult" to turn both feet in the direction of a stroke, just to protect the low back. It takes "too much attention" to mobilize different parts of your body in order to protect your wrists. It is "too hard" to take the extra step rather than leaning over and hunching your shoulders during a massage.

When psyches are not taken care of, it becomes "too much trouble" to take care of the physical self. Consequently, we settle for habitual positions or familiar movements that are "safe" even when they sacrifice physical comfort. This is a serious problem that can lead to the kinds of recurrent patterns that cause repetitive motion injuries. This chapter outlines ways in which the massage professional can foster healthier emotional and mental states. The goal is to preserve the psychological health and energy necessary to keep abreast of faults in body mechanics. Sections are dedicated to building the psychological skills that will help sustain a career in massage. The psychological skills highlighted here are *establishing clear boundaries, communicating clearly and well,* taking *time out* for yourself, finding *support,* and maintaining *interest.*

ESTABLISHING CLEAR BOUNDARIES

Because touch crosses a customary boundary (the skin) that separates one human from another, it is important that clear boundaries between client and therapist be defined and understood. There is a great potential for misunderstanding and inappropriate behavior within the confines of a massage session. For example, the professional touch of a massage practitioner can be confused with sexual touching. Or, for the client, the touch of a therapist can inadvertently evoke past memories of unhealthy touch. When our professional behavior does not convey clear boundaries to clients, the situation is likely to backfire, causing needless stress and hurt feelings all around. During massage training and in professional practice, we need to establish a safe and comfortable environment that engenders trust and mutual respect. Indeed, it is only in such an environment that therapeutic massage can be given.

It is important to adhere to boundaries whether the person you are treating is a friend, partner, family member, or clinical client. In a massage, an inequality in power exists because the therapist is in control and clothed, while the client is on the receiving end and undressed, and therefore more vulnerable. As the therapist, it is your responsibility to remain aware of this power differential and ensure that it is not abused.

You cannot maintain a safe space for clients to heal without setting limits. In order to set boundaries or limits, you first need to know what you want. Boundaries can refer to time, money, intimacy, or the kinds of bodywork services that you provide.

Knowing what you want entails discovering who you are. Exploring requires a new process of self-examination each and every day. Some days, you may be feeling more open and on other days more vulnerable. One day, your body may be performing at peak condition so that you can perform with maximum output during sessions. Another day, you may be recovering from a strained Achilles tendon and need to draw back and be more protective of the ailing leg. Healthy boundaries will have to be redrawn each day that you work and live. On a given day, notice your physical responses to your client's behavior. Are you feeling lightheaded or nauseous? Does your back or head ache? Do you have a sinking feeling in your stomach? Physical sensations may be clues that your comfort zone is being encroached upon. Check in with your heart and mind as well. Is your heart in the work you are doing? Does it feel heavy? Is a little voice whispering that something is not right with your world?

As soon as you recognize an uncomfortable feeling in connection with a client's behavior, let your client know. This gives the client an option of stopping or modifying the objectionable conduct. Even if you cannot figure out "why," when something does not seem right, speak out. If you do not know what needs to happen to make things safe again, consider these three golden rules—*stop, slow down,* and *back off. Stop* doing what does not work when it is clear that something is not working. *Slow down* rather than trying to power or fake your way through resistances. *Back off* when you cannot safely perform a technique or accomplish a goal. Take the time to figure out what you need, and do not be afraid to ask for it. When you are not specific about your boundaries, relationships with clients can become confused. Instead of an avenue for healing, the massage session becomes the scene for a melodrama where both parties are distressed or out of balance.

When you are in the midst of an emotional response, it can be overwhelming to set and enforce boundaries. You may find yourself trying to plead or justify your position if you are feeling guilty about setting a limit. When you feel afraid, angry, or guilty, some preliminary work to process your emotions is needed to help clear the confusing feelings. Once free of emotional encumbrance, you will be better able to establish clear boundaries without having to explain or justify the logic. In a more clearheaded state, you can choose (but not feel obligated) to share your reasons with the involved person.

Processing emotions may mean calling a friend, mentor, or colleague. It may be taking a class or joining a support group or seeking appropriate counseling to clear confusing or hurtful issues. Learn to identify cues that signal a need for help. Certain circumstances can actually invite boundary conflicts. Richard Beyer, a hypnotherapist who specializes in relationship issues, compiled a slate of potentially unhealthy situations (Sprague, 1994). Beyer identifies the following signs that indicate boundaries have been or are likely to be crossed:

1. Trusting no one—or, on the other hand, trusting everyone.
2. Telling everything about yourself—even to total strangers. Sharing intimate secrets with someone on your first meeting.
3. Falling in love with a new acquaintance or falling in love with anyone who reaches out to help you.
4. Being sexual, for your partner, not for yourself. Acting on your first sexual impulse.
5. Going against personal values or rights to please others.
6. Accepting food, gifts, or touch that you don't want.
7. Touching a person without permission. (Although massage clients imply a general consent to be touched when they employ you for massage, you cannot assume that clients are giving tacit permission to be touched in all areas. First-time or even repeat clients may not be comfortable with touch around the neck, inside the thighs, over the glutes, or in other areas. If you are unclear about how comfortable your client is with touch in any area, it is best to ask.)
8. Taking as much as you can get for the sake of getting.
9. Giving as much as you can give for the sake of giving. Allowing someone to take as much as they can from you.
10. Letting others direct your life or define what you want or need.
11. Believing others can anticipate your needs and expecting them to automatically fulfill them.
12. Falling apart so that someone will take care of you.
13. Cutting yourself or hitting, biting, or burning holes in your body. These are acts of self-mutilation.
14. Overindulgence in alcohol, food, or drugs. Alcoholism, bulimia, and anorexia.
15. Accepting sexual, physical, or emotional abuse from others or perpetrating these types of abuse on others.

Sometimes you may feel uneasy about your feelings or actions but cannot pinpoint exactly what is wrong. These are times when a danger of overstepping your authority is not so obvious, but it still exists. Estelle Disch, PhD, a clinical sociologist and psychotherapist, has compiled a list of queries to help massage practitioners identify whether boundary issues are interfering with the ability to work effectively (1992). "Are You in Trouble With a Client?" includes items on various aspects of the therapeutic relationship. Sample statements (to which the reader responds with a yes or no answer) include, "I often tell my personal problems to this client." "The client often invites me to social events and I don't feel comfortable saying either yes or no. "The client's pain is so deep it scares me." "This client owes me a lot of money and I don't know what to do about it." "I sometimes hate this client." Disch's questionnaire can be used to red flag issues that need attention. If you have already attempted to change the identified behaviors but still find a tendency to continue, you may need to seek outside help. Ben Benjamin (1992) suggests seeking professional supervision if your answer is affirmative to any of the questions. Benjamin also advocates supervision on a regular basis to improve the work of all bodyworkers.

Sometimes, even with the benefit of checklists and other aids, you will be confused about whether a boundary has been violated or not. This may be because the situation you are currently experiencing is confusing, or it may be because you have not had any good models for boundary setting in the past. Take heart in the knowledge that whatever your past or present circumstances, setting limits is a skill that can be practiced and improved.

Personal Space

One boundary that separates "you" from "not you" is your skin. In addition, many people are aware of a 9-foot by 11-foot (approximate) elliptical "boundary" that extends out from the body (Czimbal and Zadikov, 1991). This aura or "personal space" is generally perceived to be shorter in the front and back, and longer around the sides. Within the ellipse, it feels like "your space." Outside, it feels like shared space. It does not feel good when others enter the space uninvited. The size of the ellipse is determined by culture and past history with touch. Families who customarily touched a lot and were physically close tend to encourage a small personal space. Families who maintained more distance between one another while talking, eating, or sharing tend to create adults who surround themselves with a larger circle. You can explore your personal boundaries by answering the following questions.

1. Where is the physical boundary outside your body? What does it feel like?
2. Is the size and quality of the personal space different for other people?
3. Who do you allow inside your personal space? What characteristics do they have?
4. Have certain people crossed that boundary without permission? What did it feel like? What were the circumstances when boundaries were crossed? What did you do when someone moved into your personal space?

Exercise 9.2. Exploring Your Personal Space

You will need a partner to complete this exercise. There are two roles—boundary setter and boundary tester. Try both roles before answering the questions for discussion at the end of the exercise.

To begin, the boundary setter physically defines his or her personal space by drawing an invisible line with the hand—around the front, sides, and back of his or her body, as well as overhead (and underneath, if appropriate). The boundary tester witnesses this to clearly understand the limits of the setter's boundary. Within the line, the space belongs to the boundary setter. Outside, the space is shared with others.

In the first variation, the tester comes right up to the edge of the boundary but does not go past it. The boundary setter's personal space is like an invisible force field that repels any intruder. Before going on, both individuals should stop and see how going up to the edge feels from their individual perspectives.

Next, the tester comes up to the limit again, but this time continues right on through. Stop and think about the feeling that this situation creates.

Finally, the tester comes to the border and asks permission to go to the other side. The boundary setter must consider whether he or she can comfortably grant permission to cross. If it feels okay to revise the boundary, permission is granted. The tester then moves past the imaginary line. If the setter decides that it does not feel okay to have the tester come through, the tester must respect this decision and move back. (*Note:* It is extremely important that the setter does not grant permission to the tester just to be "nice" or because he or she does not want to hurt the other person's feelings. As stated before, both people must check in with what *they* want and need in order to set or move a valid boundary.) Both partners again stop and consider how they feel about what has transpired.

Now switch roles and repeat the entire sequence.

Questions for Discussion. Which role did you like better? Why? How did it feel to "invade" the other person's space? How did it feel to have your space invaded? How did it feel to ask permission to come closer? How did it feel to be asked for permission to change the rules? How did it feel to grant or refuse entry? How did it feel to be granted or refused permission to enter into someone else's personal space?

COMMUNICATIONS SKILLS

Exercise 9.2 is an activity that I recommend for all beginning massage students in order to clarify the personal impact of boundaries. In the massage field, conflicts about limits are likely the rule rather than the exception. Professional bodywork boundaries can be crossed in many ways. To be sensitive to client boundaries, therapists need to avoid touching without permission, pressing too forcefully when touching a client, rushing into clients' personal space without giving them time to react, or using criticism or a harsh or loud voice in the session. To be sensitive to their own needs, therapists need to speak up when clients inadvertently or consciously force intimacy that is not appropriate to the bodywork session.

Several key issues are brought out into the open with Exercise 9.2. One, of course, is the visceral effect of setting and articulating limits. Another key point is the need to take stock of "where you are" in the moment to more clearly see where you want to establish boundaries.

Permission

In the last exercise, the need for massage therapists to develop clear communication skills is brought to the fore. One aspect of clear communication is *asking for permission* before entering a space where the limits are either in dispute or unclear. Following hand in hand with asking is *waiting to receive permission* before crossing a boundary that has been previously set.

Equalizing

What happens when a therapist and a client have conflicting ideas as to where the safe line of demarcation should be fixed? When one person wishes to be in another person's personal space without receiving permission, a boundary disagreement exists. People with different-sized ellipses can get into some awkward boundary disagreements before finding a good compromise. I have actually seen "dances" between two people of different cultures and expectations across the floor. One partner continually advances because the personal gulf seems too great while the other retreats because the first person keeps getting too close.

Massage therapists pursue their practice in a variety of settings. No matter whether the venue is in a home office, a neutral environment like a day spa or health club, or in the client's business place or home, the person giving the massage is responsible for inspiring safety, respect, and comfort. This behooves all communications to be sensitive, noninvasive, and straightforward. As the practitioner, you must maintain appropriate limits while working and make sure to equalize down to a mutually shared comfort zone. When you find yourself in the receiving role, it is your job to let the practitioner know right away when bodywork is uncomfortable in any way.

A good rule of thumb when two people need to agree on a mutual boundary is to *equalize* down to the lower level of intimacy. For equalizing to occur, the person who wants the more intimate form of touch must accept the less intimate touch desired by the second party. For example, let us examine the situation in which a bodyworker, Teresa, is saying good-bye to her first-time client, Mary. Teresa wants to hug Mary, but Mary is extending her hand for a handshake. For equalizing to occur, the therapist must adjust to the lower level of intimacy and shake hands only.

Assertiveness

Let us say the tables were reversed. What if the client offers a higher level of intimacy than you feel comfortable accepting? In that case, for equalizing to occur, you need to make your wishes clear, and again a handshake and nothing more is warranted. How will you ensure that equalizing happens when the other person does not seem to care about or respect your wishes?

For instance, what if a client tries to force a good-bye hug without regard for your feelings? If clients do not like or agree with what you want and need, they may try to make you feel ashamed or guilty. They may try to bargain or accuse you of manipulating or controlling the situation. Beware! If you have not gotten completely rid of emotional baggage, these people will be able to hook into old "patterns" and deter you from establishing a healthy boundary. In these cases, it is important to learn and practice the skill of *assertiveness*. Taking care of you can mean speaking up or removing yourself from the situation. Empowering yourself can take many forms. It all depends on how much you are willing to risk and whether there is a safety issue involved. Acting assertively means learning how to stand up for your needs.

In the face of potential conflicts and limitations, it may be helpful to identify what we *can* do. Do healers have absolute "rights" that cannot be compromised? What boundaries are inviolable? *The Counseling Center* (1996) formulates some basic rights for all health care providers:

1. The right to ask questions
2. The right to not feel guilty or bad
3. The right to have and state my own opinions
4. The right to say "no"
5. The right to say how I feel
6. The right to stand up for myself
7. The right to be imperfect
8. The right to get angry
9. The right to make mistakes
10. The right to ask for what I want
11. The right to accept compliments
12. The right to not be intimidated or patronized
13. The right to slow down
14. The right to set limits
15. The right to not explain myself
16. The right to be ME

Let us begin the discussion of assertiveness with a look at how people typically react to boundary disagreements. Sometimes, as massage therapists, we view the world through rose-colored glasses and expect our world to be free of disagreements or unpleasantness. It is important to recognize that conflict is natural, even though many feelings that go along with conflict are not comfortable. Most people either avoid conflict or pretend it does not exist. One theory is that we avoid and deny because we have been conditioned to believe that it is bad to disagree. Disagreements mean arguing or fighting. When we view conflict as an avenue for problem solving rather than a synonym for fighting, attitudes toward assertiveness change.

If we attempt to put the myriad of possible reactions to conflict on a graph, most people would be surprised to see that assertiveness falls in the middle, not at the extreme. Nonassertiveness, assertiveness, and aggressiveness are characteristic responses that lie on the continuum of responses to boundary disagreements. (See Figure 9.1.)

At one end of the spectrum lies nonassertiveness. Nonassertive behavior is

Figure 9.1 Assertiveness is in the midrange of behaviors on a continuum that ranges from nonassertive to aggressive. Assertiveness maintains a balance of concern for your own rights and the rights of others.

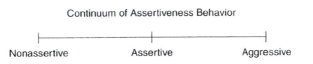

Continuum of Assertiveness Behavior

Nonassertive   Assertive   Aggressive

defined as being totally concerned with the rights of others at your own expense. People in the helping professions, such as massage therapists, can often be inclined to this extreme. At the other extreme is aggressiveness. This is defined as being totally concerned with what you want at the expense of others. Aggressive people get what they want no matter what, "come hell or high water." True assertiveness lies in the middle. It is a practice that attempts to satisfy personal needs while maintaining good relationships with others. Assertiveness is based on the premise that everyone has rights—both you and the other guy. The assertive approach to life conflicts leads to a state of health and balance. In contrast, both aggressiveness and nonassertiveness lead to imbalances that can cause serious disease states. For aggressive personalities, poor interpersonal relationships provide stress. Aggressiveness has been associated with an increased incidence of "Type A" stress-induced diseases such as coronary heart disease, high blood pressure, and ulcers (Allen, 1983). For nonassertive personalities, unmet needs become the stressors. Research (Allen, 1983) correlates nonassertive tendencies with cancer. These studies suggest that failing to practice assertive behavior can be detrimental to your health.

To determine your predisposition to act and speak confidently, take some time to respond to the "Are you assertive?" test below. The higher the score (76 is a maximum), the more assertively you usually behave. The lower the score (0 is the minimum), the more your resolution style reflects nonassertiveness. The scale does not measure aggressiveness.

Exercise 9.3. "Are You Assertive?" Test

Directions: Answer each question by marking the appropriate number from 0 to 4. Mark 0 if your response is almost never, 1 for seldom, 2 for sometimes, 3 for usually, and 4 for almost always. Answers should reflect how you generally express yourself in a given situation. In the event that a situation does not apply to you, circle the number of the response that you think would most characterize you. Answers should reflect an honest opinion of what you *do* or *would do,* not what you "wish you would do" or what you think you "ought to do."

_____ 1. When you meet a stranger in a social situation, do you initiate introductions and start a conversation?

_____ 2. Do you speak up when someone breaks in line in front of you?

_____ 3. Do you freely volunteer information or opinions in group discussions, even when you don't know the other people very well?

_____ 4. Do you dominate when you and close friends are deciding how to spend leisure time together?

_____ 5. Do you feel comfortable about returning defective merchandise?

_____ 6. Do you ask questions in class without fear that you might sound stupid?

_____ 7. Do you feel comfortable about asking reasonable favors of others?

_____ 8. If your instructor makes what you consider to be an unreasonable request, do you express your feelings and reasons to him or her?

_____ 9. If you are angry with your parents, can you tell them so directly?

_____10. Are you able to withstand purchasing things you don't really want, even if a salesman applies pressure?

_____11. Do you insist that a spouse or roommate(s) take on a fair share of the necessary chores?

_____12. When a person is overdue in returning something of value to you, do you mention it?

_____13. When talking to someone, do you find it easy to maintain eye contact?

_____14. Can you accept graciously when you are given a compliment?

_____15. Do you know what to say to an attractive person you are interested in?

_____16. If someone keeps bumping your chair or regularly talks during a movie, do you ask the person to stop?

_____17. When the food in a restaurant is not prepared or served to your satisfaction, do you demand that the situation be corrected?

_____18. Are you able to invite someone you think is attractive out?

_____19. At meals with family or friends, do you find it easy to break into or initiate the conversation?

Questions for Discussion.   Total up your points. How did you score? What does the score tell you about yourself? How can you use this information to better handle conflict situations?

_____

Behaving assertively is more difficult for some than for others. Even so, there are a number of techniques that can help everyone, no matter what the initial skill level, to practice more effective and assertive behavior. These techniques include utilizing learnable skills like assertive _body language,_ the _DESC_ form of saying what you want, the _broken record_ approach, _escalation, delaying, compromise, clarification,_ and _choosing not to assert._

Body Language.   Check for nonassertive, assertive, and aggressive cues in your habitual body postures and movements. Assertive body language can help you to say what you mean and mean what you say. Assertiveness is not only a function of what you say, but also how you say it.

If you are wondering how body language can affect the efficacy of a message, consider the following example. Suppose a student came to my office to discuss what appears to be an error in grading. During the interview, the student talked very softly without making eye contact. Instead of standing or sitting comfortably, the student constantly swayed or shifted weight. The student's voice had a whiny, hesitant sound. Under these circumstances, it might be hard for me to take any request seriously or to give it much credence.

Consider once again the same basic scenario of a grade dispute. Now, what if the student approached while I sat engrossed in paperwork. As the student stated the request, I leaned forward with glaring eyes and my hands clenched into fists. My voice rose to a shouting pitch and my finger pointed at the student. This is a pretty aggressive stance, and the nonverbal message is that this probably isn't a good time to talk.

Alternately, what if the student stated the case and I responded by adjusting my watch, tapping a pen, and looking over my glasses? Again, it would not be hard to surmise that my attention was elsewhere, and it might be a good idea to consult at another time.

If, on the contrary, both parties maintained a comfortably erect posture and established eye contact, this body language provides support for a real talk. To make the request/presentation more effective, the student could utilize other confident and straightforward body messages, such as facing straight on; speaking in a clear, steady voice that was loud enough to hear; and keeping body cues consistent with the words being spoken. It would *not* be consistent body language, for example, to say, "It makes me so angry," while smiling at the listener.

DESC.   A second tool for clearly and effectively saying what you mean is the *DESC* form of communicating. Each of the letters in the acronym represents a crucial step in the method: D stands for "describe," E is for "express," S stands for "specify," and C refers to "consequences." *D*escribe means to paint a verbal picture of the situation at hand. *E*xpress means to say what you feel about the situation. You *s*pecify several ways that you would like the other person's behavior to change. *C*onsequences are what you will do if the other person's behavior changes to your satisfaction, AND what you will do if it does not.

The form goes like this (fill in the blanks):

When you _____ (describe the situation),

I feel _____ (express what you feel).

I would like/or prefer _____ (specify how you want the other person's behavior to change).

If you do, I will _____.

If you do not, I will _____ (spell out the consequences).

Feel free to use these steps to effectively implement the DESC approach:

1. Decide what boundaries you need and want. (Are these boundaries negotiable or are they firm?)
2. Monitor whether the agreement is being kept.

3. If the agreement is not being kept, inquire why not, and decide what you need to do to enforce it (that is, what will be the consequences). This is the hard part. Consequences have to be something that you would really do. They are not what you would like to do, but if the situation came up that you would have to enact them, it would be too threatening to your relationship. For instance, what if a client keeps showing up half an hour late to sessions? In the past, you have been accommodating the late arrival and going past the time allotted to give an entire hour on the table. You feel cheated and unappreciated. What would you do? Share these consequences with the client/antagonist.

4. Enact the consequences if the situation does not change to your satisfaction.

The big advantage of this communication method is mapping out how you want to respond in a conflict situation before it actually occurs. DESC takes you out of the charged atmosphere where emotions can override intellect. In the "heat of the moment," we often speak and act before we think. DESC (*d*escribe, *ex*-plain, *s*pecify, and *c*onsequences) requires planning and practice of what you are going to say before the conflict arises.

The *broken record* approach is just what it sounds like. When someone seems not to hear what you say, simply repeat the message until it finally gets through.

Escalation is starting out with an appropriate response and realizing the option of becoming more aggressive (and loud) until the message is heard.

Delaying is a tactic to use when you do not know how to react in the moment. It postpones an argument in order to allow some space and time to elapse. The breathing room allows you to determine how you want to respond. A statement that demonstrates delaying would be, "Maybe we can discuss this issue later tonight, after dinner." One big caution in utilizing "delaying" is not to delay open-endedly. Make sure that you set a time for discussion in the future. Without a specific time for future discussion, the tactic sounds as if you are trying to avoid the issue forever.

Compromise gives the other person a way out. If you back someone up against the wall, they will react like a "caged tiger" and strike out against you.

Clarification means making sure that you understand the other guy and that he understands you. To accomplish the first part (clear understanding), ask your partner to clarify any expectations and repeat those expectations out loud (active listening). To accomplish the second part (clear communication), the DESC model can be very helpful in stating what you want clearly.

Realizing the option to *decide not to assert* is a viable alternative for assertive behavior. This might be an appropriate choice, for example, when you are in the midst of participating in a public event, like a party or fundraiser.

COMMUNICATING PROFESSIONAL BOUNDARIES

Professional bodywork policies must be decided upon, vocalized, and discussed with clients. Clear professional boundaries allow you to easily answer questions about types of services, training and experience, appointment policies, fees, client/practitioner expectations, sexual appropriateness, and recourse policy (Palmer, 1993). This goes a long way in setting up a safe professional situation.

The client should be able to find out what kinds of treatment the practitioner offers, such as whether the therapist addresses pain and other medical problems or offers a stress reduction and relaxation approach. As far as training goes, it is the consumer's right to be assured of the competence of the practitioner. It lets clients feel that they are in competent hands to know that the therapist has at least the minimum standard in massage therapy, which is currently 500 hours of training over six to twelve months. If clients thoroughly understand the therapist's policies with regard to appointments, they can avoid disappointment or surprise. Specificity about the length of each session, office hours and availability, and cancellation policies creates the basis for a good working relationship. Money is a charged issue for most people. Make sure your fee policies are clear before beginning a new therapeutic relationship. Since there is generally some anxiety about a stranger touching the body, it is helpful to review details of what to expect in a typical bodywork session. This is true not only for clients who have never received bodywork before, but also for all first-time clients. Generally, clients want to know what parts of the body you will work on, where they will be draped and covered, how undressed to get under the drape, if a shower is available, and whether you use oil, lotion, or powder.

Although it should be evident that sexual misconduct is always unethical and inappropriate in a massage situation, you should state that it is unethical and inappropriate. Some therapists do this with a statement on their intake form and/or prominently posted on the wall and/or during the interview process. It is *always* the responsibility of the health professional to ensure that sexual misconduct does not occur.

Exercise 9.4. Role-Plays

To develop the ability to apply equalizing and assertive behavior to boundary disagreements, practice role-playing these scenarios.

1. One partner is a massage student who wants to try out a deep tissue massage technique that was described secondhand but has not been demonstrated in class yet. The other partner plays her client, who fears that the student will hurt him with the new technique.

   Some possible developments of the story line include the following. Act out each option and discuss how it feels.

   a. Student/therapist continues practicing the technique despite the client's protests. Because the student/therapist has not actually been taught what to do, the student/receiver ends up getting physically bruised. In response, the student/receiver vows never to get massage again.

   b. The student/therapist does not practice the new technique but feels hurt and "not into" the massage. The bodywork is light and erratic. The student/receiver ends up thinking the student/therapist is a poor massage practitioner.

What do you think would be an appropriate response to this situation? Consider the issue with regard to each individual's perspective.

2. One partner is a massage client who becomes sexually attracted to the partner who is playing the therapist. The second partner, the one who plays the therapist, can act out the role with several variations: (a) he or she is mutually attracted to the client, or (b) the feeling is not requited. Other variations can use different combinations of genders, for example, client/male–therapist/female, client/female–therapist/male, client and therapist/male, client and therapist/female. Dramatize each option and discuss how it makes you feel. Possible plot developments include the following. Try each alternative and consider its merit.

   a. The therapist tells the client, "It is alright to initiate a sexual relationship," because the client is a regular and a big tipper and the therapist does not want to lose that client. The therapist figures he or she can just stall the issue in the future with this client.

   b. The therapist is highly insulted and angrily tells the client to leave the office and never return.

What do you think would be an appropriate response to each situation? Consider the issue with regard to each player's perspective.

3. The client presents with severe varicose veins. The situation can advance in several ways. Act out each option presented here and discuss it from both points of view.

   a. The practitioner is rushing through the massage. He or she is inattentive and nonresponsive to the client's requests to slow down and lighten up. Meanwhile, the client feels as though the practitioner is working so quickly and deeply that his or her body is not able to assimilate the work.

   b. The practitioner avoids the legs entirely and makes some comments about how ugly varicosities are. In fact, the touch over the entire body is very light and tentative. When the client comments that he or she is ticklish, the therapist acts hurt and stops the massage. From the client's perspective, the pressure is so light that it feels ticklish and uncomfortable.

4. One partner is a massage student trading with another student for the first time. The student/therapist is not very skilled at draping yet. The drape hangs loosely, and as the practitioner attempts to effleurage the leg, his or her hand catches in the drape, undoing it. The student/client is not sure about the student/therapist's intentions. He or she feels uncomfortable about the way the draping is so insecure.

   a. When the student/receiver tells the therapist about his or her discomfort, the therapist laughs it off and makes a comment about "people who are too uptight about their own bodies."

b. The receiver does not say anything, but vows never to work with this student again. Later, the receiver spreads the information that this student/therapist is unsafe to work with.

What do you think would be an appropriate response to this situation? Consider the issue with regard to each individual's perspective.

TIME OUT

Massage therapists are blessed to make their livelihood from such enjoyable and rewarding work. However, this does not preclude a need for other avenues for enjoyment in life. "All work and no play makes Johnnie (or Johanna) a dull boy (or girl)," even when the work is generally fun.

Playtime is sometimes referred to as recreation. "Re-creation" has the wonderful connotation of creating something all over again. By concentrating on having fun, we "re-create" our world and our place in it. We become ourselves again, but new. We find ourselves fresh and better able to deal with challenges of daily life and work as a bodyworker. Taking time out to play can leave us feeling that we can take on the world.

Play is not only needed for process time; it is also valuable in itself. Play lights a fire under our vitality and creativity. When I observe how children learn, I see that children learn best by playing. If that is true for young bodies and minds, why shouldn't it also be true for adults? We cannot grow as bodyworkers or learn anything new without allowing ourselves to play. Taking time out for self-nurturing is not a luxury in the field of massage therapy. It is a necessity for our mental and emotional health and peace of mind.

Exercise 9.5. Time Out with Nurturing Activities

Take some time right now to generate a list of nurturing activities that you can incorporate into your life. These should be things that you *can* and *will do.* A useful list will not include activities that you should do, or would do if the world were different. These activities are specifically for the times when your world is not a perfect place. If you are waiting for everything to fall into place before you act on your ideals, I can almost guarantee that this will not happen.

I ask massage students to generate lists like these once every semester, at least four times a year. They are especially helpful to look at right after midterms, or in the middle of winter here in the Northwest, when the skies have been depressingly damp and gray for months without an end in sight.

Ideally, your nurturing activity list will reflect activities that are fun for you, without regard to what anyone else thinks. For that reason, I think it is important to reflect and meditate about what you find to be self-nurturing. If you draw a blank about possibilities for nurturing activities, think about the following suggestions that have been generated by students of massage and health science. If you feel disconnected with what could be fun, pick a suggestion from the list and try it. It just may turn out to be fun.

1. Take a bubble bath with scented oils and herbs. Light candles around the tub and/or use Christmas lights for illumination.
2. Go for a hike. Look at your surroundings. The Northwest is blessed with beautiful forests with old growth and wild and scenic waterfalls. Heading west, the tumultuous Pacific Ocean provides a backdrop for walks. What wonders of nature (or civilization) surround you?
3. Play with children or pets. Animals and little human creatures instinctively know how to have fun. Let them show you how to play with toys or marvel at the joys in the world.
4. Put on some pleasing music. Listening to rhythms and melodies can transport people to a better plane. Play an instrument if you know how. Perhaps you have always wanted to learn how to play guitar or piano. If so, what better time than now?
5. Enjoy a cup of hot chocolate. (You can substitute herbal tea or decaf coffee, if you like.) Invite a friend to join you for conversation or enjoy the quiet inside yourself.
6. Read a book. It does not matter whether you choose fiction or nonfiction, fantasy or reality, history, sci-fi, or comedy. Books can transport you to a different time and place or simply give you a different perspective on your life as it is now.
7. Do something out of your ordinary routine.
8. Buy yourself or loved ones some flowers and let their fragrance and color fill your senses.
9. Generate your own list of nurturing activities from past experiences. What would feel entrancing and nurturing to you?
10. Consider the following poem by an anonymous author (Billard, 1996; *The Counseling Center*, 1996):

Letting Go

To "let go" does not mean to stop caring; it means I can't do it for someone else.

To "let go" is not to cut myself off; it's the realization I can't control another.

To "let go" is not to enable, but to allow learning from natural consequences.

To "let go" is to admit powerlessness, which means the outcome is not in my hands.

To "let go" is not to try to change or blame another; it's to make the most of myself.

To "let go" is not to care for, but to care about.

To "let go" is not to fix, but to be supportive.
To "let go" is not to judge, but to allow another to be a human being.
To "let go" is not to be in the middle arranging all the outcomes, but to
allow others to affect their own destinies.
To "let go" is not to be protective; it's to permit another to face reality.
To "let go" is not to deny, but to accept.
To "let go" is not to nag, scold, or argue, but instead to search out my
own shortcomings and correct them.
To "let go" is not to adjust everything to my desires, but to take each day
as it comes and cherish myself in it.
To "let go" is not to regret the past, but to grow and live for the future.
To "let go" is to fear less and love more.

FINDING SUPPORT

Just as we may be tempted to shortchange scheduling sufficient "time outs," we may neglect to call on others for help. At certain times, we may need outside help to effectively "recharge our batteries." It is important to remember that we are not in this work alone, even though sometimes it may seem as if we are. The massage trade can be very isolating. Massage therapists are generally working in one-on-one situations. Clients may be reluctant to offer more feedback or conversation than a hastily mumbled "fix me" at the outset and an "I feel great" as they leave. Before we know it, practitioners can find themselves starving for recognition. The healer's hallmark can put us in a position of constantly giving out to others. It may seem as if we never get back what we give. Massage practitioners need to make the effort to reach out to colleagues for professional support. It is helpful to think of ourselves as part of a network of health care practitioners that form a larger circle of professional support.

Referrals

Each day, a bodyworker confronts complex cases that skirt the boundaries of scope of practice. The advice of someone with a slightly different perspective can help sort out these difficult situations. On a strictly physiological level, let's use the example of a client who presents with a spasm that is not responding to massage. After three to five sessions pass without improvement, I suspect that the "knots" that I am palpating may not be muscular spasms or fascial adhesions. It is imperative that this client gets the problem checked by a qualified health care practitioner in order to rule out a diagnosis of lipomas (fat tumors) or any other contraindication for massage. So I look to my referral list and suggest that my massage client visit a physician or nurse practitioner before continuing to schedule more sessions. Consider the following typical case in which the bodyworker needs to refer. A client presents with constant pain that extends from the low back down the back of both legs. My first thought is not to jump in there to try and fix it. Instead, I remember that pains running down both legs are *not* signs of piriformis entrapment (and may be symptomatic of disc compression in the spine). Spinal adjustments are not within my area of expertise. Prudence requires a referral to a chiropractor or osteopathic physician. It is helpful to remember that the area of expertise for the bodyworker is soft tissue dysfunction (meaning problems with muscles, tendons, or ligamentous tissue). If the client's problem lies somewhere else, we need to refer. Although many people come with stories of emotional pain and suffering, it is important to remember that the body is the area of expertise for massage providers. When clients inappropriately dump on us or reenact emotional releases without an accompanying lasting physical improvement, it is time to refer to a counselor or other mental health care professional. We are doing both our clients and ourselves a disservice to keep mute about such alternative avenues for change.

It is vital for massage professionals to develop a network of referrals for clients, and for us. Good massage practitioners are health educators and advocates for the health care community. We are often the first people to spot bruises or other possible indicators of serious health problems. We may be the ones our clients reach out to first when they are undergoing a serious life transition (e.g., grief, job change, depression) that may require counseling or another type of expert help. As massage therapists, our area of expertise is soft tissue dysfunction. Abiding by the boundaries of the profession helps clients (and therapists) to feel safe.

Bodyworkers do not "heal" alone. We have a place in the health care chain. It is important to be on the lookout for providers who are equipped to handle situations that may be outside your scope of practice. Start building referral lists now. Whenever you find a competent and skilled chiropractor, physical therapist, or psychotherapist, make a notation in your Rolodex. These are people who may be able to help your clients heal. The effort you make in building a good professional referral system will come back to you. Other health care providers will begin referring back to you, and your clients will remember that you sent them where they needed to go.

Social Support

Professional bodyworkers must not only recognize the need to become health care advocates who seek out support for clients, but caring individuals who look for help for ourselves as individual human beings as well.

The names that you collect for your referral network can aid you in a professional capacity as well. We do not serve our clients well by attempting to go it alone. This is true, not only in reference to the client's healing process, but also in respect to maintaining our own optimal health and development. It is not possible to grow without the help of others. Sometimes we need inspiration. We may need an objective ear to listen to our cases. We may need a shoulder to cry on. Just as a seed cannot grow into a beautiful flower without light, water, and food, neither can we manifest our own professional potential without finding succor. A certain amount of support can be self-generated, but not all. Every time I start to think that I can carry the world on my shoulders, someone walks into my office and presents a new situation with which I need help. Beware of thinking you are the "master massage technician." Immediately the world will show you how that just is not so. We need colleagues to help us. It is not a weakness to admit that we can be vulnerable and imperfect. Realizing and accepting vulnerabilities and imperfections, along with asking for help when it is needed, are strengths.

Support fosters a sense of belonging. Having people to whom you feel close and to whom you can talk satisfies a basic human need. Research has shown that people who have someone to talk to about their problems are more healthy physiologically and psychologically (Greenberg, 1983). People who support you want to share your high points and your lows, your triumphs and your defeats. Anyone who accepts you for what and who you are can provide social support. Support can come from friends, family, and lovers, or paid support staff such as teachers, counselors, or other care providers.

To develop social support, you must be willing to reach out and ask for help when you need it. Sometimes, massage therapists are so in the habit of giving that it becomes very difficult to receive. It may be especially difficult to find yourself in a position in which you need to ask for help from others. Practice the art of social support before you get into a needy situation. Perhaps it may help to remember that learning how to receive in an open way can actually help you to model behavior that allows others (i.e., clients) to receive. Cultivate friendships in which the give and take runs both ways.

Exercise 9.6. Bull's-eye

On a piece of paper, draw a series of concentric circles forming a bull's-eye. Label the figure "My Support Relationships." The number of rings that are drawn depends on your current circumstances. Begin with three circles radiating out from the center, and as you complete the exercise, you can add more onto the outside as needed. Now identify and write in all names of individuals that appropriately belong in each section. Write the names in pencil, because relationships do change from day to day.

Starting in the core, write in the names that belong there. Core relationships are with people you would feel free to call at 3 A.M. if you needed them and who would not chastise you for doing so. If you needed something at that ungodly hour, these people would respond without reservation. These kinds of relationships are rare. Sometimes, while we are learning how to have core relationships, professional therapists may provide the center support. Sometimes, a distant family member or an old high school friend acts as our mainstay.

Do not write in names that you want to put in the center, but ones that appropriately belong. We have a tendency to want to put everyone we know in the center, but consider that it really would not feel right to have such an intimate connection with everyone with whom we come in contact. I have been told that it is a major accomplishment to fit five people in the bull's-eye in the span of an entire lifetime. Core relationships tend to be free and easy and not dependent at all. There is no constant needing with these people. A friend who lives on the other side of the continent and whom we never see and always forget to call may rightfully take a place in the core. Occasionally, we remember to send a hastily written but heartfelt card that says, "I love you so much and am so sorry I haven't written." Then another 10 years go by. An interval like that can go by because there is no need. A loving relationship is always present, and whenever the two people connect, it ignites.

Individuals who dwell in the next outward ring do pull on heartstrings. These orbits present more difficulty and more work. The circle closest to the core usually relates to romantic or family connections. We fervently wish these people could be in the core and are always trying to find some way of putting them there. And we are always getting tangled up in some way that prevents them from residing in our core. Middle rings are for less intimate relationships including professional relationships and more casual friends. Acquaintances, such as the people with whom you stop and visit when walking the dog, live in exterior circles. The outermost ring is for the mailperson, or the checkout clerk at the grocery store, and folks who smile on the street even though you do not know their names.

Take at least five to ten minutes to play with this exercise, then stop. You can continue, if need be, with the support bull's-eye again at a later time. That is why you wrote in pencil, because relationships do change.

Questions for Discussion. Were you surprised at any names that emerged in your bull's-eye? Were you surprised at the location of certain names? Did any names surface on multiple levels? Did any nonliving people reside in your circles? Did any nonhuman creatures reside there? Where did you place yourself on the circle?

This activity is designed to help you see where your relationships really are, not how you would like them to be. The "bull's-eye" helps you to sort out the connections that you need as opposed to the connections that you would like to impose. This kind of clarity can serve to lighten up all of the relationships you are currently in, from those who live in the outermost circles to the people who dwell closest to your heart.

MAINTAINING INTEREST

Even when pursuing work that we love, sometimes the repetition of a daily routine can make us feel bored or unappreciated. When we become apathetic toward our work, our body mechanics get sloppy. We neglect to exercise or stretch our bodies and are unprepared for the physical demands of massage. Physical as well as mental functions can become impaired due to unhappiness, stress, and want of diversion, entertainment, and fun. These factors combine to make us susceptible to on-the-job injury. It is crucial, therefore, that we learn how to maintain interest in our work.

Burnout

Burnout is a depletion of energy and feeling of being overwhelmed by others' problems (in Crawford, 1998). Crawford calls it an "insidious malaise of the spirit" that can take over every aspect of our lives. Some red flags that you may be experiencing massage burnout include the following:

1. You feel happier when clients do not show up for appointments.
2. You are becoming numb to the work you are doing; you are not feeling "really there" when you perform massage.
3. You find yourself being scattered; for example, forgetting appointments that you have scheduled.
4. You find your body hurting more than it used to—particularly in the wrists, arms, and shoulders or other places that are crucial for massage.
5. You find yourself in more and more situations that are filled with conflict, such as disagreements over when a client was supposed to show up or disputes about services that were or were not paid for or rendered.
6. You are tired all the time—too tired to take clients *and* too tired to enjoy a break.

More general signs of burnout include feeling unmotivated, "used up," bored, frustrated, and dissatisfied. The whole experience makes you dread seeing clients and more susceptible to injury or illness. Getting sick is "desirable" because it means you have to take a break from massage. Hopefully, you can take heed of warning signals before they mushroom into more serious consequences. Serious forms of burnout can manifest as depression, low self-esteem, fear of the workplace, and widespread lethargy. These stages can last several months to several years and require continual attention before they begin to reverse.

The nature of bodywork itself puts practitioners at special risk for these kinds of complaints. Crawford (1998) has identified several contributing factors in massage burnout:

1. Individuals who choose helping professions are statistically more likely to experience burnout. Perhaps this is because it is more difficult for those who think of themselves as "helpers" to say no. Perhaps it is because we are prone to take it upon ourselves to "fix" things that are outside of our power to change (that is, someone's health).
2. Some massage therapists have chosen the profession as a reprieve from the stress of former careers. Changing professions does not automatically make problems go away. Bodyworkers who leave other jobs because they were tired of the routine are inclined to experience dissatisfaction with massage therapy too.
3. Touching people is a very intimate act. Although this aspect of bodywork is rewarding, it can also be very stressful to connect and disconnect from many people on such a deep level.
4. People usually call massage therapists when they are in pain. The pain may be physical or emotional, or there may be elements of both. Regardless, individuals who are hurting often lash out at those who attempt to help. Even if that is not the case, it can be difficult to witness another person's suffering. Consider the example of dentists, who have the highest rate of depression in any helping profession.
5. Massage therapists often feel isolated by their work. Many operate sole practices. Self-employment can make excessive demands on time and energy. Even those who work in spa settings or in group practices generally work

without the benefit of supervision and community. Evenings, weekend shifts, and odd hours can take a toll. I tend to classify our breed as a lot of rugged individualists. Granted, working alone gives us a relative autonomy, however, it can make us prone to competition and alienation from peers.

6. Lack of monetary compensation is another factor. I have never heard of a practicing massage therapist who could not get all the work he or she wants. I have often heard of therapists who feel that they are not getting adequate pay for all of the work that they do. In addition, many therapists do not have health insurance and worry about what would happen should they be forced to take a hiatus from work. On top of these worries, new clients may fail to schedule return visits or "regulars" may cancel sessions that have been budgeted to pay bills.

Therapists need to galvanize energies and break unhealthful routines before massage burnout steals away businesses and happy lives. Figuring out how to continue to enjoy massage therapy will put a "brake" on the cycle of unhealthy habits. Begin the process by answering questions like "What made you excited about the field when you first entered the bodywork profession?" and "What made you excited about practicing massage?". It is important to discover both professional and personal motivations.

Staying Fascinated

If you are currently experiencing early warning signs of burnout, what *would* it take to recapture your interest? Are you utilizing all of your skills in your profession? Do you enjoy teaching, research, or humanitarian pursuits? Is there a new technique or specialty that you are eager to learn? Have you always wanted to get involved with a bodywork research project? If this is the kind of focus that gets you motivated, you may want to consider attending one of Tiffany Field's research workshops at the Touch Research Institute in Florida (Knaster, 1998). These three-day intensive trainings are offered at the end of each month, and are a good way to hone investigative skills.

Perhaps it sounds more exciting to spread the word about massage in the community. If so, you may want to become a member of a public-speaking support group like "Toastmasters" in order to hone your presentation skills. If you are ready to talk in front of groups now, consider registering as a member of a local Speaker's Bureau for a variety of community groups.

Perhaps you are a humanitarian who yearns to provide massage to those who otherwise cannot afford the service. Begin to make connections that enliven massage for you.

Another way to enliven a job is to incorporate more outside interests into daily duties. I have always maintained that the best massage practitioners find a way to combine their enthusiasms. Are you an athlete or dancer at heart? Do you like interacting with other physical people? Opportunities abound in this genre. Perhaps you would enjoy volunteering for the Boston Marathon or some other such athletic event in your region. American massage therapists were active in the 1996 Olympics and are gearing up for the games in 2002. Do you love to speak Spanish or sign language? If so, are you meeting and massaging people who appreciate and need bilingual skills? The more aspects of self-expression that you can bring to your sessions, the more fulfilling they become—both for you and for everyone you touch.

In addition to focusing on ways to keep the field of massage stimulating for you, it is vital to stay fascinated in the moment as you are performing your craft. "Staying fascinated" transforms massage work from mind-numbing physical drudgery to a moving meditation. If you are not intrigued with the intricacies of the bodywork session—if you are thinking about your lunch or the guy who cut you off on the way to work—you are not wholly "with" your client. On some level, the client perceives the mental distance and the experience is diminished.

Staying fascinated is not possible every single moment in massage. Neither is "perfect" body mechanics. No one can maintain optimal positioning every instant of a massage, no matter how skilled or sincere the effort. But we can make the effort to monitor and be aware of our mental and physical states. We can commit to change when we discover uncomfortable positions and movements. We can create an intention of staying fascinated with our work.

The next exercise is designed to show just how powerful an intention can be when used in conjunction with touch.

Exercise 9.7. Creating an Intention

For this activity, one partner touches while the other role is being touched. It works best when there are several dyads, so that after the activity is completed you can discuss your findings with your partner, and then compare results with other pairs. A leader writes a list of adverbs on a blackboard in front of the group. The passive members (ones that are being touched) keep eyes closed as the leader points to each descriptor on the board. As the leader indicates a word, the toucher takes on the intent described by that word. For example, when the leader points to "inviting," the touchers think of being "inviting." When the leader points to "connected," the touchers think of touching in a way that is "connected." Continue in this manner for each descriptor listed below. (You can add other descriptors, if you choose.)

Inviting(ly)	Present	Invasive
Connected(ly)	Empty	Sedating
Neutral(ly)	Self-centered	Activating

Take note of any thoughts and feelings each type of touch evokes in you, in either role. Switch roles, repeat the exercise, and discuss.

This activity and the discussion that precedes it lead to the conclusion that maintaining interest is a goal to be striven for rather than an end in itself. Staying engrossed with body mechanics and massage is a process.

The puzzle of how to stay fascinated brings us full circle to the psychological skills discussed in this chapter—maintaining boundaries, communicating well, finding support, and nurturing ourselves.

SUMMARY

This chapter describes psychological self-care skills that prepare the bodyworker for work and support-enhanced body mechanics. Skills that help sustain a career in massage include establishing clear boundaries, communicating clearly and well (asking and receiving permission, assertiveness and conflict resolution, taking time out for yourself, and staying interested), avoiding burnout, and finding support.

Clear communication means asking for permission in situations in which the limits are unclear and waiting to receive permission before crossing a boundary that has been set. Equalizing means that the person who wants a more intimate form of touch agrees to accept a less intimate touch if another desires it. Assertiveness is based on the premise that everyone has rights. True assertiveness attempts to satisfy personal needs while maintaining good relationships with others.

Taking time out leaves us fresh and better able to deal with challenges of daily life and work as a bodyworker. Establishing good referral lists can take some of the pressure off of us to "fix" everyone and everything. Finding support may mean calling a friend, mentor, or colleague. Staying interested may involve taking a class, getting new skills, sharing with others, or adapting your practice to include your special interests.

Role-playing is a good way to try out any and all of these skills and to identify special circumstances in which you will need to adapt to mental and emotional challenges.

REFERENCES

Allen, Roger, *Human Stress—Its Nature and Control* (1983). Minneapolis, MN: Burgess Publishing Company.

Benjamin, Ben, "Discovering Your Boundary Issues," *Massage Therapy Journal* (Summer 1992), pp. 31–32.

Billard, Jill, Personal communication (1996). Washington, DC.

The Counseling Center, Presentation information (1996). 97 McCain Drive, Suite B, Frederick, MD.

Crawford, Dianne Poulseno, "The Ethical Obligation to Prevent Burnout," *Massage Therapy Journal* Vol. 37, No. 1 (Spring 1998), pp. 115–118.

Czimbal, Bob, and Maggie Zadikov, *Vitamin T: A Guide to Healthy Touch* (1991). Portland, OR: Open Book Publishers.

Disch, Estelle, "Are You in Trouble With a Client?" *Massage Therapy Journal* (Summer 1992), pp. 31–32.

Greenberg, Jerrold, *Comprehensive Stress Management* (1983). Dubuque, IA: Wm. C. Brown Publishers.

Knaster, Mirka, "Tiffany Field Provides Proof Positive Scientifically," *Massage Therapy Journal,* Vol. 37, No. 1 (Spring 1998), pp. 84–88.

Palmer, David, "Defining our Profession: Strategies for Inventing the Future of Massage," *Massage and Bodywork Quarterly* (Summer 1993), pp. 28–32.

Sprague, Philip, Alchemical Hypnotherapy Workshop (1994). Portland, OR.

Chapter Ten

Adaptations for Special Populations/Conditions

Conceptual Objectives The massage student/practitioner who successfully completes this chapter (reading and exercises) will be able to:

- Explain how to modify body mechanics to optimize a massage when the client is placed in a nonprone, nonsupine position (on the side, in a chair, on a bed, in a wheelchair, on a mat on the floor).

- Explain how to modify a massage routine for special massage techniques (e.g., deep tissue, energy work, shiatsu, prenatal massage, geriatric massage, on-site chair massage).

- Explain how to modify body mechanics to optimize a massage when the massage environment changes (e.g., in cramped quarters, busy environment, increase in therapist's weight).

Practical Objectives The massage student/practitioner who successfully completes this chapter (reading and exercises) will be able to:

- Demonstrate changes in body mechanics that optimize a massage when the client is placed in a nonprone, nonsupine position (on the side, in a chair, on a bed, in a wheelchair, on a mat on the floor).

- Demonstrate changes in body mechanics for special massage techniques (e.g., deep tissue, energy work, shiatsu, prenatal massage, geriatric massage, on-site chair massage).

- Demonstrate changes in body mechanics that optimize a massage when the massage environment changes (e.g., in cramped quarters, busy environment, increase in therapist's weight).

- Demonstrate ergonomic positioning of client and therapist for specific passive stretches.

The first half of this book lays the groundwork for establishing healthy body mechanics each time that you massage. Hopefully, you are already discovering that by applying body awarenesses that you have discovered this far, basic massage becomes more productive and enjoyable to perform. Chapters 1 through 6 present all the skills you need to attend to body mechanics and create an excellent "vanilla" session. Under standard conditions, you now know how to refine your work in a way that will not hurt you or your client.

By the same token, the information presented thus far has been oriented toward a "standard" positioning for both bodyworker and client. In a "typical" massage, the bodyworker is standing, working on a massage table with the client placed exclusively in prone (face down) and/or supine (face up) positions. In reality, many situations arise day to day that call for variations on these positions. Adaptations are needed in order to achieve optimal body mechanics for these special conditions. While your body is still learning to find its own kinesthetic understanding, it is easy for awareness to be thrown off line by a novel situation. Fortunately or unfortunately, massage therapists have chosen a track where "novel situations" are not the exception, but the norm. Many massage scenarios require deviations from a standardized approach to body mechanics, even one that is built on a foundation of kinesthetic understanding. Guidelines must be flexible when massaging four patrons an hour while they are seated in a chair. Other modifications are called for when working with a patient who, for various reasons (such as pregnancy or extreme low back pain), must be treated while lying on her side. Therapists may also need to rework body alignment or hand positioning when providing sessions for clients who cannot lie on a standard massage table. Some clients may be wheelchair-bound or restricted to a hospital bed, and others may opt for sessions while fully clothed and/or lying on a cushion placed on the floor.

As I present workshops on developing body awareness and body mechanics around the nation, one question is invariably raised. "How can I tune into body awareness and maintain good body mechanics in my unique circumstances?" The comment is formed in many different ways, but the basic concern remains the same. "Kinesthetic understanding activities really helped me to become more comfortable as I massaged during this workshop, but in real life, they can't work for me because . . ." "Because my working environment discourages using good body mechanics." How is this so? "My room at the spa is cramped." "The law firm where I contract for seated corporate massage books 12 to 13 half-hour sessions each day, without rest breaks." "My clientele is limited to pregnant women, who must lie exclusively on their sides." "My practice is devoted to outcalls for frail elderly and patients with chronic degenerative diseases like multiple sclerosis, polio, and spinal cord injuries. They can't get up on a professional massage table. They can't get out of wheelchairs. How could standard body mechanics guidelines possibly work for me?"

This chapter presents and discusses ergonomic challenges to optimizing body mechanics during massage. The accompanying exercises will help you apply kinesthetic understanding of efficient body mechanics to situations other than the bodywork norm.

The first part of the chapter reviews special massage populations that necessitate a revised approach to body awareness and body mechanics. These include on-site or *seated massage, geriatric massage,* massage for clients with *spinal cord injuries, prenatal massage, shiatsu, subtle energy work,* and *deep tissue* versus relaxation massage. From a discussion of each population and their special circumstances, appropriate biomechanical changes are derived.

The second section covers actual modifications in positioning. These comprise both direct changes to accommodate therapist needs and indirect body mechanics changes that a therapist makes to adapt to an alteration in the client's orientation (on or off the massage table).

There are many instances in which the practitioner voluntarily makes a change in stance or positioning. Some altered positions are *kneeling* (as in shiatsu, but also for low back relief in Swedish massage), *sitting on a stool, sitting or standing on the massage table,* backed *against the wall* in a small studio space, and *working in a public area.*

There are also numerous occasions when novel client positioning calls for adaptations in practitioner body mechanics. One example is when the client is *seated* in an on-site massage chair or a regular office chair. For medical reasons, some individuals will be confined to a wheelchair, a hospital bed, or a regular bed. Other clients are best treated while lying on the side or lying on a mat placed on the floor.

When the client is seated, the practitioner can adjust by changing level often (i.e., moving from standing to kneeling to sitting). When a massage table is impractical for a patient, the therapist may adjust by kneeling, sitting, or bracing against the bed. When the client presents in the sidelying position, the therapist can modify direction of effort or force. When the client is lying on a futon, kneeling may be the preferred stance for the massage.

The third part of the chapter is devoted to describing efficient approaches to the application of passive stretches. This section describes techniques for stretching specific muscles in ways that require less effort from you. Ergonomically sound stretches use therapist alignment to create the levers and pulleys that move and lift the client. This transforms stretching into an activity that is not stressful on your frame.

Other available body mechanics texts focus on administering pressure to a reclining client. Some texts recommend skipping stretches entirely, because lifting is so laborious for the bodyworker. Although poorly performed movement therapies can place stress and tension on the therapist's body, stretches and range-of-motion exercises reduce spasms and increase flexibility for many clients above the effects of pressure alone. This fact makes it worthwhile to keep stretches in the massage repertoire, as long as the practitioner can save him- or herself from strain and injury. It is important to figure out how to perform range-of-motion activities in a way that is not harmful to our bodies. For these reasons, suggestions for positioning and lengthening specific muscles (e.g., iliopsoas muscle or shoulder adductors) are included in this chapter on special massage conditions.

On-Site Massage

As part of an integrated health promotion program for offices, corporations, and small businesses, *on-site massage* helps to reduce employee stress, improve employee morale, increase productivity, and lower health care costs. In on-site massage, the practitioner renders bodywork services to a client who is seated in a specially designed massage chair. It is important to realize that this situation is really a stress management technique designed for the convenience of the client. Sessions are short in duration, ranging from five minutes to a half hour. The practitioner usually has several hours of short sessions booked one right after another, with few or no rest breaks in between. Sometimes, the setting is in a corporate environment, such as a law practice or educational facility. Another on-site environment could be a chair set up at athletic events or health fairs. Once again, the objective is to work intimately yet quickly with a large volume of people. Stroking is achieved over clothing, and no oil or lubricant is used. Lotion can be applied to the arms and hands of a patron; this may be especially desirable for people who work with their hands, such as construction workers, hair stylists, or office workers. On-site chair massages often incorporate acupressure as well as effleurage (gliding), petrissage (kneading), tapotement (percussion), vibration, and friction. Chair massage also is more effective when stretching or joint movements for the cervical spine and shoulder are included in the repertoire. A session is completed in a very short time, with little space for intake and feedback about the massage.

The corporate massage therapist must be prepared to address many different needs thoroughly and yet time efficiently. Your energies will be constantly challenged to meet the changing temperaments of a variety of stressed-out folks. As many as 80 percent of these clients will never have experienced a massage before (Jedlicka, 1996). Hygienic procedures require washing hands between each client. "Handiwipes" or towelettes moistened with alcohol or a 10 percent bleach solution can serve this purpose. Between clients, you also need to change face protectors and spray down the massage chair and wipe it with a paper towel. Add to that the duties of greeting and providing a quick intake/assessment for the next person, along with receiving payment and saying good-bye to the last one. Intakes are important to rule out situations in which chair massage would be inappropriate or even harmful. Contraindications for chair massage include recent surgeries or injuries, certain medications, pregnancy, or trying to get pregnant. Meeting the many responsibilities and holding all these differing energies can be very stressful for the practitioner and wear down one's stamina.

The chair itself presents a challenge to proficient body mechanics. Practitioners must align their direction of force differently for a chair (pressure coming from the side) versus a table (pressure down into the table). It will help to move around the client to work in several orientations—from the back, from the front, and from each side of the chair. Certain massage strokes have been specifically adapted for seated clients (whether they are sitting in an on-site chair, an office chair, or even a wheelchair).

You will notice that the following techniques utilize many different parts of the body to save the practitioner's fingers, palms, and thumbs from overuse. *Forearm compression* uses the meaty part of the forearm to pump the client's muscles against bone, in a variation of palm compression. If needed, the bony side of the forearm can provide a more focused tool. *Elbow presses* get into the muscles even deeper and more precisely. Situate your elbow and circle it in the knots that need release. Percussive strokes often used in seated massage work include *closed fists* on denser muscles, *cupped hands,* and hacking (using the *ulnar side of the hand* as a striking surface). Brushing involves fast, firm strokes for finishing a sequence and transitioning to another area. Although usually performed with the palmar sides of the hands, it could be adapted for use with the *back sides* of the hands, or with the forearms.

Some strokes adapted for chair use can be very hard on the thumbs, fingers, or wrists if not performed correctly. Thumb presses use the soft pads of the thumbs to penetrate into tissue. Thumb walks use the thumbs in a rhythmic trek over a portion of the body. In both these techniques, make sure the thumb is aligned with the wrist in a straight line (see Chapters 3 and 4). Areas where different tissues meet (i.e., tendon on bone, tendon to muscle) need the extra focus of techniques like circular or cross-fiber friction. To avoid injury, make sure to keep fingers or thumbs braced. Indian burns (rotating grip around the axis of a long bone) and chucking (pumping longitudinally up the axis) are supplemental techniques for the arms that can torque your wrists if you aren't paying attention. A thumb/four-finger squeeze can be used to simulate petrissage through clothing on large muscle groups, such as the upper trapezius (at the top of the shoulder) and the deltoids (the lateral upper muscles of the arm). This type of motion requires attention to thumb and little finger muscles as they move into opposition.

The following body mechanics guidelines (established in previous chapters) apply especially to chair massage:

1. Lean with the whole weight of the body. Use the power of your legs to step into the stroke, as well as working your back, shoulders, and arms to deliver the manipulations. Although you are leaning rather than pushing, do not lean so far as to fall onto the client (that is, keep some weight under your own control). Leave some space between the two of you. When you identify a spasm, adhesion, or trigger point and focus thumb, hand, arm, or elbow pressure on it, don't push or slide past the point. Allow your focus to remain steady and your body to act as a lightning rod for conducting the power of the stroke.

2. Keep wrists and fingers loose and relaxed.

3. Keep your toes pointing forward in the direction of your work.

4. Use an open stance as a base. Slide one foot ahead and let your knee be slightly bent while the other foot is back in a lunge position. (See Figure 10.1.)

5. Move around often to discover the best, most comfortable positions for you. Try kneeling, standing, and/or sitting on a stool alongside your client. Work from several different angles and levels. A massage that incorporates changing positions and levels will feel better (more thorough and full) for

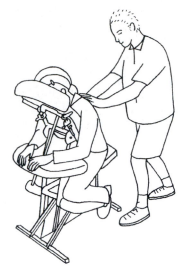

Seated Massage

Figure 10.1 Seated massage can be performed efficiently and easily when you move around often, use an open stance, keep your body aligned in the direction of your stroke, use the weight of your body in delivering pressure, and keep your wrists and fingers loose and relaxed.

the client as well as for you. As you make adjustments in your standing stance/posture, let one foot "squiggle" (slide) into the new, more stable position.

Geriatric Massage

The elderly population presents a challenge to the massage therapist's biomechanical skills. Geriatric massage requires proficiency in a broad range of massage techniques. One day, you may be easing a terminal patient's transition into death with light touch and energy work. Another session may provide sports massage to an older runner to get her ready for the next marathon. One session can concentrate on relieving the ache of arthritis while the next is devoted to restoring muscle function lost after a stroke.

You will encounter a wide variety of health conditions and complaints in the elderly population. An older massage client can usually be classified into one of the following three groups (Miesler, 1991): robust, age appropriate, or frail. Of these distinctions, the frail group provides the most challenge for maintaining good body mechanics. Robust individuals display no outward indication of impaired health. They appear younger than their chronological age, mentally sharp, and physically active (engaging in golf, walking, swimming, gardening, etc.). Age-appropriate seniors show some health impairments due to age, such as elevated blood pressure, diabetes, or some slowing down of activities. Frail persons look and feel fragile. There are clear signs of considerable health impairment, and the client is probably housebound and in some cases bedridden. Your massage assessment and subsequent plan will determine what kinds of adjustments in body mechanics you will need to make.

For robust individuals, find out if any chronic conditions are present via a good intake procedure. In many cases, you can disregard age and massage this client like any other.

For age-appropriate persons, complete the intake process and ask about tendencies to headaches, arthritic pain, or light tremors. Obtain permission to consult with the health care provider, if necessary. Miesler (1991) recommends that age-appropriate massage not last longer than 30 minutes, and that clients are not left in the prone (face down) position more than 15 minutes. When the session is complete, you will need to help the client to a sitting posture and wait at least 30 seconds before assisting him or her off the table (Miesler, 1991). These modifications provide little, if any, need to adjust your basic body mechanics.

For frail patients, realize that you may not be using a professional massage table at all. If you do use a table, you will want to help the client get on as well as off. Use plenty of pillows to prop limbs and support body parts. If you must lift clients, support them under their arms or around the rib cage and use your legs as levers to lift, rather than your back. (Make sure you review the hints for ergonomic joint movement/stretching/lifts, provided at the end of this chapter.) Using gentle pressure may call for an adjustment in your stance, so that you are not fighting with your own body to hold back. In the scant 15 minutes per session indicated by Miesler (1991), he suggests beginning with the client supine (face up) and finishing the back from a sidelying position. See the section on Massage for Pregnant Women for help in adapting your body mechanics to work with a sidelying client.

Special Situations.   The location for your geriatric sessions may require additional ergonomic modifications. For geriatric clients in general, make sure to have a footstool handy for getting on and off the massage table. If you take outcalls, impress upon customers that better results can be achieved in a quiet site. If you transport the massage table, ask clients to provide a space that is big enough to allow you to walk around the table.

If you are massaging a bedridden patient in a hospital bed, use the mechanical lifting controls to adjust the patient's height and angle of incline relative to yours. Hospital beds have side rails with a variety of release mechanisms. These releases can pinch your fingers if you are not careful when you disengage them. Ask an attendant to show you how the mechanism works. If you have a patient lying in a standard bed, you may find it best to work from a kneeling position to save your back (providing you have no preexisting knee problems). (*Note:* If you find yourself kneeling for any length of time, you may want to invest in knee pads. These can be purchased in sports stores in the roller blade section or in a gardening shop.) In a double bed, you may be able to pivot your client 90 degrees so that you can massage feet and legs from one side of the bed and neck and shoulders from the other side. To work the back, roll your client to the foot end of the bed.

For clients who must receive bodywork while in wheelchairs, have them use a pillow for draping and cushioning. The client places the pillow over the chest (for modesty in females and for comfort with males) and leans over the massage table or some other convenient ledge. This uncovers the entire back for bodywork. Sore and spasmed pectoralis muscles can be kneaded when the client leans back in the chair. To massage the extremities and head, adapt stances and strokes as previously recommended for the on-site chair work.

Positioning. When clients are not comfortable, they cannot completely relax. No matter how good a massage you deliver, an uncomfortable client gets a less effective massage. Face cradles (headrests) and bolsters (leg rolls), soft pillows, and rolled-up towels are standard positioning tools. Extra propping may be needed for obese clients or those with joint or spinal deformations. The basic propping rule is to use common sense and give the body as much support as possible. If you see an area that is not supported by the table, place a prop underneath.

Often, you will have to use resourcefulness to solve a positioning problem. Use bolsters, pillows, rolled towels or blankets, foam, or whatever you can find to furnish additional support for a painful or distorted body part. Syndromes that present challenges to positioning can indirectly affect body mechanics. Consider the following common conditions as described by Miesler (1991):

1. *Hyperkyphosis*—an exaggerated curve of the thoracic vertebrae. In the prone position, kyphotic clients may need a pillow under the lower chest. In the supine position, they may need a pillow under the head. In severe cases (i.e., ankylosing spondylitis—hardening of the connective tissue between vertebrae), the prone position cannot be employed. The back can be massaged in a sidelying position, with the head supported by a pillow and a lengthwise bolster under the top leg or the contour body cushion. You can also opt to massage the back with the client sitting on a stool and resting head and arms on the massage table, or sitting backwards and leaning over a straight-backed chair cushioned with a pillow on the chest.

2. *Scoliosis*—lateral curvature of the spine (can be either S shaped or C shaped). The concave side(s) of the curve is where the muscles are overdeveloped and contracted. The convex side of the curve is where the muscles are weak and overstretched. Often, a pillow is needed to support the weakened side.

3. *Hip pain.* Seniors with hip joint or sciatic problems may not be able to lie face down because of severe pain. If propping under the hip does not help, position your client in a sidelying position. Keep the top hip and knee flexed and forward, supported by a bolster placed lengthwise.

4. *Torticollis (wryneck).* The sternocleidomastoid muscle is shortened on one side, so that the head turns to the opposite side. Extra propping may be needed under the chest and/or face in both prone and supine positions.

5. *Obesity*—client who holds over 30 percent of his or her optimal body weight. Very obese clients may need pillows under the chest and/or head. Adjustable-height headrests may suffice for this adjustment in the prone position. With the increased width of the client, you may need to adjust the height of your massage table downward in order to maintain optimal positioning.

6. *Joints lose mobility/range of motion.* Synovial membranes dehydrate with age and lack of use. This may aggravate wear and tear on joint surfaces and lead to arthritis (inflammation of the joint). If the inflammation is not too acute or severe (i.e., not too red, hot, swollen, or painful), massage, movement, and hydrotherapy can reduce the pain and swelling associated with

these complaints. Again, it is important to communicate with the client and suggest shorter, more frequent sessions to get a cumulative effect. Avoid straining yourself to "fix" a problem in one session.

7. *Fat deposits may be lost.* This may mean padding the massage table, bed, or wheelchair. Be sure you have plenty of pillows, props, and bolsters on hand. Without them, you may find yourself in the awkward position of lifting and supporting one part of the client's body while applying pressure to another.

8. *Bone substance is lost.* This occurs mainly in postmenopausal women but can occur in men too. Osteoporosis (loss of bone) is not a contraindication to massage per se, but it requires a gentler touch and more careful handling of the client.

Massage for Clients with Spinal Cord Injuries

When massaging clients with spinal cord injuries, the therapeutic goal is to prevent atrophy, while helping to eliminate toxicity and edema (swelling) (Burns-Vidlak, 1989). Massage therapists need to maintain constant communication, describing the purpose and intent of each massage stroke and checking pressure in areas which may have limited sensation. These precautions not only assure the client, but will save the therapist from applying needless and counterproductive force.

Vibration can be extremely helpful with clients who suffer from spinal cord injuries or paralysis. Gentle vibration is safe even when administered directly over nerves, muscles, tendons, ligaments, bones, arteries, and veins. It is mild enough not to harm already compromised tissues and yet penetrating enough to affect chronically painful and inflamed soft tissues on a deep level. The main biomechanical difficulty in administering vibration for any period of time is the buildup of tension for the therapist. To release the tension buildup during prolonged vibration, use your breath. Exhale to deliver the force of the oscillations. Take a breath and pause when you feel your muscles tensing up. Then continue another round of pulsation to the damaged tissues.

Other techniques that are particularly helpful for a client with paralysis include colon massage and visualization techniques, neither of which puts strain on the therapist's muscles. Massaging the entire route of the colon and concentrating on the stomach muscles as a unit helps prevent constipation and muscle spasms in the area. Use visualization exercises to relax parts of the body below the spinal cord injury.

Massage for Pregnant Women

The most important adaptation here is to be able to massage a pregnant client in the sidelying position. I have seen the "pregnancy massage tables" with a hole cut out for the abdomen but do not recommend them. There are problems with placing a pregnant woman on her belly, regardless of whether you use one of these special tables. In the prone (face down) position, the weight of the uterus is pushed up against the inferior vena cava and abdominal aorta, which lie deep to the pregnant uterus. Although the table has a space for the belly, compression of the uterus occurs at the edges of the hole. Pressure applied to the back or buttocks can cause an increase in intrauterine blood pressure, perhaps to dangerous levels. Another reason to avoid putting your client in the prone position is that it increases the pull on uterine ligaments (particularly the round ligament, which already has to strain as the uterus expands from a pelvic to an abdominal organ). Tension on the uterine wall presents a potential for abruption of the placenta (where the placenta actually tears away from the uterus and hemorrhaging occurs) (Waters, 1995).

What about the pregnant woman who is still in her first trimester and has not begun to "show" (acquire a tummy)? Bette Waters (1995) cautions that 10 to 15 percent of all pregnancies end in miscarriage before 13 weeks' gestation (the first trimester). Although no known connection has been established between massage and miscarriage, she suggests waiting to begin prenatal massage after this dangerous period has passed. By the end of the first trimester, the prone contraindication becomes pertinent.

Neither do I use the supine position for pregnant clients. When the pregnant client is lying flat on her back, her vena cava and aorta are compressed by the weight of the uterus. This restricts blood flow to both mom and baby. (See Figure 10.2.)

For these reasons, pregnant clients are best massaged only in the following

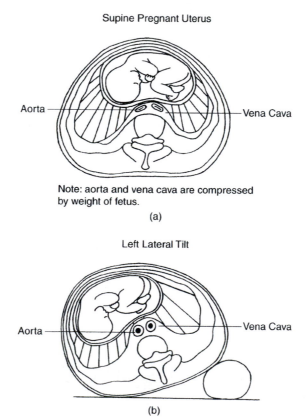

Supine Pregnant Uterus

Aorta — — Vena Cava

Note: aorta and vena cava are compressed by weight of fetus.

(a)

Left Lateral Tilt

Aorta — — Vena Cava

(b)

Figure 10.2 (a–b)   When a pregnant woman is lying on her back, the vena cava and aorta are compressed by the uterus.

positions: sidelying (particularly to the left), tilted on a 45-degree angle to the left, and in an adapted supine (sometimes called Fowler's) position.

In the left sidelying position, the weight of the pregnant uterus rests on the left abdominal wall, rather than on any major blood vessels or organs. The blood pressure is not elevated, and mother and baby receive a continuous supply of nutrients. The massage can be completed with the woman shifting to lie on her right side. Shifting can be a little awkward, especially with the pregnant woman's changing center of balance. You do not need to lift your client. I suggest that the client get on all fours in a kneeling position under the sheet. Then she can ease herself down onto her other side. Above all, be practical. Use whatever method is easiest on you and your client. If she changes sides successfully, you have both done it right.

The left lateral tilt is an alternative position that consists of placing a rolled blanket or wedge under the woman's right side, from the shoulder to the top of the iliac crest. The tilt should be enough to raise the shoulder, ribs, and thigh approximately 15 degrees. In this position, the weight of the uterus moves off of the aorta and vena cava. This position allows the therapist access to the head, face, neck, and arms while standing or seated at the head of the table. Massage and range-of-motion exercises can be performed for upper and lower extremities from the left lateral tilt (Waters, 1995). Working with a client in this position is essentially the same as working with a supine client in terms of body mechanics. You may want to slip on some clogs or use a step stool to increase your height on the elevated side.

In an adapted supine position, the client is on her back with her head elevated 18 to 20 inches above the height of the massage table. This slant is sufficient to prevent the uterus from pressing down on the aorta and vena cava. Pillows or a triangular-shaped bolster can accomplish this nicely. A sheet is placed over the wedge or bolster, with the client's weight as an anchor. Alternately, you can slide the head of the table against the wall in order to anchor the wedge, but reaching from the head of the table becomes more difficult. A bolster is placed under the knees to reduce strain on the abdominal muscles and lower back. This position can be used in the last months of pregnancy. (See Figure 10.3.)

Side positioning of the mother can significantly change the effective vectors of force in a massage. With a prone or supine client, the massage therapist is usually pressing down into the table and working in conjunction with gravity. This is not the case when massaging a sidelying client. If you are performing effleurage down the back of a client who is lying on her side, for instance, your pressure is directed perpendicular both to the table and to the force of gravity. It would be like mowing a lawn with a very steep slope. You would have to be riding sideways so as not to fall down the slope. A few easy-to-make adjustments in body mechanics can make delivering side pressure easier:

1. Use resistance provided by the client to contribute some of the pressure for strokes. Cue the client with the phrase, "push into me, move into my hands," or something similar.

2. Place your body strategically to create two-way traction. Use this kind of effort to elongate muscles instead of deep effleurage or longitudinal fric-

Sidelying Position

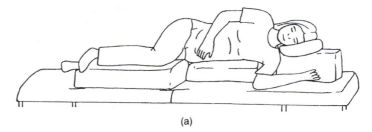

(a)

Adapted Supine (Fowler's) Position

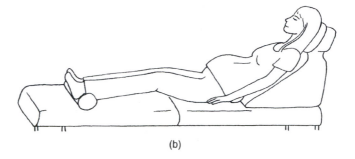

Figure 10.3 (a–b)   The adapted supine and sidelying positions prevent the pregnant uterus from compressing the aorta and vena cava.

(b)

tion. These two options are harder to achieve when gravity is working against you in the sidelying position. Line up your hands so that they are facing in opposing directions, away from each other. Then place your body directly in the center of the two forces to create the traction for a muscle release. For example, in stretching the levator scapulae, put the weight of your body between crossed hands. One hand rests on the side of the neck behind the ear and the other is on the shoulder. Lean over and press down to create a stretch in two directions at once.

3. Incorporate more easy range-of-motion movements into your bodywork. When a client is lying on her side, both the shoulder and pelvic girdles actually become more mobile. Use the handles of the scapula—place one hand in front of the shoulder and the other in back—to rotate it in the joint. You can apply similar movements to the hip joint, with one hand on the anterior iliac crest and the other over the posterior superior iliac spine. To affect the muscles of the shoulder joint, use the humerus as a lever to rotate the shoulder. To open up the sacroiliac joint, locate the anterior superior iliac crests and apply perpendicular pressure directly on top of them into the core. Make sure the hip bones are healthy and that it is not late in the pregnancy before you attempt this.

4. Use visualization and breathing cues to expedite relaxation in the client's soft tissues. Both of these tools make your job as a massage therapist much easier. Stretching is always easier to accomplish during the out-breath. Visualization is extremely helpful in allowing the woman to achieve relaxation of tight muscles and a good training tool to envisioning a healthy pregnancy, labor, and birth.

5. Employ more active resistive stretches as part of your prenatal massage routine. Muscles like the iliopsoas, quadriceps group, and adductor group need special attention in a woman who is preparing to give birth, and they actually become easier to lengthen when she is placed in a sidelying position. When the ligaments become loose late in the third trimester, use alternate kinds of work besides stretches.

Shiatsu

Some massage therapists work primarily or exclusively with an Eastern orientation to their massage. This may necessitate massaging while clients are lying on a futon placed on the floor. It is helpful to remember that in this new position, effective body mechanics still depends on alignment and how you deliver the pressure. The best advice is still to rely on body weight instead of effort. Lean to let your body work for you, rather than push or press. It may seem ironic to think of "finger pressure" (the literal definition of shiatsu) that is not pressing, but this is the essence of shiatsu. Shiatsu techniques involve leaning body weight through the fingers, thumbs, palms, elbows, knees, or feet. Originate the lean from your geographic center in the point of the tan tien or the wider area of the hara. Three additional strategies for applying pressure without pressing are: perpendicular pressure, stationary pressure, and supporting pressure (Lundberg, 1992).

Perpendicular pressure is achieved by maintaining a right angle between the client's body and your vector of pressure. Your focal point is straight in to the bone (Lundberg, 1992).

The idea behind *stationary pressure* is to lean into your body weight without forcibly moving. When hands remain still, they can better tune in to the client's energy (chi). You do nothing, since the natural response of unrestricted energy is to flow. Any extra action you coerce or compel will obscure the natural movement of chi (Lundberg, 1992).

Supporting pressure conveys caring, respect, and safety (Lundberg, 1992). Utilizing this bodywork "technique" activates a two-way process. Not only do you focus on supporting the client, but you also allow the client's weight to support your own. The degree in which you allow yourself to trust in the receiver's physical strength determines the quality of energy you can provide. Supporting pressure leads to mutual trust, which in turn creates relaxation and less need for external pressure and force. A support hand (sometimes referred to as a "mother" or "father" hand) is used to maintain connection with the client's body. Positioning your body as a brace for the client's weight may be appropriate in some situations. Whole-body contact is common practice in shiatsu, especially when the client is sitting. Supporting pressure allows ergonomically sound and easier delivery of strokes.

Other techniques that are derived from a shiatsu orientation (and that can help improve your body mechanics) include *palming, thumbing, passive stretches,* and *using elbows, knees,* and *feet. Palming* means leaning or holding with an open palm. In palming, use your open hand to cover an area on your partner's body. Let the contour of your hand mold to the shape of the body part. Hold or sink into the tissue. Tilt your whole body back, slide your hand a little further along the meridian line, and lean forward again. Palming can be administered with different parts of the hand, such as the hypothenar eminence (on the ulnar side) or the heel of the palm as well as through the center of the hand (Lundberg, 1992).

In *thumbing,* remember to use perpendicular pressure through the entire line of the thumb. This means making sure that the thumb is in a straight line with the wrist and the forearm. Skip this technique when you are feeling tired or when your sensitivity is otherwise low (Lundberg, 1992).

Use elbows, knees, and feet (Lundberg, 1992). Knees and feet, although not regularly employed by the Swedish relaxation practitioner, are regularly incorporated into Eastern massage. After adding these supplemental instruments to your repertoire, you may become more aware that fatigue occurs more readily when using thumbs and fingers alone. Elbows, knees, and feet are well suited for work on more robust (yang) clients and strong, resistive areas of the body. These tools are also excellent for working deeply into stiff and sore muscles that chronically hold on to tension. These more focused instruments allow you to sink in to areas of blocked chi in a "benevolent" way, releasing the blockage and associated pain. The heel of the hand can also be used in this way. Use your fingers to locate areas of tension, then place your elbow in the areas you have identified. Work with the length of the ulna bone, rather than the point of the olecranon process. Your knees can be a supplemental tool for the client's legs. When using knees, begin from the crawl position on all fours, and then transfer your weight slowly onto one knee, in order to control the delivery of pressure. Foot techniques are used on the receiver's feet. Stand with your heels on the prone client's feet, near the balls of their feet, facing away from their body. Alternately, match up the balls of your feet with the client as you face him or her. Transfer your weight back and forth, from one foot to another.

In shiatsu, *passive stretches* are incorporated into arm or leg circumductions, by pausing and stretching the limb at strategic points in the circle. Tractioning the whole body is also used to release chi generally and encourage relaxation. When performed without driving through resistance, stretching reveals and releases tension blocks. The shiatsu practitioner takes care to ensure that lengthening the client's muscles feels good to the practitioner too. In fact, a good reach is a point where the therapist stretches his or her own body as well. Move your whole body to follow the action of the stretch (Lundberg, 1992). (Ergonomic positioning for specific stretches is presented at the end of this chapter.)

Energy Work

Paradoxically, one of the most difficult challenges to effective body mechanics occurs in subtle energy bodywork. Energy (e.g., reiki, craniosacral, polarity, jin shin do) practitioners tend to hold their hands and body still for extended periods of time as they sense and encourage subtle shifts in temperature, cranial rhythms, pulsations, electricity, or magnetism. (This is not true for therapeutic touch practitioners who move as they smoothe through energy fields.) Because of the extended lack of movement during most energy techniques, it is imperative to settle into the most stress-free (comfortable) positions you can find. I find that tensions in my muscles can be used as signals to move away from the client's body and allow the client to integrate the work that has been done. When I continue to hold a position once I find a discomfort calling, I watch my muscles tighten and restrict the sensations of subtle physical and psychological shifts.

Other suggestions that can aid in the ergonomic delivery of energy work include using an adjustable stool, which will help you to accommodate small discrepancies in height. (Do not rely solely on height variations you can reach with the stool. Remember that standing and kneeling are options as well.) Resting the weight (of your arms) on the table when feasible (e.g., as you cradle the head) can be helpful, too.

Deeper Work

In Swedish relaxation massage, your weight moves during the execution of a stroke. In deeper work, it is imperative to be lined up in a position to deliver the pressure before contacting the client's body. When you have a deeper focus, pressure is concentrated in a smaller area and only a little movement can take you out of balance. Think of lining up your body like a cue lining up for a shot. You must consider the angle that reaches down into the target muscle as well as the direction you are moving over the surface. To do this properly means that you must adjust your position often and back away periodically to give the client time to integrate the work. Also remember to use the power of resisted stretches (see Chapter 6) to augment your deep pressure work with chronically injured tissues. These suggestions, along with leaning into your work and using alternate tools (elbows, forearms, heels, and sides of hands), have been the most helpful for me as I manually lengthen with deeper tissues.

ADAPTATIONS IN THERAPIST POSITIONING

One general body mechanics goal, whether sitting, standing, or lifting, is maintaining the four normal curves of the spine. A healthy spine has a slight forward curve in the cervical (neck) region, a backward curve in the thoracic (upper back) area, another forward curve in the lumbar (low back) region, and the slight backward curve in the sacrum bone itself. Injury is more likely to occur when the bodyworker either exaggerates or diminishes these normal curves for an extended period of time or with excessive force.

Standing—Baseline Position

For a good resting standing posture, the center of the head, shoulders, and hips should fall in a line when viewed from the side. The next exercises should help the practitioner translate the sense of standing alignment into a moving dynamic.

*Adapted from Beth McKee, Aston-Patterner®, personal communication/Body Mechanics Tutorial (1995).

**Exercise 10.1. Experiencing Weight Shift
with Effleurage in a Standing Position***

The following series of exercises reminds us that adjusting the width and length of the stance establishes a base of support. Students will practice maintaining a relaxed, supported feeling in their bodies as they move through an effleurage (long, gliding) stroke.

Body rocking—Recall the concepts of grounding originally presented in Chapter 3 (Exercises 3.13 and 3.14) as you begin to establish a base of support in the standing position. Begin your practice by shifting your weight from the back leg to the front leg in a smooth, easy flow with your arms relaxed at the sides. Rock back and forth, shifting your weight from one foot to the other and back again. Change the leading foot by taking a step either forward or backward. Repeat this several times until you are able to shift easily.

Now add some arm swings. Allow your arms to lift and reach forward as you swing forward onto the balls of your feet. Hands are full, soft, and open. Arms are extended but not locked. The legs, especially the knees, are slightly flexed and ready to move. Move your whole body in the direction you are facing, initiating the weight transfer at your ankles. Feet, pelvis, hands, and face all point to the same bearing. Your spine remains erect, and the weight shift is easy and full. You flow with your own "body rocking."

Mentally review the body rocking. Now close your eyes and imagine that a client is lying on the massage table next to you. In your mind's eye, see yourself moving into an effleurage stroke. Now begin to carry out the effleurage, remembering the guidelines you kinesthetically sensed in your body for alignment. Let your face, hands, pelvis, and toes be heading and moving in the same direction. Your arms are extended but not locked. The knees are slightly flexed and able to move readily. Feel the mobility in the hip joints. The spine is erect and elongated as you move. Allow your inner self to feel soft and open as the body carries out the transfer of weight. Feel your hands imparting the sense of freedom as you move. (See Figure 10.4.)

Questions for Discussion. Could you feel the movement originating from your pelvis? Do you realize how you can use this sensation to transform your body mechanics as you perform the effleurage stroke?

Contrast this feeling with the following experience. Lock the back leg and try to shift the weight by body rocking once again. What happens to the rest of your body? What happens to your knee, hip, wrist, elbow, and shoulder joints? Now repeat the original body rocking movement with the knee unlocked. But this time, face the table and lock your arms. With your elbows locked, extend your arms on the table and try to shift your weight. What happens? For a second variation, allow your arms to be extremely bent on the massage table and once again play with shifting your weight. What happens this time? Return to the original easy flowing "body rocking" and feel the ease of movement return.

Were you able to establish easy "body rocking" with all of your joints lined up and facing the direction and intention of your stroke? How did it feel to perform your massage from this alignment? Were you able to keep joints slightly unbent (no hyperextension of the knee or elbow, for example)? Was the pelvis loose and able to pivot freely? How did that feel to you? Do you think this will make a difference for your client? How?

Sitting

When sitting, the back should have the same four gentle curves as it does when standing. Slouching places pressure on the lower back that is 10 to 15 times greater than when you are reclining (Boehm, 1993). Because it is not feasible to sit far enough back on a stool to make efficacious use of a lumbar support cushion, it is imperative to entrain a habit of supporting your back from within. Imagine each vertebra resting easily on top of one another as you sit to feel your internal support. To prevent rounded shoulders and a forward jutting head, keep your head in line with your body as you work (head–tail line) and do not drop your head down to look at your client. Glance down rather than dropping your head. You can still keep the client in sight when your head is balanced easily on top of the cervical vertebrae. (This is helpful when working from a standing position as well.)

Starting Position for Body Rocking

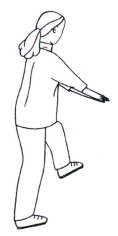

Figure 10.4   Keep your body in a straight line as you shift your weight forward and back.

Exercise 10.2. Experiencing a Weight Shift in Effleurage from a Seated Position

In this exercise, students will experience the distinction between using upper versus lower body strength as a lever for seated massage work.

Find a partner and decide which one of you will be the receiver first. The next instructions are aimed at the giver. Seat yourself on an immobile stool next to a massage table on which your client is lying down. Place yourself close to your partner, and intentionally begin with tense arms and shoulders. Use the effort of your arms and hands alone to perform some initial effleurage (gliding) and petrissage (kneading) strokes. Now sit back and relax hands, arms, and shoulders. Both giver and receiver should make a mental note on how this feels in their body, at this moment.

Then see if you can move forward into the client's body by shifting your weight forward on the chair. Pay attention to any stress and strain that you feel rising in your own body. Both partners should make a mental note on how this feels in their own body, at this moment. Now sit back and relax your upper and lower back, as well as your hands, arms, and shoulders.

Now try the exercise a third time, but this time exchange the immobile seat for a rolling and height-adjustable stool (preferably with a pneumatic adjustment), as you would find in an ordinary office chair without arms. Move along your line of effort with your entire torso and use the wheels to propel yourself further in the direction you intend to go. Make a mental note of how your body feels at this moment. Notice how the weight is balanced on the ischial tuberosities of the pelvis (the "sits bones") and how easily and effectively you can shift your weight from this balance point. It is as if you are balancing on a quadrangle made up of the two feet and two ischial tuberosities. Feet can help you pivot and change direction by scooting you on the stool, but the center of support and grounding is on the sits bones. A shift here has more effect than one initiated from the arms and hands or even from the feet.

Working in Cramped Quarters

Many therapists work in offices that are not designed to ergonomic specifications. The most common complaint I have heard about these settings are that the rooms are too small. Often, a niche barely wide enough to hold a table is carved out of a chiropractor's or naturopath's unused examination room or placed in the back of a beauty or hair salon. Many times, practitioners who take outcalls find themselves trying to find space for their tables backed up against a computer and file cabinet in the spare office room. Some suggestions that may help you adapt to these less-than-optimal conditions include the following:

1. Use all available space, including the walls. Get rid of extraneous tables to hold lotions and oils and use ledges built into the wall, or, even better, use a

holster to hold your lubricant on your body. When you find yourself backed up against a wall, use its resistance to prop or brace yourself. Some practitioners employ a half-sitting stance, propped against the wall. Another space that you can use, providing you have asked and received permission from your client, is sitting on the massage table itself. For example, when massaging the triceps on the back of the arms and the upper trapezius fibers, try perching one leg on the table next to the client's head. Your line of sight is toward the top of the table. From this position it is quite natural to let your thigh serve as a bolster for the client's arm. You can also sit on the table facing the foot of the table or facing out when massaging the client's feet.

2. The table itself can provide extra massaging space when you use the table like a footstool. To do this, lower the table height and step one foot on the table to balance. The hips sink down in the center. By shifting weight to the front or back foot, the legs can transfer your weight. Your power comes from your legs as they push against the "footstool" and floor.

Weight Change/Pregnancy

Sometimes, a practitioner must adapt body mechanics to account for a temporary gain or loss of weight. This happened to me when I became pregnant with my first son. By using the principles outlined in this book, I was able to continue working throughout my entire pregnancy. In fact, both my unborn son and I seemed to feel better after the mild exertion of performing a massage (and still do). We both loved receiving them as well. Be encouraged that you can massage, with your doctor or midwife's approval, as long as you remain comfortable and healthy, during a normal pregnancy. Some musculoskeletal changes that will affect your body mechanics during this time of shifting hormones, emotions, and mass include the following: The growing fetus places an additional strain on the lumbar vertebrae, and consequently pain is often experienced in the low back. Abdominal muscles are stretched to their limit as the fetus expands inside the womb and the pelvic muscles, which hold up the internal organs, are supporting a heavier load. The iliopsoas muscle, which flexes and outwardly rotates the hip, becomes contracted and needs to be stretched. Shoulder muscles, such as the serratus anterior and pectoralis major, are pulled forward by the expanding weight of the breasts. The result is a tendency to round the back, which can be further aggravated when performing massage.

These tendencies can be counteracted by adjusting whenever you become aware of strain and practicing the "positive pregnancy stance" as described in Exercise 10.3.

Exercise 10.3. Positive Pregnancy Stance

Stand erect with your feet slightly apart and the outer edges of your feet parallel to each other. Distribute the weight of your body evenly over the arches of your feet. Completely straighten your legs by tightening your quadriceps (front thigh) muscles. To create horizontal alignment in the pelvis, lift up your front hipbones and move your tailbone down toward the floor, as if you were tipping your pelvic bowl up. Lift your sternum (breastbone) up and slightly forward. Drop your shoulders and relax your arms. Lengthen the back of your neck and look directly forward. Ankles, hips, shoulders, and ears should be in a straight line. Adjust your standing posture as the pregnancy progresses. (See Figure 10.5.)

Adapting to Novel Client Positions

When the client is lying in a novel position on the massage table (or perhaps not even lying on a table at all), it can seem as if your smooth routines and transitions have gone out the window. The client seems like a foreign creature, and you do not have a plan for the session. Tendencies to hunch your shoulders; brace yourself against the table, bed, or chair; and stop breathing become stronger, while you are trying to figure out what to do. It is helpful to remember that all of the strokes and manipulations in your repertoire will still work when the client is in a new position. You just have to move your body into a position where it is comfortable to use them. Tuning into kinesthetic awareness can ameliorate this process. The primary purpose of the exercises in the text, particularly the exercises in Chapter 3, is to help you build the skill of kinesthetic awareness. The cardinal rule developed in that chapter applies to all variations in client positioning. When you feel uncomfortable, change something. It is a trial-and-error process. You have to feel out adjustments to make them work for you. However, in the previous section of this chapter, there are a number of suggestions to make the trial process easier. To help adapt your routine to a sidelying client, see the section on working with a pregnant client. To adapt your sessions to a client who is seated in a chair or wheelchair, see the sections concerning on-site massage, geriatric massage, and massage for clients with spinal cord injuries. To alter your routines for a bedridden client, refer to the sections on geriatric massage and spinal cord injury.

Positive Pregnancy Stance

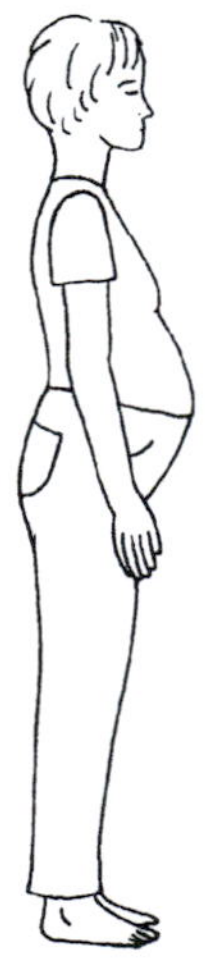

Figure 10.5 A positive pregnancy stance counteracts tendencies to round the back and feel strain in the low back.

To alter your massage for a client lying on a futon placed on the floor, see the section on shiatsu.

THERAPIST POSITIONING FOR PASSIVE STRETCHES

General rules for stretching clients are presented first, followed by specific directions for commonly used table stretches. The levers and pulleys of your body need to be in place *before* you make a move, just as you would need to get all your tools in order before executing any mechanical weight shift. Keep your dynamic alignment as you move the client through range of motion. When you need to lift, push, or pull, think about maintaining the normal curves of your spine. When lifting a heavy object, such as a long limb in a hamstring stretch, remember to lift with the legs. This means sinking down into a lunge position with both knees bent and using the legs, rather than the back, as a lever for lifting the client. Keep the back long and resist the urge to pick up the leg with a rounded back. Keeping the limb to be lifted close to your body as you lift will aid in this. When pushing or pulling something heavy, like both limbs in a quadratus lumborum stretch, bend your knees and engage your abdominal muscles to maintain spinal alignment, before you push or pull. All stretches are more easily accomplished when performed in conjunction with the client's out-breath. To get more length from the muscles that are *not* severely or acutely injured, repeat two to three times and use hold–relax (postisometric resistance or reciprocal inhibition) patterns (described in Chapter 6) rather than passive stretching alone.

Exercise 10.4. Preparation for Stretches—Self-Awareness of the Skeleton

This activity provides a kinesthetic review of the "handles" that you use to lengthen the muscles crossing joints. The handles are the skeletal bones, as well as the rough spots or indentations on the bones where the muscles attach.

The exercise is performed in a group. The leader calls out instructions, as follows: *Part 1:* Stand in anatomical position and touch the following bones and processes as they are named:

Occiput	Carpals	Medial malleolus	Clavicle	Iliac crest
Ulna	Sternum	Lumbar vertebrae	Acetabulum	Cervical vertebrae
Fibula	Tibia	Acromion process	Metatarsals	Greater trochanter
Femur	Patella	Parietal bones	Ribs	Ischial tuberosities
Radius	Scapula	Coracoid process	Metacarpals	Sacroiliac joint
Humerus	Wormian bones (sutures in skull)			Lumbar vertebrae

Part 2: Stand in anatomical position and demonstrate these drills.
Touch your left carpals to your frontal bone.
Touch your right olecranon to your left femur.
Touch your left metacarpals to your right fibula.

Touch the phalanges of your right hand to your left humerus.

Touch your right humerus to your left tibia.

Touch your calcanei to your ischial tuberosities.

Touch your olecranon processes to your floating ribs.

Touch all phalanges of both hands to your scapulas.

Exercise 10.5. Preparation for Stretching—Directional Movements

This activity provides a kinesthetic review of movements which you will use to lengthen the muscles. (See Figure 10.6.) The exercise is performed in a group. The leader calls out instructions, as follows:

Stand in anatomical position and perform the following movements as they are named.

ABduct your right leg and left arm. Now, ADduct them.

ABduct your fingers. Now, ADduct them.

ABduct your wrists. Now, ADduct them.

Rotate your arms medially (internally, in). Now, Rotate your arms laterally (externally, out).

CIRCUMDUCT your arms, one at a time.

Rotate your head.

PRONATE your forearms. Now, SUPINATE them.

FLEX your neck. Now, EXTEND it.

FLEX your spine at the waist. Now, EXTEND it.

FLEX your hip. Now, EXTEND it.

FLEX your knee. Now, EXTEND the knee joint.

FLEX your elbows. Now, EXTEND them.

FLEX your shoulder. Now, EXTEND the the shoulder joint.

DORSIFLEX your ankle. Now, PLANTAR FLEX your ankle.

EVERT your ankle. Now, INVERT your ankle.

ELEVATE your shoulders. Now, DEPRESS your shoulder blades.

PROTRACT your mandible. Now, RETRACT it.

Relax and take a few deep breaths.

Specific Stretches

Gluteal Muscles.   The client is supine (face up). The therapist is on the same side of the table as the target muscles. The therapist holds the client's posterior thigh just above the knee and moves the hip into a circle. The therapist's supporting hand is on the client's shoulder. As the limb is taken into flexion, locations where there is a glitch or stuck place in the movement should be noted. Places where the therapist or the client feels resistance are the spots to target when holding the stretch. Move the limb on a diagonal toward the opposite shoulder to focus on gluteus maximus, and more directly across the body to focus on gluteus minimus or piriformis. (See Figure 10.7.)

Hip Rotators. The client is supine (face up). The therapist is on the same side of the table as the target muscles. The therapist takes the client's hip and knee into a right angle with the table. The therapist's supporting hand is stabilizing the knee, and the moving hand is placed, palm up, just above the ankle. To stretch the lateral rotators of the hip (e.g., piriformis), pull the ankle. To stretch the medial rotators, push the ankle away. (See Figure 10.8.)

Hip Adductors. The client is supine (face up). The client's opposite leg is draped over the edge of the table, in order to keep the client from being pulled off the table. The therapist places his or her body between the target leg and the table, and is facing the head of the table. (*Note:* This positioning is the key to allowing easy, comfortable body mechanics during the stretch.) The therapist holds the client's leg just above the inside of the ankle with the outside hand and just above the knee with the inside hand. To focus on the long adductors, simply walk the leg up into abduction. To focus on the shorter adductors, keep the client's knee bent as you walk the leg out. (See Figure 10.9.)

Hamstrings. The client lies supine (face up) on the floor. The therapist performs this stretch after identifying a need during the massage and the client is dressed in shorts and top. The therapist kneels alongside the client and holds the client's leg just above the inside of the ankle with the outside hand and just above the knee with the inside hand. (*Note:* This positioning is the key to allowing easy, comfortable body mechanics during the stretch.) The therapist inches up and uses his or her body as a wedge to flex the hips and keep the knee straight. (See Figure 10.10.) (This stretch can also be performed on the table. For modesty, this is done only with client permission and with the client holding onto a secure diaper drape tucked under and around the target leg.)

Hip Abductors. (Tensor Fascia Latae and Iliotibial Band, Gluteus Medius and Minimus). The client is sidelying, with his or her back to the therapist. The client's upper hand is draped over the edge of the table, in order to keep the client from being pulled off the table. The therapist places his or her body at the waist of the client, and is facing the foot of the table. (*Note:* This positioning is the key to allowing easy, comfortable body mechanics during the stretch.) The therapist's inside hand stabilizes the client at the hip, to keep the client from rolling forward or back. The lower hand supports the client's leg just below the knee. To stretch the abductors, bring the leg back and off the table into adduction. (See Figure 10.11.)

Iliopsoas (Psoas Major and Iliacus). The client is supine and over to the side of the table enough to allow extension of the leg. The client's opposite hand is draped over the edge of the table, in order to keep from being pulled off the table.

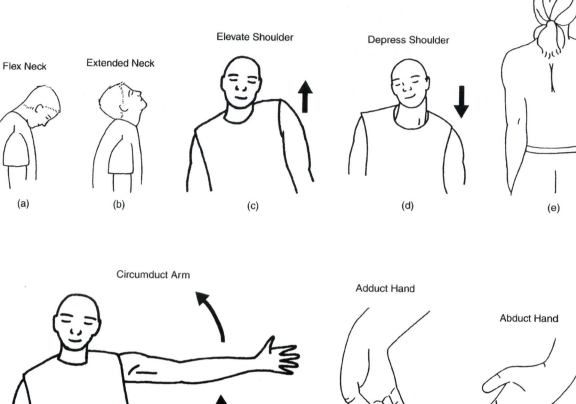

Flex Neck (a)

Extended Neck (b)

Elevate Shoulder (c)

Depress Shoulder (d)

Adduct Shoulder (e)

Circumduct Arm (f)

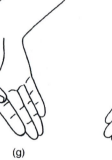

Adduct Hand (g)

Abduct Hand (h)

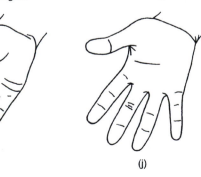

Adduct Fingers (i)

Abduct Fingers (j)

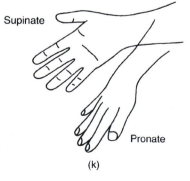

Supinate and Pronate the Hand

Supinate

Pronate (k)

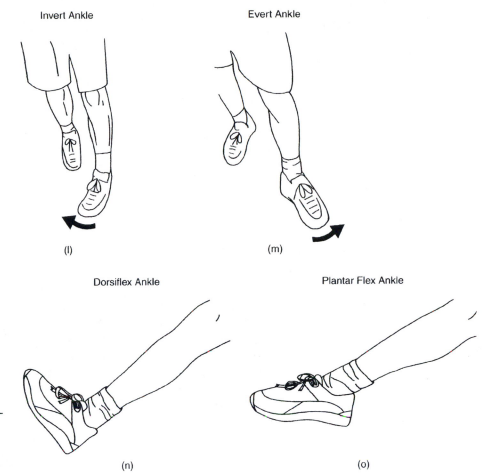

Invert Ankle

Evert Ankle

(l)

(m)

Dorsiflex Ankle

Plantar Flex Ankle

Figure 10.6 (a–o) Review the directional movements before performing any of the passive stretches described in this chapter.

(n)

(o)

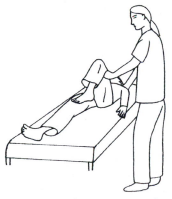

Gluteal Stretch

Figure 10.7 Move the client's hip toward the opposite shoulder for a gluteus maximus stretch and straight across for gluteus minimus and piriformis stretch.

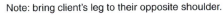
Note: bring client's leg to their opposite shoulder.

Lateral Rotator Stretch   Medial Rotator Stretch

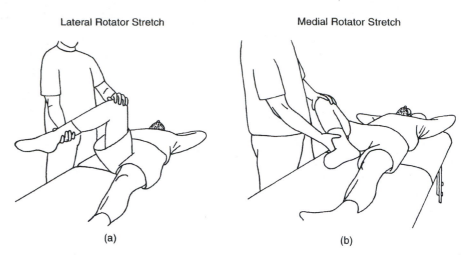

Figure 10.8 (a–b) Rotate the hip in the opposite direction of the hip rotator muscles you want to lengthen.

(a)   (b)

The therapist is on the same side of the table as the target muscle, facing the client's feet. The therapist's body is serving as a support for the client at the level of the client's waist. The therapist's upper hand stabilizes the client at the hip. The lower hand supports the client's thigh just above the knee. To lengthen the iliopsoas and iliacus, bring the leg off the table to the side, and let gravity do the work. (*Note:* This positioning is the key to allowing easy, comfortable body mechanics during the stretch.) Keep the knee as straight as possible, to isolate the target muscles from the quadriceps.

An alternate way to stretch the iliopsoas muscle is to position the client at the end of the table with the ischial tuberosities off the edge. Have the client hold one knee close to the chest and lie back on the table. Place the client's raised foot against your side and use your body to keep the client's knee close to his or her chest. This is important to keep the pelvis level. The client's other leg will be suspended, and gravity will stretch the psoas. Press on the knee to get more stretch. To switch sides, first pick up the overhanging leg and have the client hold it. Then let the other leg down while you press your side against the elevated leg. Assist the client off the table by picking up the overhanging leg and rolling both knees to the side. Let them drop to the table and help the client to sit up.

Hip Adductor Stretch

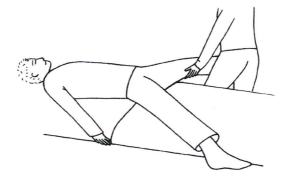

Figure 10.9 To stretch long adductors of the hip, walk the leg into abduction.

Hamstring Stretch

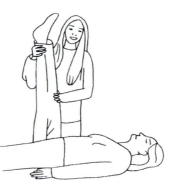

Figure 10.10 Walk the extended leg up.

Use either of these variations rather than placing the client in a prone position in which you would have to lift the leg up, rather than letting gravity do the work of lengthening the muscles. (See Figure 10.12.)

Quadratus Lumborum.   The client is prone (face down). The client's arms are draped over the edge of the massage table, in order to keep the client from being pulled off the table. The client's head is turned toward the therapist. The therapist stands on the side of the table opposite the target muscles to be stretched. The therapist stabilizes the client's hip with the upper hand, and the lower arm is wrapped around both of the client's upper calves with the fingers contacting the client's knee. The knees are bent. (*Note:* Positioning is the key to easy, comfortable body mechanics during this stretch.) Using the massage table to support the weight of the legs, draw them toward you.

An alternative is to have the client lying on his or her side diagonally across the table. The bottom leg is bent at a 90-degree angle and the top leg is extended. The client's top knee must be able to clear the back edge of the table. Stand behind the client with one hand on the greater trochanter and the other hand on the knee. Have the client hold on to the top end of the table as you press the trochanter toward the foot and the knee toward the floor. (See Figure 10.13.)

When stretching other areas of the body, it is not lifting, but rather getting your body out of line, that can provoke stress and strain. Arms and head are

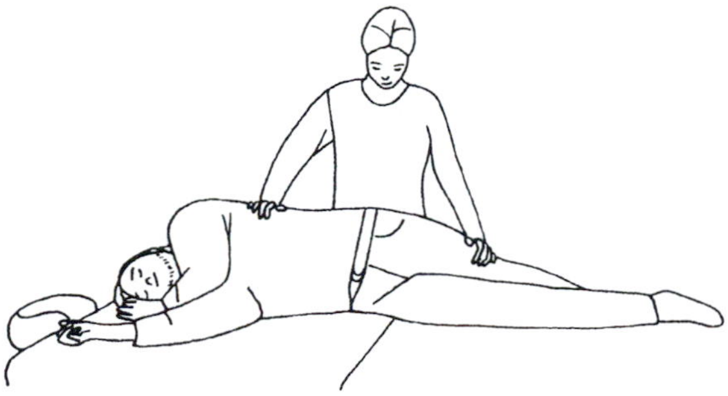

Hip Abductor Stretch

Figure 10.11 When sidelying, the force of gravity will pull the client's top hip into adduction.

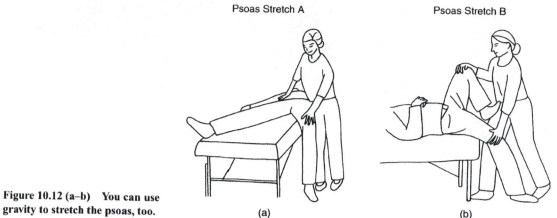

Psoas Stretch A   Psoas Stretch B

Figure 10.12 (a–b) You can use gravity to stretch the psoas, too.

(a)   (b)

QL Stretch A

(a)

QL Stretch B

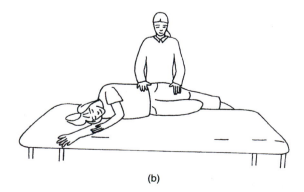

Figure 10.13 (a–b) When stretching the quadratus lumborum (QL), do not lift, but let the table support the client's legs as you slide them to the side. Use gravity for a QL stretch in the sidelying position.

(b)

lighter than legs and not so hard to lift. For this reason, the upper extremity and neck stretches will be treated in groups based on the direction of lengthening. This brevity comes with the reminder for you to sense how your body is feeling as you move the client into a stretch. If your body is not comfortable, reposition yourself until it is. Since a stretch involves sustaining a position over a length of time, it will not do to try and tough out a poor alignment for "just" the duration of the stretch. Remember that eight to ten seconds are required to maintain what flexibility a client already has, and 60 seconds are a minimum to increase flexibility.

Cervical Sidebenders. (Scalenes, Sternocleidomastoid [SCM], Levator Scapulae). The client is supine (face up). The therapist stands or sits at the head of the table. The therapist's arms are crossed. One hand supports the client's head, while the other rests on the client's shoulder. Using the massage table to support the weight of the head, draw it toward the client's shoulder, opposite of the side you wish to stretch. (See Figure 10.14.)

Cervical Extensors. (Semispinalis, Splenius Capitis, Erector Spinae). The client is supine (face up). The therapist stands or sits at the head of the table. The therapist supports the client's head with both hands. Lift the head with both hands, so that the chin comes closer to the chest. (See Figure 10.15.) (*Note:* I have also seen this stretch performed with forearms crossed under the client's neck. The advantage of this position is that the initial part of the lift can be sustained by simply straightening up off bent knees. The disadvantage is that the end of the lift requires you to scrunch up your shoulders.)

Cervical Flexors. (Scalenes, SCM). The client is supine (face up). The therapist stands or sits at the head of the table. The therapist supports the client's head with both hands. Arc your fingers under the neck and pull up, so that the chin arches away from the chest. The fingers are hooked over the client's occiput. This stretch can also be performed with a towel or scarf as an anchor. Slip the towel under the client's neck. Then, make an arc under the neck to lift it, holding the towel close on either side of the client's ears. Hooking the towel under the occiput

Cervical Sidebender Stretch

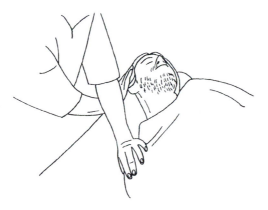

Figure 10.14 When you cross your arms, you can lean forward and use body weight to stretch the lateral flexors of the neck.

Cervical Extensor Stretch

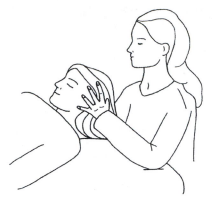

Figure 10.15 Straighten up from bent knees to supply some of the lift.

provides a wider base of support for cervical extension. (See Figure 10.16.) (*Note:* I do not teach inexperienced students the form of cervical stretching in which the client moves off the head of the table so that you are the sole support for their head. Taking the head straight down is a contraindication, it needs to be on a diagonal to avoid compressing important blood vessels. There is also the danger of dropping the client's head.)

Cervical Rotators. (Upper Trapezius, SCM, Semispinalis, Splenius Capitis). The client is supine (face up). The therapist stands or sits at the head of the table. The therapist brings the client's nose to one side. One hand is on the occiput and the other is on the forehead. To apply resistance, the upper hand shifts to the side of the jaw, along the body of the manubrium. (See Figure 10.17.) (*Note:* All of the muscles of the shoulder girdle insert on the scapula and act on it. When lengthening any of these muscles, the shoulder blade is moved. For this reason, these muscle groups are referred to as either shoulder girdle or scapular movers.)

Shoulder Girdle (Scapular) Abductors. (Pectoralis Major and Minor, Serratus Anterior).   The client is supine (face up). The glenohumeral joint should be

Cervical Flexor Stretch

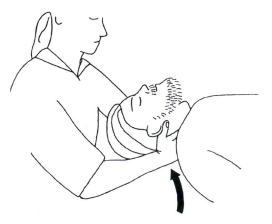

Figure 10.16 Arch the client's neck up and away from the chest to stretch cervical flexors.

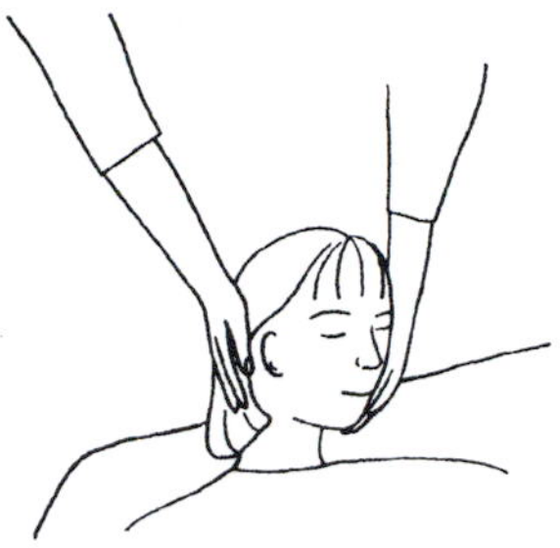

Cervical Rotator Stretch

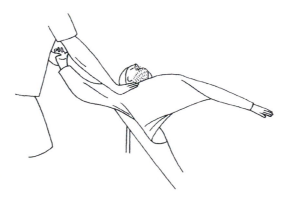

Figure 10.17 Let the table support the client's head as you rotate it.

positioned on the very edge of the massage table. The client can be asked to stabilize the stretch by holding on to the opposite edge of the table with his or her free hand. Basically, your intent is to draw one or both of the shoulders back into the military posture. (See Figure 10.18.) In one variation, the therapist stands at the side of the table, and takes the client's arm down toward the floor. This stretch can be performed at a 45-degree angle from the body, and again at 90 degrees and at 135 degrees. This helps isolate the fibers of the clavicular, sternal, and costal divisions of the pectoralis major, respectively.

Shoulder Girdle (Scapular) Adductors. (Rhomboids, Middle Trapezius). The client is supine (face up). The therapist stands at the side of the table and reaches across the client to the opposite arm. The therapist pulls the client's arm past the midline of the body, into adduction across the chest. This stretch can be combined with the shoulder joint abduction stretch for deltoids and supraspinatus, described below. To target the rhomboids and middle trapezius fibers, make sure one hand is cupping under the shoulder blade of the opposite side, and focus the pull into that area. (See Figure 10.19.)

An easy alternate method for lengthening the shoulder girdle adductors begins with the client in the prone position. Ask the client to slide the arm under his or her own body. Gravity will provide the stretch. (*Note:* If you use this option, make sure to monitor your client's discomfort level, verbally and nonverbally. The

Pec and Serratus Stretch

Figure 10.18 Keep the client's shoulder joint on the edge of the table to allow for a good pectoralis and serratus anterior stretch.

Rhomboid and Trapezius Stretch

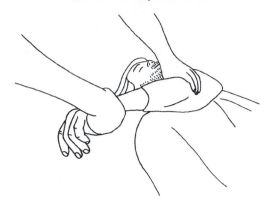

Figure 10.19   Stand at the side of the table and reach across the client to stretch the rhomboids and middle trapezius muscles.

client should stop the stretch when mild resistance is reached. If you cannot be assured that the client can do this, use the other method.)

Shoulder Girdle (Scapular) Elevators (Levator Scapulae, Upper Trapezius). The client is supine (face up). The therapist stands at the head of the table. The therapist pushes down on the client's shoulder with one hand and laterally flexes the client's neck away from that shoulder by pressing the palm of the other hand on the side of the head. (See Figure 10.20.) You can also traction the client's arm (not at the joint) down toward the foot of the table to stretch the elevators of the scapula. (Also see Figures 10.14 and 10.23) (*Note:* All of the muscles of the shoulder joint insert on the humerus and act on it. Thus, when lengthening any of these muscles, the upper arm is moved. For this reason, these muscle groups are referred to as either shoulder joint or humeral movers. Also, taking the arm into full flexion is the same as bringing the arm into abduction. An analogous relationship exists between shoulder joint extension and adduction against the body. For this reason, flexion and extension are not described with stretches here.)

Levator Scapula and Upper Trapezius Stretch

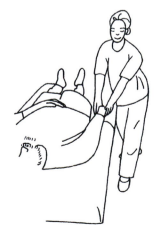

Figure 10.20   Do not pull directly on a joint when stretching the elevators of the scapula.

Shoulder Joint Abductor Stretch

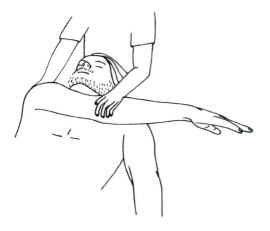

Figure 10.21 Stretching the posterior deltoids, teres minor, and infraspinatus is accomplished by bringing the client's arm into adduction across the chest.

Shoulder Joint (Humeral) Abductors (Deltoids, Supraspinatus) and External Rotators (Teres Minor, Infraspinatus). The client is supine (face up). The therapist stands at the side of the table and reaches across the client to the opposite arm. One hand is above and the other is supporting from underneath, behind the elbow. The therapist pulls the client's arm past the midline of the body, into adduction across the chest. To target the teres minor and infraspinatus, rotate the arm inwardly, as you take it into adduction. (See Figure 10.21.)

Shoulder Joint (Humeral) Adductors (Latissimus Dorsi, Teres Major, Coracobrachialis, Pectoralis Major—Sternal Division). The client is supine (face up). The therapist stands at the side of the table, next to the arm that he or she wishes to stretch. The therapist takes the arm and walks to the head of the table to abduct the arm. The therapist also moves the arm out into external rotation because all of the shoulder joint adductors internally rotate the shoulder joint. (See Figure 10.22.)

Shoulder Joint Adductor Stretch

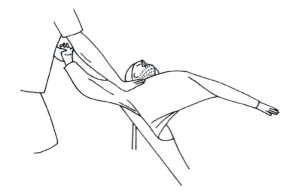

Figure 10.22 Walk the client's arm toward the head of the table to bring the adductors of the shoulder joint into a stretch.

SUMMARY

This chapter outlines situations in which modifications in body mechanics may be needed and gives guidelines for those modifications. Special situations that may call for variations in body mechanics include on-site chair massage, geriatric massage, massage for paralyzed clients, pregnancy massage, shiatsu, energy work, and deep tissue work. Special circumstances in which you will need to adapt positioning and stance include working from a seated position, working in cramped quarters, and becoming pregnant. When the client is positioned differently on the table (e.g., sidelying or in an adapted supine position) or when the client is not on a table for the massage (e.g., sitting in an office chair, massage chair, or wheelchair, or lying in a sickbed), ergonomics change as well. Appropriate adaptations are suggested for each of these situations.

Whenever possible, let the meta-principles of the MORE system (movement, observation, rest, ease and exploration) serve as a guide with alternative situations and circumstances. Include movement in your work. Observe what you are doing in this novel situation. Find a way to rest before, during, and after a session, and do not rely exclusively on fingers, thumbs, and palms. Use the rest of your body (e.g., forearms, elbows, backs of hands) as alternative tools. Keep yourself open to sense ease and exploration in your work. One guideline that prevails throughout all adaptations is the idea of lining up your body for each stroke or manipulation.

When stretching a client, your body needs to be positioned *before* you initiate the stretch. When you lift, push, or pull, think about maintaining the four normal curves of your spine. When lifting a heavy object, remember to bend, then lift with the legs. Resist the urge to pick up extremities with a rounded back. Keep the limb to be lifted close to your body as you lift. All stretches are more easily accomplished when performed in conjunction with the client's out-breath.

Ergonomically based passive stretching is presented in the third section of the chapter. Specific stretches are described in detail for therapist and client position and direction of movement.

REFERENCES

Boehm, Regi, "Integration of Neuro-Developmental Treatment and Myofascial Release in Adult Orthopedics" (1993). In John Barnes, *Myofascial Release Manual*. Paoli, PA: MFR Seminars.

Burns-Vidlak, Larry, "Massage Therapy for the Handicapped–Spinal Cord Injuries," *Massage Magazine*, Issue 22 (October/November 1989).

Jedlicka, Debbie, Personal communication (1998). Wilmington, DE: Deep Muscle Therapy Clinic and School.

Lundberg, Paul, *The Book of Shiatsu* (1992). New York: Simon and Schuster.

McKee, Beth, Aston Patterner[R], personal communication/Body Mechanics tutorial (1995). Washington, D.C.

Miesler, Dietrich, "Geriatric Massage," *Massage Magazine,* Issue 33 (September/October 1991).

Osborne-Sheets, Carole, "Massage and the Pregnant Pelvis," *Massage Therapy Journal,* Vol. 310, No. 2 (Summer 1998), pp. 88–96.

Waters, Bette, *Massage During Pregnancy* (1995). Fuquay-Varina, NC: Research Triangle Publishing, Inc.

Chapter Eleven

Stress and the Bodyworker

CHAPTER OBJECTIVES

Conceptual Objectives   The massage student/practitioner who successfully completes this chapter (reading and exercises) will be able to:

- Define stress, stressors, and the physiological stress response.

- Explain the difference between successful and not-so-successful coping mechanisms.

- Discuss viable options to improve time management.

- Explain how to set goals.

- Discuss general diet and exercise guidelines that help increase wellness and reduce stress.

- List options for coping with stress at the emotional level.

Practical Objective   The massage student/practitioner who successfully completes this chapter (reading and exercises) will be able to:

- Demonstrate and explain how to perform relaxation techniques, including progressive muscular relaxation (PMR), diaphragmatic breathing, visualization, and autogenics.

Chapter 7 reported on a variety of common injuries and repetitive stress syndromes that affect specific muscles, ligaments, or joints. In addition to these specific manifestations of stress, a generalized stress response can also strike massage therapists. The goal of this chapter is to understand and find strategies to cope with the generalized stress response, commonly referred to as *stress.*

This chapter begins with a disclaimer. Be assured that just reading this chapter will *not* manage your stress for you. You must do that for yourself. What can be achieved within the confines of the written page is to help you learn about yourself—what your stressors are and how you typically react to them. The information presented here should give you a theoretical framework of what stress is, along with some concrete coping skills and relaxation techniques. It is your responsibility to assess this knowledge, weigh the options, and choose what works best for you.

WHAT IS STRESS?

Physiologically, stress is the rate of wear and tear on the body. Hans Selye (1976) first introduced the term *stress*. Largely from the work of Selye and his predecessor, Walter B. Cannon (1932), stress has come to be defined as the body's response to any unusual demand. Seaward (1994) has expanded this definition to the following, "Stress is the inability to cope with a perceived (real or imagined) threat to one's mental, physical, emotional and spiritual well being. It is also the sum of all the physiological adaptations and responses to that threat."

Walter B. Cannon was the first physiologist to detail how the body reacts to threats. Cannon observed that animals pursued two modes of immediate action. One was to turn and fight off the attack, and the other was to flee from the danger. "Fight or flight" became the well-known label for this acute stress response (activation of the sympathetic nervous system). Hans Selye, an endocrinologist, wanted to know what would happen as a result of repeated incidents of stress. He studied the effects of chronic stress on laboratory rats and referred to the collective changes as the general adaptation syndrome. It has three stages. The immediate effects are called the *alarm reaction* (Cannon's fight or flight response). If the stress is not alleviated, the body stays metabolically activated at a lesser stage than the alarm reaction, but at a higher rate than normal. This is called the *resistance stage.* If the stress continues to a point where one or more of the organs can no longer stand the higher rate of strain and fails to function, the body reaches the *exhaustion stage.*

The physiological stimulus for the stress response originates in the brain and "travels" to the rest of the body via the hypothalamus and the pituitary gland to the target organs. The impulse reaches the organs by direct nerve contact or by secretion of chemicals directly to the organs or via the bloodstream.

A stress response is correlated with a higher incidence of many unpleasant symptoms and actual disease states, including headaches, stomach distress, infectious diseases, high blood pressure, and heart disease. Stress responses are also associated with emotional symptoms such as depression, irritability, anxiety, discouragement, worry, and burnout. Continual activation of the stress response may increase the occurrence of behavioral and performance disorders such as procrastination, increased errors in work, short tempers, poor relationships with others, sleep problems, and eating disorders.

What Is a Stressor?

A stressor is the perceived unusual demand that causes you to adapt or change. One key word to emphasize is *perceived.* A demand to adapt may be real or imagined. It may be outside the body or something originating from within. And the demand can be something you wanted or something you didn't want. For instance, let's say Jim's instructor, Linda, passes him in the hall without her customary greeting. Jim is worried that he has done something wrong. In reality, Linda just had an argument with her boss and she is preoccupied with that. Here, the stressor is not a *real* disturbance, but rather Jim's perception of the event. However, the stressor always has a *real* effect on the body. That physiological effect is stress.

Let us consider some of the more common stressors. Ask yourself which stressors are likely to disturb you and which stressors you can control. Job stressors can include unreasonable deadlines, competition, work overload, boredom, lack of fulfilling work, unclear or constantly changing tasks, clients who are unsupportive or habitually critical, fear of failing, fear of new demands, wondering why you are not getting ahead, and job insecurity.

Family stressors encompass divorce, upheavals, friction between family members, moving, sickness in the family, death of a loved one, worry over children or elderly parents, and even marriage. Marriage is a family event that is considered positive, but worries about future changes that matrimony can bring are stressors.

Economic and social strains involve the pressure to achieve and gain material wealth; exposure to conflicting values by television, newspapers, and other media; beginning and ending romantic relationships; changing or uncertain male and female roles; and a feeling of unclear values.

General stressors include illness or injuries (e.g., repetitive motion and common injuries covered in Chapter 7); unwanted noise, air, and odor pollution; excess caffeine, tar, nicotine, alcohol, and other drugs; overcrowding (traffic and fear of crime); obesity; and uncomfortable temperatures.

In sum, almost any life situation that requires a change or adaptation can be considered a stressor. Even pleasant events, like promotions, vacations, or marriage, can be stressors since they require many adjustments.

Some stressors are actually beneficial to your health. "Eustress" is good stress that arises in circumstances that the individual finds motivating or inspiring. Falling in love, embarking on a journey, and buying a puppy are likely examples of eustress. The situations are perceived as enjoyable and not seen as a threat. "Distress," on the other hand, is considered to be undesirable. It is often used synonymously with stress. Examples of distress are breaking an arm, getting fired from your job, and flunking out of school. Eustressors contribute to optimal performance. Too many stressors, whether they are positive or negative, lead to distress.

There are actually two categories of distress. One is acute (dis)stress, which appears and is very intense, but disappears quickly. Getting stopped by a policeman who gives you a traffic warning is a case of acute stress. The other is chronic (dis)stress, which may not seem to be so intense, but can last for days, weeks, even months or years. An example would be having a loud and incompetent rock band who insist on playing at all hours of the day and night move in next door.

What Happens to the Body in Stress?

When the brain interprets something to be a stressor, it sends alarm signals by nerves (quick messages) and by hormones (slower, longer-lasting messages) to all of the organs in the body. The cumulative effect of these messages is to tell the body to prepare for "fight or flight."

The fight or flight response (also known as the stress response) was identified and observed by Harvard physiologist, Walter B. Cannon. Cannon watched the cat's physiological changes when it was exposed to a dog (the stressor). The cat's senses (sight, hearing, touch, smell, etc.) became keener. The muscles tightened and tensed for action. The heart rate and breathing rate increased (so more blood and oxygen reach muscles, organs, and the brain). Stored sugar and fat entered the bloodstream (for energy to run from the dog). The digestive tract shut down (saving energy for emergency needs), and the extremities became cool and clammy (shunting blood to the core of the body).

Is this bad? The answer is an obvious no. Normally, these changes are helpful and adaptive. They prepare the body for physical activities of fight or flight and allow the body to function at peak efficiency during emergencies. This is why a mother can lift a heavy object (like an automobile) off her trapped child or why athletes exceed their normal abilities in championship games. So, stress is not necessarily bad. The body mobilizes for action, releases energy to confront the stressor, and then returns to normal.

Then what is the problem? There is no problem if you are a caveman who is suddenly confronted by a mastodon or other predator. In that instance, fighting or running for your life are the only appropriate responses. But these behaviors don't work so well when the stressor is a potential new massage client, demanding that you make space on your calendar to "fix" his or her pain immediately.

The initial stress response occurs instantly and lasts for a few minutes. Immediate effects of stress (the flight or fight response) transpire with the very next heartbeat after encountering the stressor. The first physiological responses include increased heart and breathing rates, increased muscle tension, blood pressure, and perspiration. These effects are the result of direct messages from the nerves to the organs (e.g., heart, lungs) with the release of neurotransmitters (chemicals) called epinephrine (adrenaline) and norepinephrine (noradrenaline) at the organ site.

Intermediate effects also originate in the brain and are preceded by direct stimulation of the adrenal glands (specifically the adrenal medulla), located on the kidneys. The adrenal glands release the hormones epinephrine and norepinephrine into the bloodstream. These are the same chemicals released in the immediate response; however, because they are circulating in the blood, their effects are sustained for a longer time. Intermediate effects can be noted after ten minutes and last up to two hours.

Long-term effects last long after the stressor has been confronted and dealt with. These effects can be observed after two to three hours and can last for more than two weeks. In this segment of the stress response, chemicals released from the brain stimulate a number of glands. Target organs of note are the thyroid and adrenal glands. The glands in turn release two primary hormones (chemicals) during this time: thyroxine (from the thyroid gland) and cortisol (from the outer portion or cortex of the adrenal gland). Thyroxine produces an increased metabolic rate and difficulty sleeping and concentrating, as well as a feeling of impending doom and anxiety. Cortisol is thought to be the most dangerous of all the chemicals released during the stress response. Cortisol breaks down the structure of protein and fat molecules stored in the body to get needed energy to fight off or flee the stressor. This can have a deleterious effect on internal organs as well as on the immune system. Virtually all parts of the body can be damaged if the stress is prolonged and if there is no way of using up the harmful by-products of the stress response.

Today's stressors may be clients, creditors, or even your own desires to excel. Modern dilemmas do not disappear when we fight or run away. Another complicating factor is that before one stressor is resolved, another may appear on the horizon. So stress becomes prolonged and built up. When the physiological changes don't get a chance to return to normal, the outcome can be chronic stress. Without a physical release or a break from the stress, the wear-and-tear factor can lead to our becoming ill. Some of the diseases that have been associated with chronic stress are heart disease, hypertension, diabetes, headaches, obesity, ulcers, arthritis, asthma, backaches, depression, anxiety, alcoholism, insomnia, diarrhea, constipation, colitis, hay fever, sexual dysfunction, and menstrual problems. We do not have to wait to be diagnosed with an illness, however, to detect elevated stress signals in the body. Warning signs of unresolved stress include tense muscles; edginess; inability to relax; fatigue; a pounding or racing heart; increased use of alcohol, tobacco, or other drugs; unspecific pains; nightmares; a change in appetite; the inability to concentrate; an overpowering desire to cry or run away; and feeling that there is no joy in life.

Does the content of these disease and symptom lists sound familiar? You may well be thinking that this sounds like a laundry list of typical complaints that clients come to resolve in massage sessions. Massage therapists are used to addressing the physical by-products of chronic stress through soft tissue manipulation. Perhaps you did not recognize this ramification of your work. Scheduling a massage for ourselves is one strategy for coping when we find ourselves bogged down by stress. Later in the chapter, a variety of other coping mechanisms to manage stress will be discussed.

Why Treat Stress?

In 1925, a second-year medical student, Hans Selye, observed that before many illnesses got established, sufferers complained of a cluster of symptoms. He named this conglomeration of symptoms the "syndrome of just being ill." It included being tired, experiencing changes in appetite, an increase in heart rate and blood pressure, and unspecific pains. In short, the second list of symptoms listed above describes the syndrome of just being ill. Selye theorized that it would be wise to treat stress symptoms *before* they progressed into full-blown illnesses or traumas. It is indeed true that managing stress levels now will help to ward off injury and disease. This is exactly what we purport to do for clients. Wouldn't it be wise to practice what we preach and develop strategies to reduce stress and better take care of ourselves?

Ten years after Selye's initial work, medical researchers at McGill University in Canada identified a triad of medical problems associated with acute stress. These were that the adrenal glands became enlarged and more active while stores of adrenal hormones dropped, ulcers developed in the stomach and duodenum, and the lymph system structures became smaller. This meant that the immune system was less able to fight off disease. These two complexes, Selye's "syndrome of just being ill" and McGill University's "triad," evolved into what is now known as the *general adaptation syndrome* (GAS). There are three distinct phases to the general adaptation syndrome. GAS charts the physiological process and results of human stress over time. (See Figure 11.1.)

The graph shows that humans have a great capacity for dealing with massive amounts of acute stress, but the capacity decreases as the stress continues over time. Difficulty arises when we are required to continually mobilize our bodies in response to stressful episodes. In other words, it is a physiological strain to be faced with chronic stress.

Causal Model of Stress

Can we stop the buildup of chronic stress? In order to answer this question, let us introduce a causal model of stress. The important parts of the model are the *stimulus* (stressor), the *mental* response, the *emotional* response, the *physical* response, and ultimate *disease* resulting from the stressor.

The event that initially triggers the stress reaction is a *stimulus* from the environment. The event can be anything from a loud noise (outer stimulus) to a pain in the gut (internal stimulus) to a reprimand from a colleague. Any demand can act as the initial stimulus (stressor).

In the next step, the environmental stimulus is analyzed and categorized. Here the mind labels the situation as good or bad, or harmless or threatening. This is where we decide if the situation is perceived as a threat.

If the stimulus is perceived as a stressor, emotions are evoked. Emotions can be positive, such as joy, excitement, or ecstasy, or they can be negative, such as sadness, fear, or anger.

Physical responses are instigated through a dual control mechanism made up of the nervous and endocrine systems. The nervous system uses electrical impulses from the brain and spinal cord to directly innervate selected organs in the body. The endocrine system utilizes chemical messengers called hormones that travel through the circulatory system. The electrical and/or chemical messages spark measurable changes in the functioning of targeted organs. If these physical changes (e.g., elevated pulse and blood pressure) are sustained over an extended period of time, disease will result.

Use the following example to personalize the stress model and make it more relevant to everyday experience. Joan left for work late this morning. She

Figure 11.1 A chart of the general adaptation syndrome shows three distinct stages of responding to long-term stressors. One is the alarm phase, in which resistance to disease dips and then recovers. Two is the resistance phase, in which resistance plateaus. Three is the exhaustion phase, in which resistance to disease plummets.

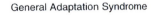
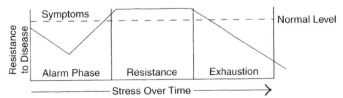

tried to get to an outcall massage appointment on time by driving 45 miles per hour in a 25-mile-per-hour zone. Joan is speeding along when she hears a siren in the distance and spots the flash of a spinning light out of the corner of her eye. She pulls over to the side of the road and stops, and a policeman walks up to the window. As she is handed a *citation,* Joan thinks, "Am I a jerk! How could I get a third ticket this year? My regular client will never reschedule. My husband will surely divorce me." That is the *mental appraisal and perception* of the event. *Emotional arousal* follows in the form of fear and self-reproach. Joan's sweaty palms; fast-beating heart; and quick, shallow breathing indicate her *physical response.* If Joan's mind, heart, and body consistently react to environmental stressors in this way, sooner or later she will get sick. Perhaps she will develop a twitch as she massages or those unexplained carpal tunnel syndrome–like aches and pains in her arms and hands. Regardless of the form of *disease,* repetitive stress creates unpleasant and costly symptoms that massage therapists want to avoid.

On the other hand, if Joan manages to interrupt the chain of events at any point, she can prevent disease and improve her all-around quality of life. How could she interrupt the stress reaction at any point in the sequence? The traffic ticket (environmental stimulus) could have been prevented if Joan got up earlier and allowed enough time for a leisurely trip. Or Joan could have accepted that she would be late and chosen to drive slower anyway. A new mental perception might be something like, "Well, I got a third ticket this morning. I'd better drive within the speed limits from now on. Even though I got the ticket, I can reschedule my client and give some compensation for the inconvenience. This was a mistake, but I am still a capable and worthwhile person. My husband still loves me, and getting a ticket is no grounds for divorce." Emotional involvement is often the hardest component to separate. Emotions erupt so quickly and forcefully, especially in the heat of the moment, that they are hard to extinguish. However, if Joan has been observing her emotions, she may be better prepared for the kind of emotions that habitually surface under stress. She can diffuse feelings after the situation has cooled down by talking with a counselor or friend or recording them in a journal. The last link in the stress chain is physical arousal. This is one of the easiest links to break. The body's response to stress can be modified with a variety of relaxation skills, such as diaphragmatic breathing, progressive muscular relaxation, or visualization. Relaxation techniques are described in more detail later in this chapter.

COPING STRATEGIES

This section reviews options for dealing with stressors to help you begin to assess which alternatives will work best for you. In numerous stress management workshops, I have asked the audience, "How do you cope with stress in your life?" The answers run the gamut from seeking a minister to zoning out in front of the television to sleeping extra hours in the day. Take some time now (before you read answers that were generated by others) to tune in and answer honestly, "how do *you* cope with stress?"

An assessment to measure the effectiveness of your baseline coping skills is provided here.

Exercise 11.1. How Well Do You Cope?*

Add 10 points if you feel that you have a supportive family.

Add 10 points if you actively pursue a hobby.

Add 10 points if you belong to a social or activity group that meets once a month.

Add 15 points if you are within five pounds of your ideal body weight, considering your height and bone structure.

Add 5 points for each time you exercise 30 minutes or longer during the course of an average week.

Add 5 points for each nutritionally balanced and wholesome meal that you consume during the course of an average day.

Add 5 points if you do something that you really enjoy that is just for you during the course of an average week.

Add 10 points if you have someplace in your home that you can go in order to relax and/or be by yourself.

Add 10 points if you practice time management techniques in your daily life.

Subtract 10 points for each pack of cigarettes you smoke in the course of an average day.

Subtract 5 points for each evening during the course of an average week that you take any form of medication or chemical substance (including alcohol) to help you sleep.

Subtract 10 points for each day during the course of an average week that you consume any form of medication or chemical substance (including alcohol) to reduce your anxiety or just calm you down.

Subtract 5 points for each evening during the course of an average week that you bring work home that was meant to be done at your place of employment.

Now calculate your total score. A "perfect" score would be 100 points. If you scored in the 50–60 range, you probably have an adequate collection of coping strategies for most common sources of stress. However, you should keep in mind that the higher your score, the greater your ability to cope with stress in an effective and healthful manner.

Over the years, health and massage students have shared many effective methods for diffusing stress. One approach is simply finding someone to talk with about the problem (this tends to be a strategy used more by women than men). Variations on this theme include calling a therapist, minister, or counselor and meditating or praying to a higher power. Another strategy is to employ relaxation techniques (such as deep breathing, yoga, and tai chi classes). A third suggestion is to avoid the situation or person that stresses you out. Other options include engag-

*From Daniel Girdano and George Everly in Controlling Stress and Tension, 3rd edition 1990 by Allyn & Bacon © Reprinted/adapted by permission.

ing in creative outlets (such as writing in a journal, dancing, creating music, or art), exercising (to use up the by-products of the stress response), and helping others.

Not-So-Successful Strategies

A number of "okay but not so successful" coping strategies have also been cited in workshops. These not-so-great methods include watching television, smoking, drinking alcohol, picking a fight, or sleeping excessively. These "okay but not so successful" techniques provide ways to temporarily withdraw from the stressful situation. They give you some "time out." What they do not do is help to reduce the bodily buildup of stress in the body. Indeed, "OK, but . . ." techniques may actually create more stress by-products in the body. Let us see how each of the "OK, but . . ." examples may not be such an effective way to cope.

Begin with an American cultural habit—watching TV. Two common types of programming that are popular on TV are soap operas and sports events. When watching TV programs the body is passive (thus the term "couch potatoes"), while the mind is emotionally involved in the outcome of the melodrama or game. The mind gets no chance to let go and renew and refresh. And the body stays in one position for a long time, so it gets no relief from feeling cranky and crabby. There is no avenue (neither fight nor flight) to release the by-products (stress hormones) of the stress response.

A second example of a not-so-successful stress management strategy is smoking cigarettes (or cigars or chewing tobacco). Smoking tobacco is essentially an act that places you at risk for nicotine addiction. Cigarettes may make you feel better in the short run (since the nicotine offers a quick physiological high and the physical act of smoking gives a time out from stressors). But when the nicotine effects wear off, the body wants to feel good again. Over the long term, the body's dependence on the nicotine "high" causes wider mood swings and offers no lasting solution to stress.

Consuming sugar and products loaded with sugar is another not-so-successful answer to a stressful situation. Sugars are simple carbohydrates that break down rapidly to provide energy and as such provide a quick rush (not unlike you would experience from imbibing nicotine). The quick increase in blood sugar makes you feel better immediately, but a quick decrease in blood sugar and a corresponding downswing in mood follow the short-lived positive effect. Over the long term, the body's dependence on the sugar "high" causes wider mood swings and offers no lasting solution to stress.

Indulging in alcohol and other drugs leads down the familiar path of dependence and addiction. Fluctuations in mood become more likely. Relying on foreign substances (such as the bottle) to cheer you up creates a whole slew of secondary problems. These include, but are not limited to, decreased communication in the family (and subsequent loss of social support), ignoring job or work requirements, and putting relationships with friends second to a relationship with the bottle.

Successful Coping Strategies

In contrast, successful coping techniques put a "brake in the wheel" of the stress response before the cycle rolls around to disease. It may be helpful to consider the full stress response as a pattern or habit that you want to break. Consider applying the steps outlined in Exercise 6.8 to your unwanted stressful habits. This involves asking yourself to:

1. Increase awareness of your stress response.
2. Generate alternatives to your habitual stress response.
3. Recognize that stress responses are ways in which humans adapt to stress.
4. Discover what you need to clear the energies and blocks set up by your particular habitual response to stress.
5. Ask yourself what you need and whether you are ready to let go of this particular response to stress.

Successful approaches stop harmful stress reactions by changing the environment directly or your perception of the situation (mind), the feelings that accompany a situation (emotions), or the physiological backlash (body) that can proceed from a stressful encounter. Successful coping techniques interrupt the stress progression before it leads to disease. Using the causal model of stress can generate alternatives for making positive changes at any level of the stress response.

Manipulating the environment means taking steps to avoid or minimize stressors. Skills such as time management or conflict resolution can help reduce stressors such as not having enough time or constantly being assailed by conflict. Conflict resolution was addressed in Chapter 9 and time management is discussed below.

Time Management. Time represents a common source of stress for most people. You often hear the expression, "There aren't enough hours in the day." In a Cathy cartoon scenario, the boss stacks extra work up on top of Cathy's already "too much to do" load. She tells the boss that she cannot possibly do all the extra work, whereas he contends that it is a simple matter of time management. When she gets back to her office, she looks at the pile of papers and yells, "Go slower!" Cathy tries to squeeze out enough time to do all that she needs to do by commanding time to "go slower!" Cathy cannot actually change the march of time itself—time is a finite resource. However, she can utilize the resource of time more efficiently.

Time management may conjure up a picture of a rigid efficiency system, in which every minute of the day is scheduled and there is no room for error. Service jobs, especially in the field of massage therapy, are fraught with last-minute changes. If your concept of time management is incompatible with a flexible schedule, think again. First, time management involves little more than a collection of simple, easily implemented but powerful ideas to help you manage your time. Second, downtime, or relaxation time, to just goof off is built into the system. It is not humanly possible or desirable to work all the time. Third, the time management techniques presented here are merely suggestions, not prescriptions for a new life. Use the options that are doable and discard the others. Adopt only the recommendations that work for you.

Time management techniques that are suggested here are *setting goals and priorities, utilizing to do lists, limiting interruptions, doing it now,* and *investing time* up front. It also makes sense to *evaluate tasks only once,* make use of *the circular file* (trash can), and check into *delegating* as a more efficient use of your time.

An important preparation for efficient time management is setting goals. It is all too easy to get so bogged down doing unimportant tasks that immediately confront you that you lose sight of what you really want to do. Setting goals and priorities reminds you to spend more time on the things you really want to do. Unless goals (the things you really want to do) are written down, they usually never get done. Working toward goals makes us feel like we are growing. It brings satisfaction and reduces anxiety.

Effective time management begins by asking the question, "What do I really want out of life?" Take some time now to stop reading and answer this question, by writing down some short- and long-term goals that you have for yourself. This process will tell you more about the real priorities in your life. Goals provide a benchmark to compare what you want to do with what you are doing. The activity can help you identify areas to be accentuated, deemphasized, or left out of your life. View these lists as challenges rather than burdens. By working through the process, you may find that some things you thought were goals were not really what you wanted at all. Identifying aims does not mean that you are stuck with the goals or that you must continue to pursue objectives that bring only suffering and pain.

On the contrary, goal setting is simply a stress reduction tool. The goals that you discover are merely there to help. You are not meant to be a slave to goals. You can always revamp, modify, and change objectives as much you want. In other words, goals are not to be taken too heavily or seriously, but they must be important enough to you in order to hold real value.

Rules for Establishing Effective Goals

1. Cultivate the habit of positive self-talk. In the field of psychology, positive self-talk is known as cognitive restructuring, cognitive relabeling, or cognitive therapy (Ellis, 1962). It is the same as affirmations, or efforts to "make firm" your aspirations (Gawain, 1978). We actually are always talking to ourselves, telling ourselves what we should, ought to, or must do. Replace the "shoulds, woulds, coulds, or musts" with what you actually do want instead. Own and take responsibility for what you want.

2. Write or think of goals in the present tense. Instead of saying, "I will get a wonderful new job with health benefits and security," say "I now have a wonderful new job with health benefits and security." The mind can be very literal in its interpretations. If you phrase goals to happen in the future, the mind cannot grasp that you will actually ever reach them.

3. Affirm what you want, rather that what you do not want. For example, it would be better to say "I wake up refreshed and on time every morning," rather than "I no longer get to work late every day."

4. The acronym KISS (keep it short and simple) provides another guideline for effective affirmation or goal setting. The clearer the statement, the stronger the feeling and the stronger the impression it will make on your

mind, body, and soul. Affirmations that are long and wordy end up not being clear. Statements that are theoretical in nature don't really mean anything in the physical world.

5. Keep your self-talk noncompetitive. It does not help to compare yourself to others. Neither is it effective to initiate goals for others that they do not aspire to. For example, a nonproductive goal would be "My son is now making $95,000 per year." Save your goals and aspirations for yourself.

6. Try to create a feeling of belief or an attitude that your goals can indeed be reached. This may mean setting aside some time to suspend and deal with doubts and hesitations so that you can put your full mental and emotional energy into manifesting your goals. (Use Exercise 11.2 on emotional resistances.)

7. Remember that affirmations are not meant to contradict or change your feelings. It is important for you to experience those emotional reactions and not deny that they exist. Resistances are telling you something concrete, something tangible, that you can work against to achieve your goal. (Use Exercise 11.2.)

Choosing goals may bring up emotional resistance. For example, you may feel depressed or overwhelmed at the thought of trying to set goals. You may find yourself eating, talking, or sleeping excessively in order to distract yourself from your aims. Or you may hear "inner voices" telling you that you "cannot" possibly do that, you "should not" be doing that, or you "ought to" be doing something else. All of these are emotional responses. They are means to avoid getting what you really want. It is important not to repress these kinds of responses, but to observe them as objectively as you can in order to learn from them.

Exercise 11.2. Working with Emotional Resistances*

Choose a goal. (If you have not recently thought about what goals you would like to set, do so as a prerequisite to this exercise.) Write this goal 10 or 20 times in succession in first-, second-, and third-person grammar. (For example: I, Marian, am an influential and well-rewarded health and massage educator and writer. You, Marian, are an influential and well-rewarded health and massage educator and writer. Marian is an influential and well-rewarded health and massage educator and writer.)

Make sure that you are not just writing out phrases by rote. Think about the meaning of the words as you are writing (or typing) them. Notice whether you feel doubts or negative thoughts about what you are producing. Whenever you become aware of a negative thought, however slight, write out the reason why the affirmation cannot work or be true (e.g., "I'm not good enough." "I'm too old." "No one will hire me.", etc.). Then go back to writing the affirmation (Gawain, 1978).

When you are finished, review the list and your responses to it. Doubts and negative self-talk will have composed a list of reasons that

*Adapted from "Writing Affirmations" in *Creative Visualization* by Shakti Gawain (1995). New World Library: Novato, CA.

you use to keep yourself from getting what you want in this particular instance.

With these new awarenesses in hand, generate some fresh goals to help you counteract the negative fears and beliefs. You may want to stick with your original objective if it still seems effective, or modify it slightly to accommodate any newly discovered beliefs.

Getting the Most out of Goals

1. Choose goals that you are pretty sure that you can accomplish. Do not take on too much at once. Set goals that feel good to you and ones that you can succeed in. The exception here is when you feel thoroughly ready and willing to tackle a big challenge.

2. When you find that you have *not* accomplished one of your goals (which will inevitably happen, sometime in life), do not criticize or blame yourself or assume that you have failed. Instead, acknowledge that you have not reached the goal and reassess whether it is still a goal for you. It may no longer be appropriate, viable, or even desirable.

3. When you do accomplish a goal, find a small but significant reward. Even a small prize makes an impression on your mind. For example, you can take a bubble bath or go thrift store shopping when you finish writing that proposal for on-site massage. Inappropriate rewards are ones that you would regret later. For example, charging a diamond necklace on credit with money that you do not have or gobbling up an entire cheesecake while standing in front of the fridge is not the best reward.

Just as it is helpful to make long-range goals, it may be useful to set tangible short-term objectives. To implement this suggestion, at the beginning of each week, it may be helpful to plan events for each day. You can start to set priorities on the lists by labeling high priority goals as "A." These are responsibilities that must get taken care of, like paying the electric bill before the power is cut off to the massage studio. Chores that are less important and less urgent are "B" tasks. "C" items are things that it would be nice to do, but even if they do not get done, it really does not matter in the long run. These are tasks that can wait. Depending on your temperament, it may also be helpful to jot down a list of things "not to do," such as watching five hours of television or stopping at a fast food restaurant for dinner.

Most people spend 80 percent of their time on B and C activities and only 20 percent of their time on things they themselves regard as high priorities. This phenomenon gives rise to what is known as the 80/20 rule (Lakein, 1973). As time management experts put it, we derive 80 percent of our rewards from only 20 percent of our activities (the A's). The majority (80 percent) of our time (spent on B's, C's, and other junk) yields only 20 percent of our rewards. That says that you need to identify and concentrate on the 20 percent of activities that will reap the big 80 percent dividend first.

Cross off all the C items from your lists. You have already identified them as items that can wait. Next, go back over your items, assigning the B's to either an A (high priority) or C (things that can wait) category. Now, cross off all your newly defined C's, too.

Once you have established some priorities in this way, it is important to revise them on an as-needed basis. Pretend you are 99 years old and looking back on your life. What really mattered? What were the important things? Compare these priorities to the way your time is now spent. Figure out small changes that help steer you in the direction that you wish to go. Would you like to spend more time with family and friends? Perhaps you could order a pizza or make dinnertime a family project. Sometimes, we think that we do not have the energy to try anything new, and yet it is the very act of trying something different that gives us a burst of energy. Periodically, review and revise your lists to see if your expectations are reasonable. This is how to set realistic and achievable goals.

What if there really is not enough time to get everything done? Then you must decide what things will get done now and where you will cut corners. Making these kinds of tough choices will, in itself, reduce stress. Letting everything slide until time runs out does not solve the problem; it creates more pressure. On the other hand, decisions and choices foster a sense of control. In turn, a sense of control reduces the feeling of stress.

Other tips to save time to concentrate on A's include evaluating tasks once, using the circular file, limiting interruptions, doing it now, and investing time up front.

Reading the mail offers a good example of how we can evaluate tasks only once. Many of us open our mail, read through it, and set it all aside in one pile to act on later. Time management experts recommend not to pick up a paper until you are ready to do something with it (Lakein, 1973). And do not put a paper down until you have acted on it in some way.

Some tasks do not even deserve a "once over." For these "treasures," do not hesitate to use the circular file (the trash can). Junk mail, for example, can be filed straight away in the garbage.

It is an inevitable part of life that throughout each day, you will be interrupted from what you have set out to do. Rather than fighting delays, it helps to recognize and plan for them by setting aside time for interruptions. You can also limit delay time by allotting certain hours when you will not accept phone calls, visitors, or last-minute clients.

Procrastination is a strategy that does not work. Problems usually do not go away by themselves. They usually just get worse if we put them off. On the other hand, once you get unpleasant tasks like chart notes out of the way, then you can relax without guilt. With these tasks, it is more important to finish than to worry about doing it perfectly. And if a task seems overwhelming, try breaking it up into smaller tasks and take it one step at a time.

Some time management gurus also include delegating among their time management tips. This is okay as long as you evaluate whether the delegation will really save time. Some questions to ask are: "Will an extra person help?" "Will a group effort help?" "Is someone besides you able to do the work?" "Are you truly delegating or just shirking responsibility?"

Finally, it is important to recognize that it takes time to make time. Planning, making lists, and setting goals all take time. The bottom line is that you need to invest time initially in order to get the maximum rewards for your time later.

Cognitive Restructuring. *Managing the mind* can be difficult to do. In essence, changing a response at the mental level involves changing your perception of a situation from one of crisis to opportunity. The Chinese symbol for crisis is the same as the symbol for opportunity. Crisis can afford opportunity. To perceive this, you must learn to see the difficulty as a challenge and get rid of your inner judge. This change in perception is a skill that can be taught, and *is* taught under the names of cognitive reappraisal or cognitive therapy (Ellis, 1962).

How a situation is perceived may be even more important than the situation itself. Cognitive restructuring, cognitive reappraisal, cognitive therapy, relabeling, and attitude adjustment are all names to describe how to change the way that you think or respond automatically to certain stimuli. The technique for positively changing our perceptions is modeled on Albert Ellis's "rational emotive therapy" (RET) method. It involves learning to see stressors as challenges rather than threats. Since cognitive therapists believe that you do not have an emotion unless you have a thought first, the process also requires you to evaluate and replace negative self-talk, also known as irrational thoughts. Ellis (1962) says that people can retrain themselves to favorably alter negative or stress-producing perceptions (irrational thoughts) into healthier and more rational self-talk.

Self-talk includes the thoughts, attitudes, beliefs, and words that pass through the mind, often unconsciously. Excessive negative self-talk is based on distorted thinking. It can be irrational and harmful to self-confidence and self-esteem. Negative self-talk is the chatter that automatically pops into the mind and tells you how horrible a situation is, how terribly you are going to do on a test, or what a horrible person you are for having conceived of such an ugly thought. Negative self-talk is the automatic punishment you think you deserve when something "bad" happens. A negative perception of an event elicits mental upset, which can then domino into the chain reaction of a stress response. The chief characteristic of excessive negative self-talk is that it tends to be incorrect and irrational. It may include the following misconceptions:

1. *Catastrophizing*—seeing the worst in every event (e.g., when you expect the worst, it will come; "Isn't this awful?").
2. *Minimizing and maximizing*—ignoring the positive and emphasizing the negative.
3. *Polarized thinking*—seeing things as black and white, with no middle ground for compromise (e.g., considering a situation to be all good or all bad; either you are perfect or you are a failure).
4. *Overgeneralizing*—believing that because something happened once, it will always happen. (e.g., "I *always* do, feel, think, act . . . this way," or "Anyone who smokes can't be trusted.").
5. *Self-referencing*—believing that people are watching you and counting every mistake.

6. *Filtering*—looking only at facts that would support a negative outcome and not considering those that would appear more positive (e.g., "I would have enjoyed the vegetables, but the chicken was burnt.").

7. *Mind reading* (e.g., "I know how you feel about me.").

8. *Control, change, or fairness delusions* (e.g., control: "I am helpless, a victim of fate," or alternately, "Everything is my fault or because of me."; change: "I can change what my sister does."; fairness: "Life should be fair."). To put it bluntly, sometimes life stinks, and you have to pick up the pieces and go on from there.

9. *Blaming* (no matter whether it is yourself or others whom you blame).

10. *"Ought to's, have to's, or should's"* (these are power-sapping rules—replace them with more empowering "I choose to's").

11. *Emotional reasoning* (e.g., "I feel stupid, therefore I must be," or "I feel boring, therefore I must be boring.").

12. *Justifying*—having to be right.

Use the following script to practice breaking away from a negative emotional response and exercising cognitive restructuring skills instead.

Exercise 11.3. RET Practice/Cognitive Restructuring

"A" is a real event, behavior, or attitude of another person. For example, "A" is the announcement of a new test by the massage therapy board in two weeks.

"B" is your self-talk about what will happen. (For example, "I can't remember any anatomy. I'm going to fail and lose my license.")

"C" is your emotional reaction. (For example, "I am anxious, worried, and unhappy.")

A more rational solution to this dilemma would be as follows.

I cannot change "A," the environment. The test will happen, no matter what.

But I do want to change "C," my emotional response. I want to feel better.

In order to positively affect my emotional response, I must change "B," my perception of the event.

More adaptive options to replace the irrational thoughts could include the following:

1. There is a lot of material to study. So I must plan well. The week before the test, I will review all the material for the test. I will be ready for the test and I will do well.

2. I'm not dumb and stupid because I have passed other tests. I can pass this test too.

3. I have the old exams so I know what type of questions to expect. There won't be any surprises. I've studied and I will do well.

4. My friends have taken the course and said that the instructor grades fairly. If I put the work in, I can pass.

Changing habitual negativity requires restructuring thoughts by enacting these steps:

1. Become *aware* of events that cause you to think negative thoughts. Also become aware of events that cause you to become worried, anxious, scared, or nervous.

2. Consider why you feel that way and *observe without judging* the thoughts that pass through your mind.

3. *Rethink* new thoughts that are more realistic. Avoid the characteristics of negative self-talk. Learn to recognize distorted thinking and channel it into more positive thoughts.

4. *Act* on the new thoughts. Look at the situation to see the effect of your actions. Do a reality check to see that what you are feeling is really accurate.

To put these activities into practice, choose a situation that is particularly bothersome to you. Be aware of the negative self-talk related to it and write it down on a piece of paper. Then try to reappraise the event. Use the information to help you learn more about yourself and help you to eliminate your stressors.

Communication. As indicated earlier, the *emotional response* is probably the hardest level to change in the heat of a stressful scene. Feelings tend to explode so quickly and powerfully that they are hard to stop once they have started. However, this does not mean that it is impossible to put a "brake on the wheel" at the emotional level. Communication with others helps us let out bottled-up emotions after the stressful episode and helps us prepare for emotional situations that tend to recur again and again. It does not matter who you talk with as long as you feel safe, supported, and heard. A confidant can be a friend, minister, counselor, member of the family, even a relative stranger who is in a supportive frame of mind.

Diet. *Physiological responses,* by contrast, are easier to change. The body, just by virtue of its mass, is slower and more substantial than thoughts and emotions. Thoughts and emotions are intangibles that are difficult to grasp or hold onto. They come up so quickly, like lightning, and can overpower you, before you know what is happening. But the body is more adaptable and tractable. You can literally "get a hold" on it with stress management techniques. Relaxation techniques, which are body-based, work even when the mind is in disbelief. Basic self-care measures of eating right and exercising prudently help prepare the body to adapt to change (stress) more easily. Although this is not a treatise on nutrition and/or fitness, some general diet and exercise recommendations are in order.

Following are general recommendations derived from the American Health Association and commonsense guidelines. First, several categories of foods should be a part of our everyday diets. These types of foodstuffs are proteins, carbohydrates, fats, vitamins and minerals, and water. Proteins make up the outside layer of all body cells; they also make many of our hormones (chemical messengers), and they help us fight infection and disease. Carbohydrates provide quick energy and are the body's preferred (most readily used) fuel. Fats carry certain vitamins and comprise other important hormones. They are also helpful to maintain healthy skin and hair. Vitamins and minerals enable the body to utilize the fats, proteins, and carbohydrates that are ingested. Water is needed to digest (break apart) nutritive substances and to flush toxins out of the systems. Human bodies must have all of the nutrient types to survive and thrive. Therefore, it makes no sense to eat diets made up of only one or two foods. In other words, the miracle "grapefruit and donut" diet is not a recommended regimen.

Another general guideline is to reduce salt intake. The human body needs about 1/2 gram of sodium per day on average, but 2 to 3 grams is a safe and adequate dosage. In contrast, most Americans eat 20 to 30 grams of sodium per day (Snodgrass, 1989). Excess salt in the diet contributes to higher blood pressure and stomach cancer and tends to swell and put a strain on every cell in the body.

A third general nutritional principle is to limit intake of simple sugars. Simple sugars taste sweet, as opposed to complex carbohydrates, which taste starchy. White bread and table sugar are examples of simple carbohydrates, whereas whole wheat pasta and grains are complex carbohydrates. Many processed foods include a lot of simple sugars, because they make "food" more palatable to consumers. Read the labels.

Decreasing your intake of saturated fats and cholesterol is another good idea. In general, you can spot saturated fats because they are solids at room temperature (e.g., butter and margarine), whereas unsaturated fats are liquids at room temperature. Once again, beware of processed foods. They often are high in fats, which are cheap and help to hold flavor in foods. Saturated fats and cholesterol tend to constrict blood vessels and put a strain on the heart. It is hard to pump blood-borne nutrients through a lining of plaque. In addition, plaque can form clots that can dislodge and land in the heart to create a myocardial infarction (heart attack), or clots can travel to the brain to cause a cerebrovascular accident (stroke).

Put a limit on caffeine and related substances. This means drinking less caffeinated coffee and sodas. Related substances are theobromine, which is found in chocolates, and theophylline, which is found in black tea. (Herbal teas are usually free of these elements.) Theobromine, theophylline, and caffeine are all pathomimetics or drugs that imitate the stress response. Also beware of over-the-counter (OTC) drugs that include caffeine as an ingredient. Caffeine is a common additive in OTC stimulants, pain relievers, diet aids, diuretics, and cold remedies.

In fact, it is a good idea to reduce your intake of all additives. Read the labels. If you cannot understand what the ingredient is, let that be a red flag. Long names like polysorbate-80 are a sign that this is probably not a natural food. (My friend, Dietmar, makes it a rule not to buy products with more than six ingredients. He also rejects foods with ingredients that are too complex to pronounce.)

In addition to all of these suggestions about "what" you eat, consider also "how" you are eating. By that I mean, are you eating while angry or upset? Are you grabbing fast food on the way to work and gobbling it down between clients or are your taking the time to truly be thankful for and enjoy your meal?

Exercise. Can you say enough about the beneficial effects of exercise? Exercising uses up the toxic products (e.g., steroid hormones) of the stress response. By doing so, exercise favorably alters the way your body handles stress. For example, a person who is under a regular exercise regimen has a heart that does not beat as fast and has hormones that do not pour out so quickly in response to stress. Participating in physical activity provides a "time out" from stressors, and produces endorphins (enkephalins—natural "high" painkillers) that make it easier to flow with changes. Exercise increases energy and stamina. It reduces appetite and aids in weight management. Exercise has also been shown to reduce depression (Corbin and Lindsay, 1988). To maintain a fitness regimen, choose an exercise (or exercises) that you like to do and find someone you would like to do it with. The best-laid exercise plans will not last long if you choose to jog because its good for you but hate to run.

Relaxation Techniques. Relaxation is the opposite of stress. What does that mean? When the body is stressed, the heart pumps faster, the senses focus harder, and the breathing gets faster and shallower. Relaxation is the opposite of all that. In a relaxation response, the cardiac and respiratory pulses slow down and become easier. The extremities get warmer because the blood is getting to all parts of the body as the blood vessels dilate and become more relaxed. In more general terms, relaxation means that the mind and body are calm. It does not mean that the mind is dull or comatose. On the contrary, the mind is focused and alert (Benson, 1975).

What people do for recreation is often not relaxation. Relaxation is not the same as being passively entertained. Lying on the couch watching football keeps the body quiet but the mind is kept busy with an emotional involvement in the game. Passive entertainment of this kind arouses the mind and prevents both body and mind from finding the freedom to restore and renew.

Lying in bed while worrying is also not a means for true relaxation. This is another case in which the body is held captive in stillness while the mind is actively running around in circles. Neither the body nor the mind has an opportunity to replenish reserves.

Extra sleep is another coping strategy that has been incorrectly associated with the parasympathetic state of rest and repose. Although sleep is essential to good health, excessive sleep is not the same as relaxation. Electroencephalograms (EEGs), which measure brain wave activity levels, show that sleep is illustrated by a wave that alternates between a low-level frequency and a very fast-paced high frequency. This is in contrast to both wide-awake EEGs (beta waves) that have a high, fast-pitched pace and relaxation (alpha waves) EEGs that have a slower, steadier pace.

Using tranquilizing drugs is another strategy that is really not relaxing. Alcohol, the most prominent tranquilizer, numbs the central nervous system. This physiological change makes you less responsive to stressors. Contrast the dulled sensation of a drinker with the relaxation response, which leaves the body and mind calm and clear without clouding the senses. True relaxation helps people react more quickly and adaptively to stress.

A prominent myth about relaxation is that it will reduce productivity: "I can't take the time out to relax!" Actually the opposite is true. Relaxation will actually increase productivity because your energy resources will no longer be wasted on anxiety and worry. You can then accomplish goals more quickly and efficiently.

Another myth is that relaxation will require a new lifestyle or philosophy. Again, nothing could be further from the truth. Relaxation techniques take only a few minutes one or two times a day, plus a dedication to practicing a calm attitude for that time. In reality, you do not even have to believe in the efficacy of the techniques for them to have a positive effect. Test this claim for yourself by sampling the relaxation techniques canvassed in this chapter. A wide variety of relaxation techniques are available to help counterbalance stress. No one technique is "better" than another. Use whichever ones work best for you.

One of the automatic physical responses to stressors is increased muscle tension. A simple, easy way to loosen up tight muscles and combat stress is to practice *stretching* exercises. It helps to develop a regular time for stretching and to supplement this time when your muscles are feeling particularly tight and achy from a heavy massage load, for example. The exercises specified in Chapter 8 take only a few minutes and can be done at home or at work during breaks between sessions or during lunchtime. You might wish to check with a medical professional before starting any stretching regimen.

Exercise 11.4. Progressive Muscular Relaxation

What if you are so strained that you can't remember how it feels to relax? Progressive muscular relaxation (PMR) is a technique that can help you actually feel the difference between tension and relaxation. There are three steps to the technique: (1) Contract an area and sense how it feels, (2) release the tension and pay attention to that feeling, (3) concentrate on the difference between the two sensations. You can practice PMR while sitting or lying down or even, in an abbreviated form, while waiting in a supermarket or post office line. It does help if you have a quiet place in which to attune to your body sensations. Work through each of the major muscle groups of the body. I prefer to move from the feet up to the top of the head, relaxing muscles, organs, and tissues in the feet, legs, thighs, pelvis, chest, shoulders, arms, hands, back, neck, face, and skull. For each area, tighten the body part, release the tension, and then notice the difference.

Here is the basic procedure to implement PMR. Tighten your hand muscles to make a fist. Notice how that feels. Your muscles become taut and strained, and your hand may even be trembling a bit. You may feel some tension extending into the rest of your hand, wrist, and forearm. Hold the tension, feel it, and record how that feels. Relax your fist slowly and let the tension slip away. You can imagine invisible strings connecting the fingers to the palm feeling as if they are loosening as well as letting go. (If you prefer, relax the hand quickly, all at once, as if someone just released the pressure on a balloon.) You may notice that your hand feels lighter than before and you may sense less pressure in the area.

Make a mental note of the difference between how your hand felt when it was tensed and how it feels now that you have released the tension. Did you feel throbbing or other sensations? Did the sensations you felt when tense dissipate when you let go? Does your hand tingle or feel warm when you are relaxed? Do you feel the blood coursing through?

Exercise 11.5. Diaphragmatic Breathing

Probably the most basic relaxation technique is deep breathing. It is a skill that can be practiced anywhere and anytime. One of the body's automatic responses to stress is rapid, shallow breathing. Breathing slowly and deeply is one way to stop the stress reaction and replace it with a relaxation response. The idea is to inhale deeply and allow your lungs to breathe in as much oxygen as possible.

Sit or stand in a comfortable, aligned posture (see Chapters 2 and 3) and rest your hands on your belly. Inhale slowly and deeply through the nose, letting your belly fill as much as it comfortably can with each breath. Resist the temptation to be a "backward breather" (someone who tightens the stomach when breathing in).

When you have expanded as much as possible, hold your breath for a few seconds before continuing. Now with hands still resting on the belly, exhale slowly through your mouth, with your lips slightly pursed, as if you were going to whistle. Pursing the lips helps you to control the speed of exhalation. As you breathe out, feel your stomach flatten as the diaphragm returns to its rounded position under the lungs. When your lungs feels empty, begin the cycle again. Repeat three or four times or as long as you feel comfortable with the practice.

Clearing your mind is a way of giving yourself a mental break from the stressors that plague you. It forms the basis for more complex skills such as meditation. Concentrating on one pleasant thought, word, or image allows your worries to slip away. Prepare by reducing distractions, noise, and interruptions as much as possible. Allow yourself to focus on the word "peace" or the picture of a sailboat drifting with the tide, or whatever image feels relaxing to you. If other thoughts enter your mind, just take note of the distraction and begin to focus on the relaxing image again.

Set aside five to ten minutes each day to clear your mind. Stretch and exhale as you complete the routine. Regular practice can help you feel refreshed, energetic, and ready to tackle your next stressor.

Exercise 11.6. Visualization

If clearing your mind is a sort of mental retreat, visualization is like a "mental vacation." It is granting permission and providing a structure for daydreams. Unlike trying to focus on one single image, visualization allows your imagination and subsequent feelings of relaxation to run free.

Visualize yourself comfortable, calm, supported, and relaxed now. Picture a peaceful scene that has a particular appeal for you. The scene can be an actual physical place or one where you like to go in your mind. Imagine all of the details. Are you lying on a warm beach with the sun beating on your back? Do you hear waves lapping on the sand? Is there an ocean scent in the air? Do you see sailboats on the horizon? Just by using the imagination, you can give yourself a vacation whenever and wherever you want. Use this technique when you feel the need to relax and find a respite to enjoy life again.

Autogenics is based on suggesting to your body it might like to feel. Sit comfortably, loosen any tight clothing, and close your eyes. Begin with a relaxing thought, such as "I feel calm" or "my mind is at peace." Then, bring your attention to your right hand and repeat a mental cue, such as "my right hand feels warm and heavy" until it actually begins to feel warmer and heavier. As you focus on the phrase, try to imagine your arm actually getting heavier and warmer. Repeat the mental suggestions with attention on the arm, shoulder, and so on until you have covered the entire body and/or feel completely relaxed. Practice for five to ten minutes to start. Open your eyes, breathe deeply, and stretch. Notice how you feel as you finish the exercise.

To review, you can successfully cope with stress and stop its progression at any point in the stress cycle. There are options for changing and challenging the environment, perceiving the situation differently with the mind, harnessing the emotions, and grounding the stress experience with the body. In the myriad of stress reduction methods, the easiest ones to adopt tend to be strategies that involve the body.

SUMMARY

The goal of this chapter is to understand and find strategies to cope with the generalized stress response, commonly referred to as *stress*. Stress is the body's response to any unusual demand. The physiological rate of wear and tear on the body is also referred to as stress. Seaward's (1994) expanded definition of stress is the inability to cope with a perceived threat to mental, physical, emotional, and spiritual well-being and the sum of all the physiological responses to that threat.

(continued)

A stressor is the perceived unusual demand that causes you to adapt or change. Stressors for a bodyworker could be a client who is consistently late or one who pays with a bad check, working too long in a cramped studio without a break, or tingling and numbness in the hand and arm.

Successful coping techniques provide ways to withdraw from the stressful situation. They give you some "time out." By doing so, successful techniques help to reduce the buildup of stress in the body. You can successfully stop the progression of stress by avoiding the stressor in the first place, changing the way you think about the stress, changing the way your emotions come into play, or altering your bodily responses to stress. Skills that will serve you in developing successful coping strategies include time management, setting goals, reaching out for support, engaging in creative projects, maintaining a healthy body through good diet and exercise habits, and relaxation techniques.

Relaxation reduces the energy wasted on anxiety and worry. Relaxation does not require a new lifestyle or philosophy. Relaxation techniques take only a few minutes one or two times a day, plus dedication to practicing a calm attitude. You do not even have to believe in the efficacy of the techniques for them to work. Some of the relaxation techniques explained in this chapter include stretching, progressive muscular relaxation (PMR), diaphragmatic breathing, clearing your mind, visualization, and autogenics.

REFERENCES

Benson, Herbert, *The Relaxation Response* (1975). New York: Morrow Press.

Cannon, Walter, *The Wisdom of the Body* (1932). New York: W.W. Norton.

Corbin, Charles, and Ruth Lindsay, *Concepts of Physical Fitness with Laboratories* (1988). Dubuque, IA: Wm. C. Brown Publishers.

Ellis, Albert, *Reason and Emotion in Psychotherapy* (1962). New York: Stuart Press.

Gawain, Shakti, *Creative Visualization* (1995). Novato, CA: New World Library, www.nwlib.com.

Girdano, Daniel, and George Everly, *Controlling Stress and Tension: A Holistic Approach* 3rd edition (1990). Needham, MA: Allyn & Bacon.

Lakein, Alan, *How to Get Control of Your Time and Your Life* (1973). New York: The New American Library, Inc.

Seaward, Brian Luke, *Managing Stress* (1994). Boston: Jones and Bartlett, Inc.

Selye, Hans, *The Stress of Life* (1976). New York: McGraw-Hill.

Snodgrass, Jeanne (1989). The George Washington University ELDERHOSTEL Consumer Health Class, Washington, DC.

Chapter Twelve

Conclusions

CHAPTER OBJECTIVES

Conceptual Objectives   The massage student/practitioner who successfully completes this chapter (reading and exercises) will be able to:

- List five or more benefits of using good body mechanics.

- Define *body mechanics, ergonomics,* and *self-care.*

- Describe the difference between a series of actions and lived movement.

- Explain the six levels of understanding for body mechanics and self-care.

MAJOR CONCEPTS

If there is an overall conclusion to be drawn from this work, it is that, above all, bodyworkers need to listen to their own bodies. The best way to maintain good *body mechanics* and avoid injury is to pay close attention to how you feel as you work. This is true also when preparing or recovering from a massage workday. Learning how to attend to the bodyworker's physical and psychological needs is at the heart of the issue and is the essence of *self-care.*

The primary guidepost for listening was delineated by the *MORE* system (movement, observation, rest, and ease and exploration). When performing massage, keep your body moving. Movement prevents your body from getting stuck in harmful positions, habits, and patterns. When you remember to observe your body, do it without judging. It is important to rest your body when it hurts or feels fatigued. Hopefully, among the many restorative alternatives provided in this book, you could identify the stretches, movements, and practices that achieve constructive rest for you. Regarding rest, it is also important to remember to use the "rest" of the body, besides overworked thumbs, fingers, and palms that often bear so much of the brunt of our work. Ease is achieved by thinking of and embodying answers to the internal question, "What could be lighter or softer?". Ease requires a choice to ask these questions during a massage, rather than "how can I fix this?" or "how can I power through?". Exploration means learning how to stay or become fascinated with your work. These four guiding principles involve a considerable amount of intent on the part of the therapist. But considering the alternatives of injured bodies and shortened careers, who can say that attention to MORE is not worth the effort? The payoff is increased job satisfaction and, as a by-product, increased life satisfaction.

With the overall MORE principles in place, subsequent chapters focused on analyzing specific methods for incorporating movement, rest, ease, and exploration in your massage, along with what to observe as you work. Chapter 3 allowed you to derive ergonomic suggestions based on Western ideology about physics. This chapter encourages you to look at the way physical bodies work from the inside. This approach led to observations on alignment and its effect on weight, mass, lifting, and leveraging. In Chapter 4, kinesthetic study was assimilated and incorporated from Eastern bodywork. The investigations of traditional Chinese medicine and ayurvedic principles led to additional standards of homeostasis, centering, and leaning, and understanding these concepts as manifestations of energy flow. Chapter 5 focused self-observation specifically on how you move (or do not move) in a session. Where you start, how you progress, and where you are moving to can change your actions in minute ways that shape the bodywork session and your body's reaction to your work. As an outgrowth of the exploration into movement patterns, Chapter 6 focused on a discussion of the process of release for patterns that are no longer useful or wise. When massage therapists release habits and focus on listening to the body instead, they can limit damaging actions and begin the process of recovery even during times of physical stress. Major repetitive stress injuries and other common injuries that afflict bodyworkers and their early warning signs are described in Chapter 7, along with self-care strategies for prevention. If a bodywork injury occurs, self-care strategies for rapid and more thorough recovery are presented. Chapters 8 and 9 dealt with physical and psychological preparation for massage. These preparations also need to correlate with what the body tells you about its needs. Physiological preparations described in Chapter 8 include stretching, strengthening, and toning your muscles. Psychological preparations in Chapter 9 covered learning enough about yourself and your work to establish clear boundaries and to communicate them well, even in the face of conflict. When you listen and respond to inner reactions to small encroachments on time and space, you can prevent them from becoming large "headaches." Chapter 10 highlighted instances in which body mechanics need to be tempered by limitations in either the client's body (human factors), the positioning of the client (situational factors), the setting for the massage (environmental factors), or the therapist's own physical constraints (also human factors). Chapter 11 applies the same identification and healing strategies to stresses that may be more mental, emotional, or even spiritual in origin. All in all, the overriding message of the text is to pay attention to yourself as well as to your clients. This implies a process of learning to love yourself at least as much as you love massage.

Definitions Revisited

In the very beginning of the book, definitions were given to help guide the exploration into body mechanics and self-care. Let us now revisit the definitions of body mechanics, ergonomics, and self-care, to allow you to see if your understanding of the terms has been shaped through your process of study and self-examination.

Body mechanics is the study of how forces act on the human body. Body awareness incorporates the study of body mechanics with the internal study of how the body feels as it acts. An unvarying protocol for a body mechanics dilemma cannot work in isolation of situational and human factors. Body awareness is incompatible with treating human bodies as machinery with interchangeable transmissions, crankshafts, and gears.

Ergonomics is the use of tools in a way that helps the human body to do the required work, as opposed to refitting the body to fit the tools at hand.

Self-care is the art and science of maintaining good health, so that you can perform your work as a massage therapist easily and well. This means taking care of the heart, mind, and soul. Thus, psychological self-care strategies, such as finding social support and setting clear and safe boundaries for yourself and for clients, are as important as a standard regimen of exercise, good nutrition, and adequate rest. This involves preparations before a client session and recovery after, as well as taking care of yourself during the massage session.

Good preventive health care certainly involves self-care *during* the massage (e.g., shaking hands out that feel cramped or changing positions when your body says it hurts). However, reliable self-care does not begin when the client gets on the table and end when the client gets off. It is essential to plan *beforehand* (e.g., developing coordination, stretching and strengthening routines) to prepare your body to meet the demands of the session. It is also crucial to maintain health care habits after the massage is complete (e.g., icing to relieve inflammation and stretching to counteract the effects of habitually curling the upper back). Self-care means learning to cope with *stress* in ways that help you avoid chronic diseases. Successful coping mitigates the debilitating results of the stress response. Self-care becomes a process that begins to shape the massage therapist's way of life. If you cannot care for the quality of your own life, how can you offer good care to others?

APPLICATIONS

Proper body mechanics and self-care techniques (both physiological and psychological) promote ease in working with clients and help you avoid occupational injury, stress, and burnout.

Once you identify a sensation of discomfort, you need to make appropriate changes to feel better during the massage. Some exercises in this text have enhanced the ability to sense the moment when a body position or technique is not comfortable or effective. Others provided alternatives to unhealthy patterns. It is now your responsibility to choose which body mechanics options work best for you. Increased self-awareness and attention to self-care is conveyed to clients. You end up helping clients more while reshaping your massage into a craft that is more effective, potent, and prosperous.

The process of "letting go" of harmful patterns or learning to relax has been addressed with simple techniques such as stretching, breathing with attention, and guided visualizations. These processes may have already been familiar, but a reminder of the potency and applications of relaxation and self-care techniques can be empowering.

Sometimes, despite the best understanding and intentions, the bodyworker can get hurt. This text provided a basic understanding of the etiology and treatment options for overuse syndromes and common injuries that can affect bodyworkers, such as thoracic outlet syndrome, carpal tunnel syndrome, low back pain, temporomandibular joint disorder, headaches, sciatic pain, and knee and other joint dysfunctions. It also provided some strategies for preventing the recurrence of repetitive stress conditions.

The text developed basic body mechanics skills by providing a theoretical framework and a kinesthetic experience of the theory. Although ideally suited to a classroom environment, where exercises can form the basis for class experiences and discussion, the information presented here can provide a rudimentary curriculum for a body mechanics study or support group. If you prefer to work individually, the exercises can be run through at your own pace (as long as you find a partner(s) to assist in the group explorations). The aim of this book is to stimulate bodyworkers to kinesthetically understand, that is, to feel in their own bodies, techniques and practices that are most ergonomically suited to individual bodyworker needs.

Kinesthetic Understanding

One thing *Body Mechanics and Self-Care Manual* does not do is present an unvarying protocol for "correct" body mechanics. You are not told that "60 degrees of abduction in the shoulder girdle is the only correct way to hold your hands," or "55 inches from the floor is the right table height," or "slide exactly two feet down the table to execute the best massage stroke." Techniques that are copied undeviatingly from others will not feel right inside. They do not even make theoretical sense. Expert techniques need to be analyzed and revised by your own "insperts" (the experts inside you). Techniques taught by rote tend to mold you into a preplanned shape that does not work for everyone. Doing things the way others tell you to do them without understanding *why* creates fear and hurt. On the other hand, learning by imitation, when accompanied with a mo-dicum of innovation, creates therapists who can adapt prepatterned body movements into an individual massage style.

A core concept that is presented in *Body Mechanics and Self-Care Manual* is the idea of kinesthetic understanding. Kinesthetic awareness is self-movement that is observed and felt kinesthetically. Kinesthetic awareness plus conceptual understanding of how the body can optimally move yields kinesthetic understanding. The process is very different from the common practice of moving on "automatic pilot." How often have you been driving in a car and suddenly noticed that you did not remember crossing the last three intersections, let alone whether the light was green or red? In a massage, how often have you come into awareness that you have been effleuraging one leg and cannot remember what strokes, if any, were applied to the other limb?

Kinesthetic understanding arises from "lived movement," a notion introduced by Erwin Straus (1966). There is a huge difference between mechanical movement and movement that is lived. Lived movement is one of the defining characteristics of living beings. Straus cites the case in which you are crossing an open field in the dark and see something huge and black looming up ahead. It looks as if it is moving by itself and can feel the sense of shock permeate your body. Then, with a wave of relief, you see that the thing really is not moving at all—that it is, in fact, lifeless. This kind of experience is what Straus calls lived movement. Lived movement arises from the unique experience of a living being, and it has a plot with a beginning and an end.

If I intend to soften an adhesion that I have located in the psoas, I must take a certain number of steps. The path and my plan of action have a unity. If I simply considered the process as an array of mechanical motions, what is the basic unit of action? Is it the application of seven grams of pressure, the contraction of one of my arm muscles, or the twitch of a single muscle fiber? Following the procedure of analysis and division, there is no clear trail of movement or an experienced change of place. There is simply a summation of distinct events that displace the body from one point to another in space. Once the act is divided up in this way, we are no longer speaking of a massage therapist that is self-motivated and responsible for his or her actions.

There is nothing in muscular contractions or intercellular changes that corresponds to lived movement and the feeling of the movement. Reducing the explanation of a lived movement to a summation of motions makes the human experiences of walking in a meadow or massaging a client nothing more than appearance and illusion.

For these reasons, the exercises presented in each chapter are crucial for understanding the heart of the text. The explorations must be applied and practiced to yield any true knowledge. The activities cannot be skimmed and marked with a mental note to come back later.

Notice the skills that grew as you worked through the exercises in this book. New or rediscovered competencies in body awareness will allow you to more rapidly be conscious of positions and movements that do not work for you. You then create your own brand of body mechanics. You need not abandon certain types of massage because they are too difficult on your body. You can instead mold your discernment, intention, and body weight to the type of work that you want to do. Mindfulness when performing deeper, focused work will yield different insights about what feels right than a cognizance when practicing subtle energy techniques will.

All human bodies are shaped by a past, present, and future; the particular events and influences of each moment in time are unique for each individual. Each body builds its own life history with special combinations of activities and experiences. Whenever possible, the text supplements universal "rules" about how bodies function (derived from physical sciences, Eastern disciplines, and movement reeducation theory) with trial-and-error narratives and exercises to help you discover what can work easily and well in your massage practice. The book (and specifically Chapter 10) adapts the "most body-wise movements" to a variety of body types. Massage therapists (and clients) come in all shapes and sizes. It is a crucial apperception in this work that each human frame is unique and exquisite in its integrity.

Although all living creatures have an experience of life, only adult human beings can have a deep experience and know that they are having it. This body mechanics text asks readers to pause and reflect in the moment on the meaning of each massage movement. When you practice this new form of body-wise, self-aware, self-correcting body mechanics, which is more correctly termed *body awareness,* see if you can feel the new life infuse into your hands as you work.

METAPHOR FOR UNDERSTANDING

I would like to end with a metaphor derived from tai chi lore (Keller, 1998). To me, it illustrates how best to utilize *Body Mechanics and Self-Care Manual.* In the tradition of tai chi (Chapter 4), the world is a duality of yin and yang. In bodywork, yin corresponds to the intent or spirit of the work. It is the inner mind and underlying structure behind an individual's practice of the massage. (The inner mind and underlying structure will be different for every massage, as it lives in every moment.) Yang is the outer manifestation or the movements (of tai chi or of bodywork) expressed through the fascia. In other words, yang corresponds to the actions of the bones, tendons, and ligaments. Another way to express the duality is that yang is seen in the structure of the body, while yin is detected in the functionality. You may have heard the principle that form follows function. I have heard this position expressed in other vernaculars (e.g., "ontogeny [the development of a single organism] follows phylogeny [evolutionary development])" or "structure and function are interrelated"). What these proverbs say is that the body is formed by what it does. It follows that massage therapists are quite literally shaped by the way we work. If you perform bodywork in a way that demonstrates concern and respect for yourself, you have mastered the concepts of good body mechanics and self-care described in this book and your body will thrive. Not only will self-care nourish you, but also it will change your physical structure in a way that will enhance the way you function. The ability to massage well will improve as a direct result of body awareness and self-care. Conversely, when you neglect physiological and psychological well-being, the body's structure is changed in a negative way. Bodyworkers cannot perform all the manipulations or stretches or even achieve the same pressure with strokes when suffering. Massage therapists owe it to themselves and their clients to attend to body mechanics. This requires mindfulness in your work during a massage session, but also in how you prepare for a session, and in how you deal with the changes that a session causes in us. *Body Mechanics and Self-Care Manual* stresses the importance of being an advocate for your own health and well-being. It is the responsibility of each massage therapist to prepare and renew physically and emotionally for the challenging role of a massage practitioner. As "helpers," bodyworkers must avoid the trap of giving so much that important signs of physical and emotional needs are missed or ignored.

Levels of Knowledge

Muscle or Ox Level. Another part of the tai chi metaphor explained above (Keller, 1998) is the notion of levels of knowledge. This book presents a great deal of information that can be utilized on many levels. Each level represents a step to process and use the information on body mechanics and self-care in progressively more efficient ways. The first level of knowledge is on the muscular plane, or as the Chinese elders say, at the *level of the ox*. The ox is an animal that powers through duties (daily chores) with sheer brute strength. Ox allows the muscles to take on work and, by force and effort, complete tasks. The work gets done but not very efficiently.

Techniques. The next step up is the *level of technique*. Techniques can show more efficient ways of using the muscles so that the same task can be achieved with less effort. This book is chock full of guidelines (e.g., keep the head and tail in dynamic alignment) that make for safer and more efficient body mechanics. A warning is not to use technique as your primary level of learning. Sometimes, new practitioners become fixated on the level of technique. They flock to classes and workshops that offer set protocols for dealing with clients. Their business cards are filled with lots of specialties, including craniosacral, myofascial, and deep tissue techniques, when the average client does not look for more than massage. It is true that having more tools in your massage toolbox will definitely come in handy with a variety of somatic problems. It certainly is helpful to have lots of options at your disposal when you meet up with a "pesky muscle" that does not want to release. However, there is more to massage than technique alone. A little technique goes a long way when you have deeper listening qualities to back it up. If you do not apply the higher levels to your bodywork, you will need a lot more techniques in your pocket in order to get the job done.

Jing—Structure and Connections. Moving past techniques is the *level of jing*. Jing here refers to the fascia, including bones, ligaments, tendons, and other connective tissues that give structure and shape to the body. Connective tissue (CT) is a fascinating substance. CT possesses some amazing properties, including thixotropy and piezoelectricity. Thixotropy is the phenomenon that CT becomes more fluid when stirred up and more solid when it is not moved. When we move, soft tissues soften and become more pliable and adaptable to change. This is one of the aims in massage therapy for clients. Why not make it so for ourselves, the therapists, too. Piezoelectricity literally is the synthesis of two words: pressure and electricity. CT has the remarkable ability to act like a crystal in that when it is pressed (as in massage), a spark of electricity results. Electricity (through neuronal connections) is the major mode of sensory and motor communication within the human body (Juhan, 1987). Some researchers believe that lines of electrical communication continue through the fascia (Gerber, 1988) as well as meridians, the channels of energy described in Chapter 4.

The majority of human body tissue is connective tissue (Tortora, 1994). Because it is so prevalent, everywhere in the body, CT acts like a continuous body stocking (Juhan, 1987). For example, if you pull on a sweater or body stocking at the shoulder, the action will snag up the entire sleeve. In fact, any place that you touch or alter will affect any other part.

I used to think that all connective tissues did was connect. Although it is true that connective tissues do "connect" (a tautology), by virtue of the connections the tissues are responsible for much, much more. Let me elaborate:

1. Because CT surrounds every organ, every muscle, and every nerve cell, and because it is what binds muscles to bones and bones to other bones and organs to body cavities, CT creates the structure of the body. Because the tendons that connect muscle to bones are CT, CT acts as the cables, pulleys, and levers that transfer muscular contractions to bones. Without the CT, muscles would contract, but they wouldn't be able to move the skeleton.

2. CT cables and sheets provide tension to support the skeleton so that it can bear weight. They act much like the sails and sheets (ropes) on a ship. If there were no CT, the skeletal system could not support itself and would fall under its own weight. But if you took away from the human body all of the tissues except for the CT system, the form of the human body would be preserved.

3. CT is the fibrous bed for all blood vessels, lymph vessels, and nerves. It keeps these circulatory, lymphatic, and nervous system byways in their channels. In other words, CT provides the boundaries that define these byways. It allows the systems to perform their individual functions and express their individualities.

4. Since CT connects the vessels, nerves, muscles, and organs, it transfers the beneficial effects of movement to vessels and internal organs. This is the way that massage and movement exercise (such as stretching or walking) keeps the veins from pooling blood.

5. Because blood and lymph are types of CT, they provide the major delivery system in the body. As massage therapists well know, circulation of blood is the pathway for nutrients to every cell. Both lymph and blood circulation provide the path for toxins to leave the individual cells.

6. By virtue of the fact that blood and lymph are CT, CT provides the major repair system in the body. Fibroblasts manufacture collagen (a type of CT) to wall off and limit the harmful effects of wounds. This protects the rest of the body from toxicity. Blood chemistry creates the inflammatory response whereby blood and lymph fluids deliver the antibodies and white blood cells that work to fight off infection in the human body (Juhan, 1987).

When your work carries an awareness of structure and connection within the body and between your body and that of the client, you have reached the *level of jing,* where massage moves to a higher plane. *Body Mechanics and Self-Care Manual* pointed toward many of the fascinating structural relationships that are affected by both habitual and unpatterned movements. The book has also attempted to point out dynamic connections between identifiable structures within the body. Through psychological exercises, the book helps establish connections between the metabolic processes churning inside of you and the outside world. True attention to body mechanics reveals mind–body connections. True attention to body mechanics and awareness also uncovers deeper person-to-person connections between practitioner and client.

Chi—Energy.   The fourth level of comprehension in the model is the *level of chi.* Chi, you may remember from Chapter 4, is the life force or energy that resides in all living things. Chi can get blocked up in certain areas, causing too much energy circulating in one region, while not enough available in another. The idea is to create balance so that enough life force is available for the whole body. When you listen to energy flow in your body, and attempt to maintain your fluidity like a well-oiled machine, you are working on the chi level.

Yi—Mind and Intent.   The fifth step is the *level of yi,* or mind and intent. When you are clear about what your goals are with each stroke, you are incorporating yi. Knowing where you are moving, what structures you intend to affect, and why you have chosen each manipulation requires greater awareness than we have devoted in any of the previous levels. Intent also involves making the space to listen to how the client's body chooses to heal. When yi manifests as part of your massage, there is no stroke or movement that is extraneous or just "fluff and buff." Massage becomes therapeutic in every sense.

Natural Level.   The top step in the tai chi model is the *natural level.* This is the place where natural movement just flows. This is the level where all the rules and awarenesses have been so incorporated into the massage that your massage just flows. Natural level is exemplified by the tiger, who does not think about techniques, energy, or connections—he or she just does. All practitioners have moments of natural massage, when everything seems to fit together and have a purpose. The principles of good body mechanics are so embodied that you are not even consciously thinking about them. You find yourselves in a mindful state—the state that Trager calls "hookup"—and both you and your client know that this is a really good session. This is what bodyworkers would like to achieve in every massage, and although it seems to be effortless, it really is the culmination of a lot of hard work and effort. Natural body mechanics and self-care is the outgrowth of continual dedication to self-study and observation, not in an egoist way, but for the purpose of being the best we can be. A session composed of natural body mechanics gives your clients and you a taste of just what a human can be. Indeed, the goal is to be a human "being"—to be here now, to be what we are meant to be. Body mechanics and self-care in massage therapy provide an inroad into the greater human experience. The journey and process of seeking natural body mechanics is truly my wish for all readers of this book. I am truly grateful for the opportunity to have walked this part of the path with you. Thank you.

SUMMARY

> This chapter reviews the contents of each chapter and the importance of supplementing reading with *kinesthetic experience.* Another way of understanding kinesthetic experience is what Straus terms *lived movement.* There is a vast difference between mechanical movement and movement that is lived. It is the contention of this text that body mechanics can never be wholly understood as a series of prescribed positions.
>
> The final chapter also revisits key terms such as *body mechanics, body awareness, ergonomics,* and *self-care,* as they are used in the text.
>
> *(continued)*

Body mechanics is the study of how forces act on the human body. Body awareness incorporates the study of body mechanics with the internal study of how the body feels as it acts. Ergonomics means allowing your body to find tools that help you, rather than adapting your body to fit a so-called tool. Self-care is turning our concern and interest to maintaining one's own good health, in order to perform bodywork easily and well. Self-care is important during the massage, as well as preparing your body for its work before a session and taking the time to "re-create, refresh, and renew" after each massage.

This book presents information that can be utilized on many levels of understanding. Each level represents a step to process and use the information on body mechanics and self-care in progressively more efficient ways. The techniques presented by the text provide information at the level of the "muscles or ox." Without subsequent steps to comprehension, techniques alone provide only a limited understanding of good body mechanics. Supplementing the first level is the level of jing or connective tissue. This is the level of structure, boundaries, and at the same time the freedom to express oneself more fully as a massage therapist. The next level of comprehension is the level of chi or life force or energy. Working with an awareness of energy levels makes it easier to adapt your massage to change. Overlooking chi is the level of yi or inner intent. Knowing what you want makes it easier to accomplish your goals. The highest level of awareness is the natural plane where good body mechanics are so embodied that we do not even need to think about them. On this plane, you naturally find yourselves in a mindful state. We all have experienced this feeling in massage, in which each movement contributes to the well-being of the client and yourself. This is the goal. The aim of one well versed in the principles of good body mechanics and self-care is to massage and live life "naturally."

REFERENCES

Gerber, Richard, *Vibrational Medicine* (1988). Santa Fe, NM: Bear and Company.

Juhan, Deane, *Job's Body* (1987). Barrytown, NY: Station Hill Press, Inc.

Keller, Wayne (1998). Personal communcation, Portland, OR.

Straus, Erwin, *Phenomenological Psychology* (1966) New York: Basic Books.

Tortora, Gerard, *Introduction to the Human Body—The Essentials of Anatomy and Physiology,* 3rd ed. (1994). New York: HarperCollins College Publishers.

Selected References

The principles utilized in this text are drawn from established practices for organizing the human body, mind, heart, and spirit. These well-known disciplines include hatha yoga, tai chi, Trager work, Bartenieff Fundamentals, shiatsu, and traditional Chinese medicine. It is important to note that all of these disciplines have emerged with the recognition that to obtain any real knowledge about the body, one must examine one's own physical self. Above all, one must take these self-observations and compare and contrast them against any stated "rules."

Throughout the text, books and articles that have sparked my thinking and influenced the development of the ideas and exercises are listed at the end of each chapter. In this section, the most influential references are presented for your continued learning.

Corbin, Charles, and Ruth Lindsey, *Concepts of Physical Fitness with Laboratories* (1988). Dubuque, IA: Wm. C. Brown Publishers.

Dixon, Marian Wolfe, "Awareness: A Bodylesson for Bodyworkers," *Massage and Bodywork Journal* (Spring 1996) pp. 20–22.

Dixon, Marian Wolfe, *Bodylessons* (1992). Portland, OR: Rainbow Press.

Dychtwald, Ken, *Bodymind* (1986). Los Angeles: Jeremy P. Tarcher, Inc.

Evans, Maja, *The Ultimate Hand Book* (1992). San Francisco: Laughing Duck Press.

Feldenkrais, Moshe, *The Potent Self* (1985). New York: Harper & Row.

Feldenkrais, Moshe, *Awareness through Movement* (1977). New York: Harper & Row.

Gardner, Howard, *Frames of Mind: the Theory of Multiple Intelligences* (1983). New York: Basic Books.

Gawain, Shakti, *Creative Visualization* (1995). Novato, CA: New World Library, www.nwlib.com.

Gerber, Richard, *Vibrational Medicine* (1988). Santa Fe, NM: Bear and Company.

Greenberg, Jerrold S., *Comprehensive Stress Management,* 2nd ed. (1987). Dubuque, IA: Wm. C. Brown Publishers.

Hanna, Thomas, *Somatics,* 4th printing (1991). New York: Perseus Books.

Juhan, Deane, *Job's Body* (1987). Barrytown, NY: Station Hill Press, Inc.

Lundberg, Paul, *The Book of Shiatsu* (1992). New York: Simon and Schuster.

Lusseyran, Jacques, "Sense and Presence," in *And There Was Light,* Vol. XI:2 (1987). New York: Parabola Books.

Millman, Dan, *Body Mind Mastery* (1999). Novato, CA: New World Library, www.nwlib.com.

Newton, Isaac, *Principia* (1686). Translated by F. Cajori (1934). Berkeley: University of California Press.

Noble, Elizabeth, *Marie Osmond's Exercises for Mothers and Babies* (1985). New York: New American Library.

Pert, Candace, *Molecules of Emotion* (1997). New York: Scribner.

Rolf, Ida, *Rolfing* (1989). Rochester, VT: Healing Arts Press.

Samskrti and Veda, *Hatha Yoga Manual I,* 2nd ed. (1985). Honesdale, PA: The Himalayan Institute.

Samuels, M., and N. Samuels, *Seeing with the Mind's Eye* (1984). New York: Random House Inc.

Satchidananda, Yogiraj Sri Swami, *Integral Yoga Hatha* (1970). New York: Holt, Rinehart and Winston.

Schneider, Meir, *The Handbook of Self Healing* (1994). London: Penguin Books.

Schultz, R. Louis, and Rosemary Feitis, *The Endless Web* (1996). Berkeley, CA: North Atlantic Books.

Seaward, Brian Luke, *Managing Stress* (1994). Boston: Jones and Bartlett Publishers.

Straus, Erwin, *Phenomenological Psychology* (1966). New York: Basic Books.

Tart, Charles, *Open Mind, Discriminating Mind* (1989). New York: Harper & Row.

Tortora, Gerard, *Introduction to the Human Body—The Essentials of Anatomy and Physiology,* 3rd ed. (1994). New York: Harper Collins College Publishers.

Upledger, John, *Your Inner Physician and You* (1997). Berkeley, CA: North Atlantic Books.

Vander, A. J., J. H. Sherman, and D. S. Luciano, *Human Physiology: The Mechanisms of Body Function* (1980). New York: McGraw-Hill.

Index

Page numbers followed by e indicate exercise. Page numbers followed by f indicate figure.